REF
RC   Genes and cancer.
268.4
.G425
1990

$49.50

DATE		

DISCARD

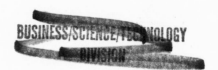
© THE BAKER & TAYLOR CO.

Genes
and
Cancer

Genes and Cancer

Edited by

DESMOND CARNEY
Department of Medical Oncology
Mater Misericordiae Hospital
Dublin

and

KAROL SIKORA
Department of Clinical Oncology
and ICRF Oncology Group
Royal Postgraduate Medical School
Hammersmith Hospital
London

JOHN WILEY & SONS
Chichester · New York · Brisbane · Toronto · Singapore

Other Wiley Editorial Offices

John Wiley & Sons, Inc., 605 Third Avenue,
New York, NY 10158-0012, USA

Jacaranda Wiley Ltd, G.P.O. Box 859, Brisbane,
Queensland 4001, Australia

John Wiley & Sons (Canada) Ltd, 22 Worcester Road,
Rexdale, Ontario M9W 1L1, Canada

John Wiley & Sons (SEA) Pte Ltd, 37 Jalan Pemimpin 05-04,
Block B, Union Industrial Building, Singapore 2057

Library of Congress Cataloging-in-Publication Data

Genes and cancer/edited by Desmond Carney and
    Karol Sikora.
        p. cm.
    Includes bibliographical references.
    ISBN 0 471 92583 7
    1. Cancer—Genetic aspects. 2. Oncogenes. 3. Cancer—Molecular
aspects. I. Carney, Desmond. II. Sikora, Karol.
RC268.4.G425   1990
616.99′4042—dc20   90-11951
                                                    CIP

British Library Cataloguing in Publication Data

Genes and cancer.
    1. Man. Cancer. Genetic factors
    I. Carney, Desmond II. Sikora, Karol
    616.994042

    ISBN 0 471 92583 7

Phototypeset by Dobbie Typesetting Service, Tavistock, Devon
Printed and bound by Courier International, Tiptree, Colchester

Contents

F Tumour Biology

Contributors

J. R. ADAIR   Celltech, Slough, Berkshire, UK.

P. ALEXANDER   Cancer Research Campaign Medical Oncology Unit, Southampton General Hospital, Southampton, UK.

R. B. ARLINGHAUS   Department of Molecular Pathology, The University MD Anderson, Cancer Centre, Houston, Texas, USA.

R. H. J. BEGENT   Cancer Research Campaign Laboratories, Charing Cross Hospital, London, UK.

A. C. BLACK   UCLA School of Medicine, Center for the Health Services, Los Angeles, California, USA.

M. BRADA   Academic Unit of Radiotherapy and Oncology, The Royal Marsden Hospital, Sutton, Surrey, UK.

D. N. CARNEY   Mater Misericordiae Hospital and Saint Luke's Hospital, Dublin, Ireland.

I. S. CHEN   UCLA School of Medicine, Center for the Health Services, Los Angeles, California, USA.

L. B. CHEN   Dana–Farber Cancer Institute, Boston, Massachusetts, USA.

N. CORBALLY   Mater Misericordiae Hospital, Dublin, Ireland.

D. CUNNINGHAM   Department of Medicine, Royal Marsden Hospital, Sutton, Surrey, UK.

J. DENEKAMP	The Gray Laboratory, Mount Vernon Hospital, Northwood, Middlesex, UK.
S. ECCLES	Institute of Cancer Research, Sutton, Surrey, UK.
M. ELLIS	Imperial Cancer Research Fund, Lincoln's Inn Fields, London, UK.
A. A. EPENETOS	ICRF Oncology Group, Department of Clinical Oncology, Royal Postgraduate Medical School, Hammersmith Hospital, London, UK.
G. EVAN	Imperial Cancer Research Fund, St. Bartholomew's Hospital, London, UK.
W. GULLICK	MRC Cyclotron Building, Hammersmith Hospital, London, UK.
A. L. HARRIS	ICRF Clinical Oncology Unit, The Churchill Hospital, Oxford, UK.
D. W. HEDLEY	Department of Medicine, Princess Margaret Hospital, Toronto, Ontario, Canada.
T. HICKISH	Department of Medicine, Royal Marsden Hospital, Sutton, Surrey, UK.
V. HIRD	ICRF Oncology Group, Department of Clinical Oncology, Royal Postgraduate Medical School, Hammersmith Hospital, London, UK.
Y. IKAWA	Tsukuba Life Science Center, Laboratory of Molecular Oncology, The Institute of Physical and Chemical Research, Wako, Saitama, Japan.
Y. ITO	Department of Viral Oncology, Institute for Virus Research, Kyoto University, Kyoto, Japan.
N. D. JAMES	Department of Clinical Oncology, Hammersmith Hospital, London, UK.
S. B. KAYE	CRC Department of Medical Oncology, University of Glasgow, Glasgow, UK.
J. KEMSHEAD	ICRF Paediatric and Neuro-oncology Group, Frenchay Hospital, Bristol, UK.

N. LEMOINE — ICRF Oncology Group, Department of Clinical Oncology, Royal Postgraduate Medical School, Hammersmith Hospital, London, UK.

A. McCANN — Mater Misericordiae Hospital, Dublin, Ireland.

R. J. OWENS — Celltech, Slough, Berkshire, UK.

K. PATEL — ICRF Paediatric and Neuro-oncology Group, Frenchay Hospital, Bristol, UK.

J. PLUMB — CRC Department of Medical Oncology, University of Glasgow, Glasgow, UK.

B. A. J. PONDER — CRC Human Cancer Genetics Group, Department of Pathology, University of Cambridge, Cambridge, UK.

A. QAYUM — Department of Clinical Oncology, Royal Postgraduate Medical School, Hammersmith Hospital, London, UK.

C. D. REDDY — The Wistar Institute, Philadelphia, Pennsylvania, USA.

E. P. REDDY — The Wistar Institute, Philadelphia, Pennsylvania, USA.

E. RIVERS — Dana-Farber Cancer Institute, Boston, Massachusetts, USA.

R. ROBERTS — Department of Biochemistry and Molecular Biology, University of Manchester, Manchester, UK.

J. D. ROSENBLATT — UCLA School of Medicine, Center for Health Sciences, Los Angeles, California, USA.

M. SATAKE — Department of Viral Oncology, Institute for Virus Research, Kyoto University, Kyoto, Japan.

K. SEMBA — The Institute of Medical Science, University of Tokyo, Tokyo, Japan.

P. W. SHEPPARD — Cambridge Research Biochemicals Ltd, Harston, Cambridge, UK.

K. SHIGESADA — Department of Viral Oncology, Institute for Virus Research, Kyoto University, Kyoto, Japan.

K. SIKORA — Department of Clinical Oncology, Hammersmith Hospital, London, UK.

J. F. SMYTH   Department of Clinical Oncology, University of Edinburgh, Western General Hospital, Edinburgh, UK.

N. K. SPURR   Imperial Cancer Research Fund, Clare Hall Laboratories, Potters Bar, Herts, UK.

P. STROOBANT   Ludwig Institute for Cancer Research, Middlesex Hospital, London, UK.

K. TOYOSHIMA   Department of Oncology, Institute of Medical Science, University of Tokyo, Tokyo, Japan.

J. WAXMAN   Department of Clinical Oncology, Royal Postgraduate Medical School, Hammersmith Hospital, London, UK.

N. R. WHITTLE   Celltech, Slough, Berkshire, UK.

Acknowledgement

The authors would like to thank Lederle Laboratories UK for allowing them to draw upon a number of articles, first published in *Cancer Topics*, as a basis for this book. *Cancer Topics* is published six times a year and is supported by an educational grant from Lederle Laboratories. It is available free of charge on request from the local Lederle office.

Foreword

WALTER BODMER

Cancer is essentially a genetic disease at the cellular level. The ideas underlying this fact go back to Boveri's suggestion in the early years of this century that chromosomal abnormalities were the basis for cancer. But it is only over the last ten or fifteen years, following the molecular biology revolution, that it has been possible to add substance to this idea. The study of oncogenic viruses has led to the discovery of the oncogenes, those normal genes which when mutated are key steps in the cancer process. The dominant oncogenes seem mainly to be connected with the control of growth through growth factors and their receptors, and the genes which control their expression and signalling from the surface to the nucleus. Recessive or suppressor oncogenes have been discovered through the study of inherited cancer susceptibilities following Knudson's fundamental idea that genetic changes in the germ line which may give rise to inherited cancer susceptibility can also be critical steps at the somatic level in the development of sporadic cancers. Genetic changes also underlie the development of drug resistance and, through differences in DNA repair processes and metabolizing enzymes, may also determine response to drug treatment.

The advances that have come from the applications of molecular biology to cancer in our fundamental understanding of the cancer process will surely lead to major new insights for better and more specific approaches to prevention and treatment of cancer. Another major novel route to cancer diagnosis and treatment comes through the development of monoclonal antibodies. These remarkable reagents can be made to pick out differences between different cell types, and possible differences between tumours and normal cells, which can form the basis for *in vivo* imaging of cancers with radioactively labelled antibodies as well as for targeting radioactivity or cytotoxic drugs or toxins. The ability to engineer antibodies at will, for example to 'humanize' mouse antibodies or to recombine antibody and toxin genes or add sequences that aid the attachment of labels and drugs, considerably enhances the potential for monoclonal antibody diagnosis and therapy.

The rate of advance of our knowledge about cancer is extraordinary and depends on an understanding of basic molecular biology and genetics and, through this, of the details of oncogenes, growth control, tumour biology, drug resistance and monoclonal antibody based diagnosis and therapy. This book provides a comprehensive yet digestible and comprehensible survey of these major areas of cancer research. The authors are all experts in their respective fields working at the forefront of new developments. There can be no doubt that this will be an important handbook for all those who wish to keep up with the current dramatic advances in our understanding of the cancer process at the molecular level.

Introduction

DESMOND N. CARNEY
KAROL SIKORA

Despite tremendous efforts, there has been little improvement in the overall survival of patients with cancer over the last 30 years. Whilst changes in the management of certain tumours, including lymphomas, leukaemias and testis, have produced dramatic improvements in survival, these tumours are rare and so have contributed little to the overall picture. Although there is no doubt that a combination of reducing smoking and changes in diet would significantly result in a lower cancer incidence and therefore increased survival, it is likely that prevention strategies are going to have little immediate impact in the overall mortality of cancer as we enter the next century. Thus there is a need for the identification and application of new therapeutic strategies.

For many cancers a number of factors have been identified which are of prognostic importance. These include patient performance status, disease extent and response to cytotoxic therapy. It is clear, however, that considerable heterogeneity in tumour response is observed, even among patients with a similar tumour. These data suggest that biological properties of the tumour cells themselves may be of prognostic importance. These properties include: the expression of drug or radiation resistance genes; specific and nonspecific chromosomal abnormalities; and alteration in the expression of a range of oncogenes.

Cancer therapy can now benefit from the explosion of knowledge that has occurred in modern biology over the last two decades. Our understanding of the function of genes and proteins, the control of gene expression and our ability to assay specific molecules has improved out of all recognition from the technology of a decade ago. If we can identify differences between normal and malignant cells, then we may be able to develop better markers of tumour load and uncover new biochemical systems with which to tamper in order to inhibit growth. The new technology has

Genes and Cancer. Edited by D. Carney and K. Sikora
Published 1990 by John Wiley & Sons Ltd

not only allowed a greater understanding of growth control through the discovery of specific segments of DNA involved in this process, but also given us new pharmaceutical agents in a highly purified form ready for clinical trial.

GROWTH CONTROL GENES

The original evidence that specific genes have a role in carcinogenesis came from the RNA tumour viruses. These small entities possess only three genes: two coding for structural proteins and the third for reverse transcriptase—the enzyme that produces a DNA copy of the virus allowing incorporation of the virus into the host DNA. The addition of a fourth gene gives these viruses the ability to induce tumours rapidly *in vivo* and also to transform cells *in vitro* (transformed cells lose contact inhibition and pile up on the plates instead of forming the usual single layer, i.e. they grow in an unregulated fashion). These transforming sequences were termed viral oncogenes (v-*onc*). Surprisingly it was subsequently shown that viral oncogenes share common sequences with cellular genes, which were thus termed cellular oncogenes (c-*onc*).

This raised the chicken-and-egg problem of which came first. Do viruses cause cancer or have the viruses hijacked cellular genes involved in cell growth control? Several factors indicate the latter explanation. Viruses carrying v-*onc* genes reproduce less efficiently than 'normal' viruses. The extensive involvement of c-*onc* genes in normal cellular growth and differentiation indicates the likely origin of oncogenes. Cellular oncogenes do not usually possess transforming potential in their native state and are termed proto-oncogenes to distinguish them from genes with the ability to transform. The confusing nomenclature of oncogenes has arisen because the viral genes were named after the tumours in which they were first described. For example, v-*src*, one of the first genes studied, causes sarcoma in chickens, while v-*sis* causes a sarcoma in monkeys.

ONCOGENE FUNCTION

The control of cell growth and development is a complex process. Oncogene producers have been shown to be involved at each level of this process, and it can be seen that alterations to this finely balanced system could result in unregulated cell growth, i.e. transformation (Figure 1).

Growth factors

Growth factors are extracellular proteins that act as growth modulators. They have several properties that indicate an involvement in carcinogenesis. Some growth factors will transform normal cells *in vitro*. Conversely, in some systems the induction of cell transformation can result in an increased production of growth factor. The observation that growth factors can both initiate and be a product of transformation suggests the possibility of self-perpetuating, positive-feedback loops, with unregulated cell division as the consequence. This phenomenon, termed autocrine

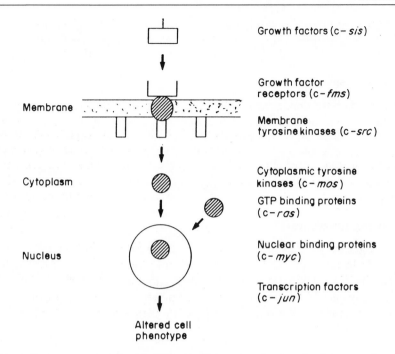

Figure 1. Some components of cell control that may be involved in transformation

secretion, has been implicated in various situations involving rapid growth, such as wound repair and embryogenesis as well as malignant transformation. Both transformation and growth factor stimulation result in similar biochemical changes, such as increased tyrosine phosphorylation and altered cellular lipid metabolism. One human oncogene, c-*sis*, has been shown to code for a known growth factor—platelet-derived growth factor (PDGF).

Growth factor receptors

There are several oncogene-encoded proteins that form part of a cell surface receptor. The presence of the appropriate growth factor switches the receptor 'on' with the resultant increase in tyrosine kinase activity within the cell. The kinase can also be regulated by an internal regulatory region, allowing responses to intracellular events. The consequences of the increased kinase activity are unknown but such activity is a hallmark of transformed cells.

Small alterations in the receptor can produce defects in the regulation of tyrosine kinase activity. An example of this is c-*erb*B1, which codes for the cellular receptor of epidermal growth factor (EGF). The equivalent viral gene, v-*erb*B, which has transforming activity, codes a receptor with a truncated external receptor. In addition, there are alterations in the regulatory region internally. Transformation can occur by the viral gene product assuming a 'locked-on' configuration, tricking the cell into rapid growth.

A second mechanism is alteration in tyrosine kinase activity. An example of this is the c-*fms* oncogene, which codes the receptor for the colony-stimulating factor

CSF-1 in differentiating macrophages. The transforming viral gene v-*fms* possesses enhanced kinase activity compared with its cellular counterpart.

Intracellular messengers

The best candidate for oncogene involvement at the level of intracellular messengers is the *ras* family of genes. The gene products have structural similarities to proteins termed G- and N-proteins that control adenylate cyclase activity. Products of *ras* genes have also been shown to have GTPase activity. These proteins are all thought to be important in the 'second messenger' system and thus provide a link between events at the cell membrane and the nucleus.

Nuclear acting oncogenes

Several oncogenes, such as *myc*, *myb* and *fos*, code for nuclear-associated proteins. Their precise localisation and function are unknown, but these oncogenes are involved in the control of gene expression, acting to initiate the production of growth factors, for example. More recently transcription factors, which control the binding of RNA polymerase to DNA and hence regulate gene expression, have been found to be oncogenes.

ONCOGENES AND CANCER

It is clear that oncogenes are involved at crucial points in cell growth. For oncogenes to have clinical relevance, it is necessary to demonstrate that oncogene products are essential for the production and maintenance of the transformed state in human cancer.

Assays have been developed to evaluate oncogene activity in human tumours. DNA can be examined for multiple copies or abnormal forms of suspected oncogenes. mRNA can be analysed for abnormal transcripts or for inappropriate quantities of a normal transcript. The protein products of oncogenes can be looked for, in either inappropriate forms or quantities, using suitable monoclonal antibodies. Finally, the putative oncogene can be 'implanted' into suitable cell cultures to look for its transforming potential—the transfection assay.

Gene amplification

Several tumour types have been shown to contain amplified oncogene sequences by Southern blotting. Breast and stomach carcinomas often contain amplified c-*myc* sequences. Tumours containing such abnormalities tend to carry a poorer prognosis. The best correlation between oncogene amplification and clinical outcome is found in neuroblastoma. Multiple copies of the N-*myc* gene—up to 300—are found in this rare childhood tumour. Such amplification is associated with a shorter progression-free survival, advanced stage and a tendency to metastasise. The function of the product encoded by the N-*myc* gene is not known and so the physiological mechanisms behind this correlation remain a mystery.

Gene rearrangement

The relocation of oncogenes within the human genome may well alter their control processes. Evidence for such movements comes from the study of those tumours where karyotypic abnormalities have been found, and from more subtle genomic shifts detected by hybridisation. The Philadelphia chromosome is found in most patients with chronic myeloid leukaemia and is characterised by the translocation of the c-*abl* oncogene on chromosome 9 to an area of chromosome 22 termed the breakpoint cluster region (*bcr*). The hybrid transcript encodes a novel protein with enhanced tyrosine kinase activity. Recently it has been shown that the majority of patients without the karyotypic change still have a shift of the c-*abl* gene into the bcr locus so providing evidence of a uniform molecular abnormality in this disease. Other examples of clinically relevant gene rearrangements include c-*myc* in Burkitt's lymphoma and the *bcl* shift in B-cell lymphoma. The exact mechanisms by which such gene movements are responsible for the development of a tumour are still unclear.

Mutation

Small changes in the structure of a gene can result in altered protein structure and function. The discovery that a single base pair change could result in altered *ras* function has led to a detailed study of *ras* mutants in human tumours. Initially such mutants were detected by the relatively cumbersome transfection assay. The recently developed polymerase chain reaction technique, which allows the expansion and analysis of small segments of genome, is ideally suited to the evaluation of mutant *ras* genes in clinical samples. Large series of leukaemias, colorectal, pancreatic and thyroid tumours have now been analysed. Several interesting observations have been made relating the likely aetiological factor in thyroid cancer to genetic changes. Exactly how the mutant *ras* gene product is involved in malignant development remains to be elucidated.

Another example of a single amino acid mutation resulting in an active oncogene product is the c-*neu* gene in the rat. This gene, which is closely related to human c-*erb*B2 gene, encodes a surface receptor with considerable homology to the epidermal growth factor receptor. The protein straddles the cell membrane with a ligand-binding external domain. Mutation of amino acids within the intramembranous portion can under certain circumstances lead to constitutive transformation. This rather puzzling observation has been rationalised by molecular modelling studies. The introduction of a novel amino acid which allows increased receptor dimerisation through hydrogen bonding within the hydrophobic environment of the cell membrane can lead to the continued activation of this receptor. In this way such mutants produce receptors in a locked-on configuration sending a positive signal to the next stage of the cell's transduction apparatus. Interrupting receptor aggregation may well have potential as a novel therapeutic strategy.

Increased transcription and expression

Several studies have now evaluated the role of increased oncogene transcription and expression in a variety of human tumours. In many cases a correlation has been made to the clinical behaviour of the tumour. The best studied example is breast cancer, where the expression of *erb*B1 and c-*erb*B2 clearly correlate to degree of progression, disease free survival and absolute survival. Another example is invasive cervical cancer where c-*myc* mRNA and protein product have been assayed. Here increased expression has been related to poor prognosis whatever the stage of the primary tumour. A major problem is the relatively short half-life and difficulty in precise quantitation of oncogene transcripts. The development of new monoclonal antibodies for the assay of oncoproteins in clinical samples is yielding more detailed information.

Tumour suppressor genes

It is now clear that the defective expression of certain genes can result in tumour development. Under some conditions the fusion of benign and malignant cells will result in the loss of the features of neoplasia. The discovery that inherited and acquired defects at a certain position on the long arm of chromosome 13 led to the mapping and eventual cloning of the retinoblastoma gene (*Rb*). The defective expression of this gene at a critical stage of childhood retinal development leads to a high risk of this exceedingly rare retinal tumour. The defective function of the *Rb* gene has now been implicated in breast cancer and a range of common human tumours.

The gene for familial polyposis coli fits a similar model. This gene was mapped to the short arm of chromosome 5 by genetic fingerprinting of patients and relatives. Minisatellite DNA probing demonstrated that further mutation to homozygosity at this site results in progression to adenocarcinoma. Mutations are present at this locus in 30% of sporadic colorectal cancers, suggesting that defective gene function at this site is important in many tumours not necessarily arising in patients with a background of polyposis.

CLINICAL POTENTIAL

The discovery of oncogenes and the development of suitable assays for clinical use has led to a greater understanding of malignant disease. We are now beginning to evaluate their diagnostic and therapeutic potential.

Diagnosis and prognosis

Monoclonal antibodies directed against oncogenes or their products may prove to be valuable as a diagnostic tool. Released oncogene products could be useful tumour markers for screening, diagnostic or follow-up purposes. Immunocytochemical techniques have already shown potential in a variety of malignancies, including breast and cervical carcinomas, and monoclonal antibodies linked to radionuclides have been used to localize tumours. Finally, patients at risk of developing a malignancy may well be identified by recognition in their DNA of sequences associated with likely oncogenic change. Techniques such as these would provide an accurate risk assessment before the development of clinical disease.

Treatment

The discovery of a novel set of growth control proteins provides new targets for the development of antineoplastic agents. Growth factors and their surface receptors are accessible to pharmacological and biological manipulation. Autocrine loops can be interrupted in several ways: by decreasing growth factor secretion using suitable inhibitors, such as somatostatin; by mopping up excess growth factor using antibodies; by preventing the binding of growth factor, using analogues that displace active growth factor from its receptor or using anti-receptor antibodies to prevent access. At a receptor level blockade of function can occur by the use of suitable ligand analogues which interfere with signal transduction. The experience with LHRH analogues suggests that down-regulation of surface receptors is possible even in a clinical situation. The mechanism for this well-documented effect is not clear. The activation of a receptor results from the binding of ligand to the external domain and then the aggregation within the cell membrane of groups of receptors. This aggregation could potentially be blocked by small peptides that mimic the intramembranous portion of the receptor and sterically interfere with aggregation.

Inside the cell the signal to grow can be interfered with in several ways. Tyrosine kinase inhibitors have been developed; these include suicide peptides that bind and are phosphorylated by the enzyme, but covalently link to it so destroying reversibly enzyme activity. Nucleoside analogues that bind to the *ras* gene product but prevent further activation are also being investigated. The nuclear oncoproteins also provide fertile ground for the search for inhibitors with therapeutic potential. The mechanism by which c-*fos*, c-*myc* and c-*jun* bind to DNA or other nuclear structures is currently being elucidated. Once these mechanisms are understood, low molecular weight compounds could well be developed to interfere with this binding and shift the partition between nucleus and cytoplasm, so altering growth control.

A major problem in the clinical use of these types of growth control agents will be to determine the best way to obtain selective tumour destruction. Clearly these products have a normal physiological role in the maintenance of cellular activity and interference is likely to have profound effects on normal structure and function. Most likely, the only way to determine how best to harness such compounds will be by painstaking clinical trials—the same way that successful combinations of cytotoxic drugs were discovered.

In the future it is likely that the clinician will be able to manipulate in a sophisticated manner the control of abnormal growth in a variety of cellular systems. This seems the most promising avenue for the therapeutic innovations that will be in use in the early part of the next century.

Oncogenes

1 Oncogenes as Clinical Tools

WILLIAM GULLICK

KAROL SIKORA

Oncogenes are a family of unique sequences of DNA whose abnormal expression is associated with the development of malignant cell behaviour. They were first demonstrated in rapidly transforming RNA viruses, but their significance lies in the discovery that they are derived from normal cellular DNA. Infection of cells, in culture or *in vivo*, by a retrovirus containing an oncogene, leads to uncontrolled cell proliferation and differentiation arrest, the hallmarks of malignancy. The exact mechanism by which this is achieved remains unclear, but sequence homology of oncogenes with growth factors and their receptors, together with functional characteristics pointing to a role in cell-cycle control, provide intriguing leads in the study of the signalling mechanisms that regulate cell growth. Over the last few years there has been intense interest in the clinical potential of information gleaned about the structure and function of these fascinating genes.

NEW TECHNOLOGY

A variety of techniques have been used to explore the molecular biology of these genes and their proteins. Techniques such as Southern blotting, polymerase chain reactions, DNA sequencing, dot-blot hybridization, Western blotting, and immuno-histology have allowed the analysis of DNA, RNA and protein in clinical samples from patients with a variety of neoplasms. A major problem is that the reagents for such exploration are only just becoming available. Monoclonal antibodies constructed against a variety of oncogene products are commercially available for only a small number of gene products. It is likely that over the next few years such reagents will allow the dissection of the full catalogue of 40 or more oncogenes.

Genes and Cancer. Edited by D. Carney and K. Sikora.
Published 1990 by John Wiley & Sons Ltd.

Already, there are hints that the information provided from such analyses can give us a molecular 'blue-print' for a cell and allow the prediction of the likely course of disease in an individual patient. The temporal and spatial expression of these genes produce the molecular framework on which the destiny of the tumour, and hence the patient, lies. They also provide novel targets for pharmacological and immunological attack.

DNA

Karyoptic abnormalities were noted in various cancers several decades ago. The refinement of modern molecular biology has allowed the examination of specific segments of chromosomes for amplification by Southern blotting and for mutation by the techniques of polymerase chain reaction analysis or cloning and sequencing. Table 1 lists genes that have been found to be amplified in certain tumours. For some tumours there is a correlation between amplification and clinical outcome. The tightest example is in neuroblastoma (Table 2) where disease-free and absolute survival is strongly correlated to amplification of the N-*myc* gene. A weaker, but equally interesting, correlation has been observed with the *erb*B1 and c-*myc* genes in breast cancer. Related to c-*erb*B1, which encodes the receptor for epidermal growth factor, is another gene: c-*erb*B2. It has structural homology to c-*erb*B1, but codes for a different receptor whose ligand has yet to be identified. Amplification and expression of this gene may correlate with prognosis in breast cancer. Studies are in progress to evaluate the long-term prognostic significance of these abnormalities.

Table 1. Oncogene alterations in human tumour biopsies

Gene	Tumour	Amplification	Rearrangement
c-*myc*	Breast	+	−
	Burkitt's lymphoma	−	+
	Stomach	+	−
N-*myc*	Neuroblastoma	+	−
	Retinoblastoma	+	−
	APML	+	−
	Breast	+	−
L-*myc*	Lung	+	−
	Breast	+	−
c-*abl*	CML	−	+
c-*myb*	AML	+	−
	Colon	+	−
c-*erb*B1	Breast/lung	+	−
	Glioma/bladder	+	−
c-*erb*B2	Breast	+	−
	Stomach	+	−
	Salivary gland	+	−
	Kidney	+	−
Ki-*ras*	Colon	+	−
	Ovarian	+	−
N-*ras*	Breast	+	−
gli	Brain	+	−

Table 2. N-*myc* gene amplification in neuroblastoma

Stage	
I	0/8
II	2/16
III	13/20
IV	19/40
IVS	0/5

DFS at 18 months

N-*myc* copies

1	70%
3–10	30%
Greater than 10	5%

Why gene amplification should result in a change in the physiology of the cell remains unclear. The main problem is that the function of the proteins coded for by most of these genes is not known.

Mutations at certain sites within oncogenes can also lead to growth abnormalities; a good example is the c-*ras* gene family. Here, mutations create proteins which are less able to hydrolyse GTP. Although GTP binding is one of the functions of *ras*, its other functions remain a mystery.

Specific chromosomal translocation is a common feature of certain tumours. An example is Burkitt's lymphoma which almost invariably carries a translocation involving chromosome 8;14. The break-point in chromosome 8 is at the site of the c-*myc* oncogene. In the more common follicular lymphoma, translocations between chromosome 14 and 18 have been noted. The break-point region has been cloned and designated *bcl*-2. This region may well be an oncogene. The Philadelphia chromosome in chronic myeloid leukaemia is a chromosome 9;22 translocation. Here, the c-*abl* oncogene, which is related to the v-*onc* of the murine Abelson leukaemia virus, is moved from chromosome 9 into a fragmented segment of chromosome 22. Examination of the break-point shows that it always occurs within a 5.8 kb segment designated *bcr* (break-point cluster region). An mRNA transcript has been detected in CML cells that is a fusion product of the c-*abl* and *bcr* regions.

Furthermore, the protein product of this message has a molecular ratio of 210 000 and appears to have deregulated tyrosine kinase activity. By constructing antibodies against this protein, new diagnostic and, possibly, therapeutic agents may become available.

RNA

Over the last four years an intensive investigation of oncogene transcription in clinical samples has been carried out. Large numbers of tumours have been collected, RNA isolated, and the number of copies present per cell estimated using hybridization. The simplest and most commonly used method has been dot blotting. Problems abound, however. First, RNA degrades very rapidly, even from the time of surgical clamping. Furthermore, RNA is difficult to process because of its instability. Dot-blotting techniques can be tremendously variable and, critically, depend on the quality and length of the specific probe used. For these reasons, much of the literature is difficult to reproduce and the results must be viewed with some scepticism. The biggest single series was of 54 tumours probed with 15 different oncogene probes. No obvious pattern of gene expression to any specific tumour or particular aggressive state of the tumour was obtained.

Correlations between outcome have been claimed for c-*myc* and c-*ras*, in colorectal and breast cancer. However, careful study of DNA, RNA, and protein in the same tumour samples is badly needed to clarify the problems.

PROTEIN

The evidence implicating oncoproteins in growth control was strengthened by the determination of the function of several oncogene products. The v-*sis* gene product, p28 v-*sis*, has been shown to have homology to 109 amino acids of the B chain of platelet-derived growth factor. This important protein is involved in wound healing and the control of growth. The c-*erb*B1 gene, the progenitor of the v-*erb*B oncogene, has been found to encode the epidermal growth factor receptor. When epidermal growth factor binds to its receptor on the cell surface, it activates the protein kinase activity of the cytoplasmic domain of the molecule so culminating in growth

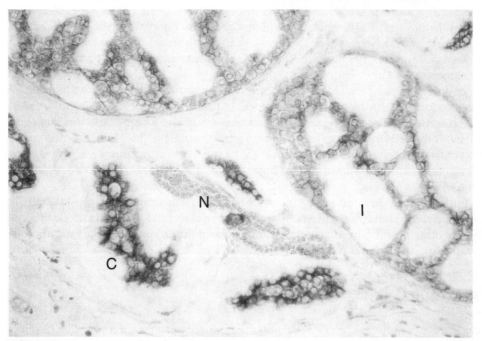

Figure 1. Detection of oncogene product by immunohistology. Paraffin-embedded section of human breast adenocarcinoma stained with a polyclonal rabbit antibody raised to a synthetic peptide from the human c-*erb*B2 oncogene product. N, normal ductal tissue; I, ductal carcinoma *in situ*; C, invasive colloid mucinous carcinoma

potentiation. Presumably, aberrant production of the internal portion, with a 'locked-on' configuration as encoded by the v-*erb*B oncogene, can result in growth without the requirement for exogenous epidermal growth factor. Recently, it has been demonstrated that simple over-expression of the EGF receptor can also lead to cell transformation. A third oncogene implicated in growth control is c-*myc*. This $62\,000M_r$ protein binds in a curious way to the matrix of cell nuclei. It has a very short half-life of 20 minutes and has been implicated in the control of the cell cycle. The level of c-*myc* RNA increases promptly when cells are stimulated into divisions.

In order to examine the relevance of oncoproteins, antibodies have been constructed to synthetic peptides. Such peptides are chosen from hydropathic plots of the predicted amino acid sequence of the oncogene product. The hydrophilic sequences are likely to be on the outside of the molecule and therefore to constitute antigenic determinants. Polyclonal and monoclonal antibodies are now available to several oncoproteins. These reagents can be used in immunohistology and Western blotting (Figure 1). Correlations between prognosis and gene expression have been made for c-*myc*, N-*myc*, c-*ras*, c-*erb*B1, and c-*erb*B2 in several tumours.

Although histology is good for giving geographical information about the distribution of oncoproteins in normal and malignant tissues, it is bad for quantitation. Sensitive flow cytometric assays have been developed to precisely quantitate oncoproteins in nuclei isolated from wax-embedded tumours. Correlations are apparent between differentiation state and clinical outcome with the concentrations of p62 c-*myc* and other proteins in lung, colonic, testicular, and cervical cancer.

TUMOUR MARKERS

Sera from patients with various tumours have been found to contain circulating oncoproteins at a higher concentration than normal. Unfortunately, the results in one large series are not clear cut. This study looked at proteins immunologically related to c-*ras*, c-*sis*, and c-*src* gene products, in the urine of patients with several tumour types. More recently, p62 c-*myc* concentrations have been found to be elevated in patients with colorectal and breast cancer. Antibodies to oncogene products have also been used for immunoscintigraphy. Tumour localization has been successfully obtained using an antibody against c-*myc* in small cell lung cancer, and to epidermal growth factor receptor in patients with gliomas. There is little evidence that such scans are any more sensitive than conventional radiological procedures, but they may be of value in finding out more about the tumours' responses to drugs or radiation and thus have clinical utility.

RISK PREDICTION

Restriction fragment length polymorphism (RFLP) analysis has been used successfully for the diagnosis of genetic disorders from trophoblast samples in the early stages of pregnancy. It is also the basis of genetic fingerprinting; a technique which has recently resulted in a successful criminal conviction. Briefly, it involves taking a sample of DNA from a patient, usually from peripheral blood lymphocytes, cleaving

Table 3. New targets for anti-cancer drug development

Gene product	Agents
Growth factors	Agonists Antagonists Antibodies
Receptors	Down-regulators Signal interference
Protein kinases	Suicide peptides
GTP binders	Nucleoside analogues
Nuclear oncoproteins	Analogues Blockers Partition shifters
Transcription factors	Blockers

it with restriction enzymes at defined sites, running the DNA on an electrophoretic gel, and probing with a relevant probe. DNA sequence differences will produce different patterns of probe binding. The recognition of polymorphic patterns in populations, after restriction enzyme digestion, is the basis of RFLP analysis. RFLPs have been observed to occur round the c-*ras* gene locus. Certain patterns are found to be more likely to be associated with leukaemia, lung, and colon carcinoma. Here, the perfectly normal genome of the individual has surrounding sequences that make him or her more vulnerable. It is conceivable that in the not too distant future, RFLP analysis will enable prediction of high cancer risk.

THERAPY

The discovery of oncogenes has clearly given tremendous impetus to the understanding of the biology of cancer. It also provides new targets for developing pharmacological agents (Table 3). Growth factors, growth factor agonists and antagonists, and antibodies to the receptors for growth factors are clearly fruitful areas for new drug design. Furthermore, nucleoside analogues of guanosine triphosphate may successfully inhibit the *ras* protein, even though its function is as yet undefined. Many oncogene products such as tyrosine kinases exert their effects by phosphorylating tyrosine on diverse proteins. Several agents are available which can block this activity. The most intriguing are suicide peptides containing tyrosine. These molecules mimic the kinase's natural substrate and bind with high affinity to the enzyme, irreversibly destroying it. Such peptides are arousing intense interest in the drug industry, but as yet have not entered clinical trials.

SUMMARY

Recent advances in molecular biology thus seem poised for exploitation in the clinic. We will undoubtedly learn much more about the biological basis of cancer.

Therapeutic gains will come from the application of our increasing knowledge of oncogenes and the function of their protein products in growth control. The design of suitable molecules to inhibit these will almost certainly produce the systemic agents of the future.

FURTHER READING

Brodeur, G. M., Seeger, R. C., Schwab, M., *et al*. (1985) Amplification of N-*myc* in untreated human neuroblastomas correlates with advanced disease stage. *Science*, **224**, 1121–1124.

Downward, J., Yarden, Y., Mayes, E., *et al*. (1984) Close similarity of epidermal growth factor and v-*erb*B oncogene protein sequences. *Nature*, **307**, 521–527.

Gullick, W. J. and Venter, D. J. (1989) The c-*erb*B2 gene and its expression in human tumours. In: J. Waxman and K. Sikora (eds) *Molecular Biology of Cancer* pp. 38–53. Blackwell Scientific Publications, Oxford.

Lemoine, N. (1990) The *ras* oncogenes in human cancer. In: M. Sluyser (ed.) *The Molecular Biology of Cancer* pp. 143–170. John Wiley, Chichester.

Slamon, D. J., de Kernion, J. B., Verma, I. M. and Cline, M. J. (1984) Expression of cellular oncogenes in human malignancies. *Science*, **724**, 256–262.

Varley, J. M., Armour, J., Swallow, J. E., *et al*. (1989) The retinoblastoma gene is frequently altered leading to loss of expression in primary breast tumours. *Oncogene*, **4**, 725–730.

Wilkins, R. J. (1988). Genomic imprinting and carcinogenesis. *Lancet*, **i**, 329–331.

Woolford, J., Rothwell, J. and Rohrscheider, L. (1985) Characterisation of the human c-*fms* gene product and its expression in cells of the monocyte-macrophage lineage. *Mol. Cell. Biol.*, **5**, 3458–3466.

2 The c-*ras* Oncogenes and GAP

NICHOLAS R. LEMOINE

The *ras* oncogenes have assumed great importance in the molecular pathology of neoplasia and are probably the most intensively studied of the oncogene families. Abnormalities of these oncogenes are more frequently detected than any other in human tumours and also occur in many experimental models. The abnormalities are usually point mutations, but occasionally gene amplifications occur. A great deal of information about the structure and biochemical function of their encoded proteins has been accumulated, and more recently interpretation of their biological functions and interactions has been possible.

THE *ras* PROTO-ONCOGENES BELONG TO AN OLD-ESTABLISHED FAMILY

The three *ras* genes found in mammals—Harvey-, Kirsten- and N-*ras*—are members of a multigene family that is ubiquitous and highly conserved in eukaryotes, including yeast (see Figure 1). It can be seen that the protein sequence of each of the three *ras* oncogene products comprises four distinct domains: the first 80 amino acids are identical in Ha-, Ki- and N-*ras*, while the second domain of 80 amino acids shows rather less conservation (70–80%). The third region, which occupies the rest of the molecule (except for the last four amino acids), is the hypervariable region, in which there is wide divergence between the sequences of the *ras* proteins, allowing experimental production of antibodies specific to individual *ras* proteins. The C-terminus of four amino acids is a highly conserved motif (CAAX, where C is cysteine, A is any aliphatic amino acid—most often leucine, isoleucine or valine, all of which are hydrophobic residues—and X is any amino acid).

Genes and Cancer. Edited by D. Carney and K. Sikora
©1990 John Wiley & Sons Ltd

ras proteins / ras-related proteins — sequence alignment

		GXXXXGK (10-16)				DXXGXE (57-62)		
ras proteins								
HUMAN/RAT Ha-ras-1	MTEYKLVVV	GAGGVGK	SALT QL I QHHFVDE	YDPT I EDSY	R KQVV I DGETCLLD I L	DTAGQE	EYSAMRD QYMR	TGEGFLCVFA I WWTKSFED I HQYREQ I
HUMAN Ki-ras-2A	- - - - - - - -	- - - - - - -	- - - - - - - - - - - -	- - - - - - - -	- - - - - - - - - - - - - - - - - -	- - -	- - - - - - - - - - -	- H -
HUMAN Ki-ras-2B	- - - - - - - -	- - - - - - -	- - - - - - - - - - - -	- - - - - - - -	- - - - - - - - - - - - - - - - - -	- - -	- - - - - - - - - - -	- H -
HUMAN N-ras	- - - - - - - -	- - - - - - -	- - - - - - - - - - - -	- - - - - - - -	- - - - - - - - - - - - - - - - - -	- - -	- - - - - - - - - - -	S - - A - HL
ras-related proteins								
HUMAN R-Ras (26 aa) SETH- - - -	- G - - - -	- - - - - - F - SY - SD	- - - - - - - -	T - ICSV - - I PAR - - -	- - -	-FG - - - - E	- - - - A- H - - -L - - - - -DRQ - - NEVGKLFT - - -
MOUSE R-Ras (26 aa) GETH- - - -	- G - - - -	- - - - - - F - SY - SD	- - - - - - - -	T - ICSV - - I PAR - - -	- - -	-FG - - - - E	- - - - A- H - - -L - - - - -DRQ - - NEVGKLFT - - -
HUMAN Rap1A/Krev1	-R - - - - -L	-S - - - - -	- - -V - FV - G I - EK	-VFEN -	- - -EV - CQQ - M -E -	-T-	QFT - - -	L - -KN - Q - - AL - YS - TAQST - N - LQDL - - - -
HUMAN Rap1B	-R - - - - -L	-S - - - - -	- - -V - FV - G I - EK	-VFEN -	- - -EV - CQQ - M -E -	-T-	QFT - - -	L - -KN - Q - - AL - YS - TAQST - N - LQDL - - - -
HUMAN Rap2	-R - - -V - L	-S - - - - -	- - -V - FVTGT - I EK	-VFEN -	-E I EV - SS PS V -E -	-T-	QFAS - - -	L - IKN - Q - - IL - YSLV - QQ - - Q - - KPM -D -
SIMIAN Ral	MAANKPKGONSLALH-V IM	-S - - - - -	- - -L - FMYDE - -ED	-E - -KA - - -	- - K - L - - -EVQ I - -	- - -	D - A - I - -	- S - TEME - - - - - - AA TAD F - - -
Aplysia Rho	MAA I RK - - - I -	-D - AC - -	TC - L -V FSKDQ - PEV	-V - -VFEN -	- AD I EV - - KQVE - ALW	- - -	D - DRL - PLS - PD - DVILM	- - S - DSPD - L - W - PEKWTPE
HUMAN RhoA	MAA I RK - - - I	-D - AC - -	TC - L -V FSKDQ - PEV	-V - -VFEN -	V AD I EV - - KQVE - ALW	- - -	D - DRL - PLS - PD - DVILM	- - S - DSPD - L - W - PEKWTPE
HUMAN RhoB	MAA I RK - - - - -	-D - AC - -	TC - L -V FSKDQ - PEV	-V - -VFEN -	V AD I EV - - KQVE - ALW	- - -	D - DRL - PLS - PD - DVILM	- - SVDSPD - L - W - PEKWTPE
HUMAN RhoC	MAA I RK - - - I -	-D - AC - -	TC - L -V FSKDQ - PEV	-V - -VFEN -	I AD I EV - - KQVE - ALW	- - -	D - DRL - PLS - PD - DVILM	- - S - DSPD - L - W - PEKWTPE
RAT Rab1/MOUSE ypt1 (7aa)YDYLF - -LL I	-DS - - - - -	- -C - LLRFADDTYTES	- I S - -GVDF	K I RT I EL - -K - I K - Q -W	- - - - -	RFRTITS	S - Y - GAH - I IV - YDVTDQE - - NHVK - WLQE -
RAT/HUMAN Rab2 MAYAYLF - L I I I	-DT - - - - -	- -C - LL - FTDKR - QPV	H -L - MGVEF	GARM IT - - - KQIK - Q -W	- - - - -	SFRSITR	S - Y - GAA - A - L - YD - TRRDT - NHLTTWL - DA
RAT Rab3 (19 aa)DYM F - Y I I I	- MSS - - - - -	TSFLFRYADDS - TPA	FVS - VGIDF	KV - T YRNDKRIK - Q -W	R - RT IT	A - Y - GAM - - I LMYD -T - EE - HAVQDWST - -	
RAT Rab4 MSETYDFLF - FLV I	- MA -T - -	- -C -LH -F - EKK - K- D	SNH - GVEF	GQ - I INVG - KYVK - Q -W	RFRSVTT	S - Y - GAA - A - L - YD -TS RETYNALTN WLTD	
RAT BRL-ras LL - V I I L	-DS - - - - -	TS - MN - YVNKK - SNQ	- KA - GADF	LT - E - MV - DRLV IMQ -W	RFQSLGV	AFY - GADCC V L - DVTA PWT - KTLDSW - (10	

	120			140		160	180	189
	KRVKD	SDDVPMVLVG	NKCD	L AARTVESRQAQDLARS YGIP YI	ETSAK	TRQGVEDAFYTLVRE I RQHKLRKLNPPDESGPGCNSCK		CVLS
ras proteins								
HUMAN/RAT Ha-ras-1								
HUMAN Ki-ras-2A	-----	------E---	----	--- PS---DTK- ----- F-	-----	---------R--------YR-K-I SKEEKTPGCVK I K-		--IM
HUMAN Ki-ras-2B	-----	------E---	----	--- PS---DTK- ----- F-	-----	----D----------K-EKMSKDGKKKKKSK T-		--IM
HUMAN N-ras	-----	----------	----	--- PS---DTK-HE--K- ----- F-	-----	-----YRMK---SS-DGTQ-C-GLP		--VM
ras-related proteins								
HUMAN R-Ras	L----	R--F-V----	--A-	-- ESQ-Q-PRSE-SAFGA -H HVA -F	-A---	L-LN-DE--EQ---AV-KYQEQE-P-SPP-A-RKKGGGCP		---L
MOUSE R-Ras	L----	R--F-I----	--A-	-- ENQ-Q-LRSE-SSFSA -H HMT -F	-A---	L-LN-DE--EQ---AV-KYQEQE-P-SPP-A-RKKDGGCP		---L
HUMAN Rap1A/Krev1	L----	TE--I----	----	-- EDE-V-GKE-G-N---QWCNCA FL	-S---	SKIN-NEI-D---Q- N--T PVEKKPKKS		-L-L
HUMAN Rap1B	L----	T---I----	----	-- EDE-V-GKE-G-N---QWCNCA FL	-S---	SKIN-NEI-D---Q- N--TPV-GKARKSS		-Q-L
HUMAN Rap2	I----	R YEK--VI---	--V-	-- ESE-E-S-SEGRA--EEW-C-FM	-----	SKIN-DEL-AE I-Q MWYAAQ-DKDDPCCSA		-N IQ
SIMIAN Ral	L--E	DEN--FL---	--S-	-- EDK-Q-SVEE-KNR-DQW NVN-V	-----	--AN-DKV-FD-M----AR-MEDSKEKNGKKKRKSLA-RIRER		-C I L
Aplysia Rho	--	RHFCPN--I I---	--K-	-- -ND-TKRE-MKM KQE△L	-C---	-KE--R-V-E-AT-AAL-V-KK-KGG		--VL
HUMAN RhoA	--	HFCPN--I I---	--K-	-- -ND-HTRRE--KM KQE△M	-C---	-KD--REV-EMAT-AAL-A RRG-KKSG		-LVL
HUMAN RhoB	--	HFCPN--I I--A	--K-	-- -SD-HVRTE--M KQE△L	-C---	-KE--REV-E-AT-AAL-K RY GSQNGINC		-KVL
HUMAN RhoC	--	HFCPN--I I---	--K-	-- -QD-HTRRE--KM KQE△L	-C---	-KE--REV-EMAT-AGL-V RKN-RRRG		-P I L
RAT Rab1/MOUSE ypt1	D-Y A	-EN-NKL--	----	-TTKKV-DYTT-KEF-D- L--- FL	-----	NEKN--QS-M-MAA--KKRMGPGATAGGAEKSNVKIQ(7 aa)GGG		-C
RAT/HUMAN Rab2	RQHSW	-NMVIM-I-	--S-	-ESR-E-KKEEGEAF--E H-LI FM	-----	-A SN--E--INT AK--Y EK IQ EGVFD I NNEAN-IK IG(19 aa)GGG		-C
RAT Rab3	-TY S W	-NAQVL--	----	MEDE-V-S-ERGRQ--DN L-FE FF	-A---	DNIN-KQT-ER--DV-CEKMSES-DTA-PAVT-AKQG(13 aa)		-AC
RAT Rab4	A MLA	-QN IVI I-C-	--K-	-D-D-E-TFLE-SRF-QE NELM FL	-----	-GEN--E--MQCA-K-LNK IESGELD-ERM-S-IQYG(20 aa)		-GC
RAT BRL-ras	aa)	-PENF-F-VL--	--I-	-- EN-Q-ATKR--AWCY-KNN-- -F	----L	EA IN--Q--Q-IA-MALKQETEVELYNEF PEP I KLDK(10 aa)		-SC
		WKXD			EXSAX			CAAX
		116-119			143-147			186-189

Figure 1. Similarity of primary sequences of *ras* proteins and *ras*-related proteins. Blank spaces have been introduced to demonstrate optimal alignment, and identical residues are shown as a dash. The regions involved in nucleotide interactions are boxed with fine rules, the 'effector' region is boxed with a heavy rule. The C-terminal CAAX motif (residues 186–189) is also boxed. The region recognised by the rat monoclonal antibody Y13-259 is shaded. Residues 12, 13 and 61 are marked in italics. The cysteine residues in the C-terminal region (residues 180–184) which may be palmitylated to modulate biological activity are underlined

Other members of the family include *rho* (found in *Aplysia*, humans and yeasts), R-*ras* (in mammalian cells), *ral* (in primate cells), *rap1* and *rap2* (human cells), *rab1*, 2, 3 and 4 (rodent cells), BRL-*ras* (rat cells). Although these *ras*-related genes show close similarity of sequence in the regions responsible for guanine nucleotide binding, there is wide diversity in other areas. Only some members of the family (R-*ras* and *rap*) possess a sequence similar to the so-called effector region of *ras* p21 proteins (and therefore by inference act through a similar effector pathway), and none but Harvey-, Kirsten- and N-*ras* have the epitope recognized by the monoclonal antibody Y13-259 (Figure 1).

The *ras* genes encode 21 kDa proteins that are synthesised in the cytoplasm and then modified and translocated for attachment to the inner surface of the plasma membrane. The essential modification has been elucidated very recently and involves farnesylation of the cysteine residue of the motif followed by carboxymethylation and proteolytic cleavage of the terminal tripeptide. Palmitylation of other cysteine residues immediately upstream of the motif (Figure 1) influences the affinity of membrane binding and may be involved in modulation of the biological activity of individual *ras* proteins. The run of six lysine residues in Ki-*ras* 2B C-terminus also promotes membrane association. All the *ras* and *ras*-related proteins are able to bind, exchange and hydrolyse guanine nucleotides, although the GTPase activity of *ras* proteins activated by mutation is variably impaired. Hence, they show several features in common with the G proteins, such as visual rhodopsin, and are assumed to be involved in signal transduction. The regions of the molecule involved in the association with GTP/GDP are shown in Figure 1. Interpretation of the significance of activating mutations has been greatly enhanced by the analysis of the three-dimensional crystal structure of ras·GDP by Kim's group at the University of California and ras·GTP by Wittinghofer at Heidelberg. Mutations which occur *in vivo* to activate the transforming activity of *ras* protein occur in loop 1 (positions 12 and 13), which is in direct contact with the phosphate groups of the bound guanine nucleotide, or in loop 4 (position 61), which is immediately adjacent to this primary loop (Figure 2). Wittinghofer has recently shown that amino acid substitutions at positions 12 or 61 interfere with the coordination of a water molecule critical to the nucleophilic attack of GTP and hence reduce GTPase catalytic activity.

It has been a matter of some contention that the transforming activity of particular mutant *ras* proteins does not correlate with the relative reduction in intrinsic GTPase function of the isolated protein, but this has been resolved following the discovery of a second protein, GTPase-activating protein or GAP, that influences *ras* catalytic activity. Two forms of GAP have been isolated from human material, both derived from one specific mRNA species by differential splicing, but only one form is expressed in adult tissues. It is a cytoplasmic protein of 120 kDa that stimulates the GTPase activity of normal *ras* proteins more than 100-fold, but which is unable to raise the catalytic activity of mutant *ras* proteins at all. Several groups have shown that GAP interacts with the *ras* p21 proteins at their effector regions (residues 32 to 40 in Figure 1, and sleeve A in Figure 2). Binding of GAP to this region also occurs in mutant *ras* proteins, but stimulation of GTPase activity and hence switch-off of the signal associated with ras·GTP complex only occurs with normal *ras*. There is also evidence that various lipid molecules, particularly phosphatidylinositol

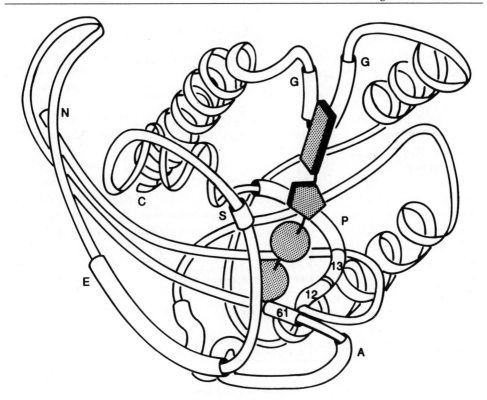

Figure 2. Backbone structure of human c-Ha-*ras* p21 protein·GDP complex, as determined by Kim and colleagues at the University of California. The flow of the backbone is shown as a continuous ribbon. The guanine base, ribose sugar moiety and the phosphates are represented by the stippled rectangular block, pentagonal block and spheres respectively. The regions binding the guanine base (G), ribose sugar (S), phosphates (P), neutralising antibody Y13-259 (A) and the so-called 'effector' domain are shown as sleeves over the ribbon backbone. Residues 12 and 13 (which form part of the phosphate-binding region on loop 1), and residue 61 (on loop 4) are those affected by point mutations and are indicated by numbered sleeves

phosphates and arachidonic acid derivatives, can influence the modulation of *ras* GTPase activity by GAP.

The fact that GAP is bound at the 'effector' region of *ras* p21 suggests that it is the downstream target for *ras* signal transduction. Because this effector region is conserved between all the various *ras* proteins and a single GAP species is responsible for the interaction, this would imply that all the signals are channelled through just one downstream route. However, it has been proposed that the carboxy terminal region of the *ras* proteins, which is quite distinct for each member of the family, could also be involved in transmission of signals, which would allow a more flexible system in which individual p21 proteins can use separate pathways. Weinberg's group at the Whitehead Institute in Massachusetts have identified a putative 60 kDa target protein, distinct from GAP, by covalent cross-linking, but this has not yet

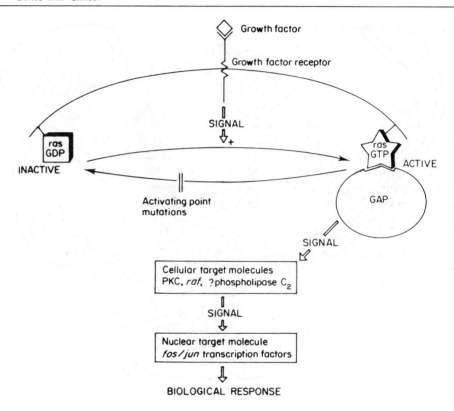

Figure 3. Schematic model for *ras*-associated signal transduction pathway. The stimulus for GDP/GTP exchange leading to activation of *ras* p21 is assumed to be a signal from a membrane-associated growth factor. Association of ras·GTP with GAP both transmits the signal (to a cellular target molecule) and inactivates ras·GTP by stimulation of *ras* endogenous GTPase activity (blocked by *ras*-activating point mutations). PKC is protein kinase C

been characterised in detail. It is also quite possible that bound ras·GTP influences the interaction of GAP with its cellular target molecule (Figure 3).

The connections both upstream and downstream of *ras* and GAP are currently rather vague, with experimental evidence often confusing and even contradictory. Much of this evidence is derived from microinjection studies of the neutralising antibody Y13-259 into normal and transformed cells. Treatment with this antibody is able to reverse the features of transformation by *ras* oncogenes, and also a number of membrane-associated tyrosine kinase oncogenes such as *fms, src* and *fes*. In addition, DNA synthesis and early increase in c-*fos* expression stimulated by serum, or purified epidermal growth factor or platelet-derived growth factor, can also be blocked by microinjected Y13-259. Such experiments have been interpreted as evidence that *ras* proteins lie downstream of membrane-associated growth factor receptors and tyrosine kinase oncogene products in the signal transduction cascade. The biological effects of the serine/threonine kinase oncogenes *mos* and *raf* are not blocked by microinjected Y13-259, and transformation either by *ras* or other membrane-associated oncogenes results in phosphorylation of the *raf* oncogene product and stimulation of its kinase activity. Hence, these cytoplasmic oncogene products probably lie downstream of *ras* proteins.

It now appears that some of these confusing results might be resolved by a model in which GAP, rather than *ras* p21, is the active participant in these pathways. It has recently been reported by McCormick and collaborators that GAP binds in stable complexes with the protein products of c-*abl*, v-*abl*, *abl*-*bcr*, v-*src* and v-*fms*, and can be phosphorylated by these kinases. There is some evidence that GAP serves as a negative regulator of c-*abl* tyrosine kinase function, analogous to its down-regulation of the active ras·GTP complex. GAP also binds tightly to PDGF receptor after PDGF-catalysed phosphorylation. The phosphorylated form of GAP is reported to have a much lower GTPase-stimulating activity on ras·GTP, which would in turn enhance the signal generated from this complex. Obviously, there is potential for interplay between the various pathways linked by association with GAP, and the situation probably varies between different cell types. A general scheme, proposed by McCormick is illustrated in Figure 4. Recent evidence from immunoprecipitation studies with anti-GAP antibodies suggests that GAP may form complexes with the protein product of the *raf* oncogene and phospholipase C_2, which implicates these molecules as potential steps in the signal transduction pathways routed via GAP.

It is in the area of second messenger molecules that the most confusing results have been found, with different groups publishing frankly contradictory data. A consensus

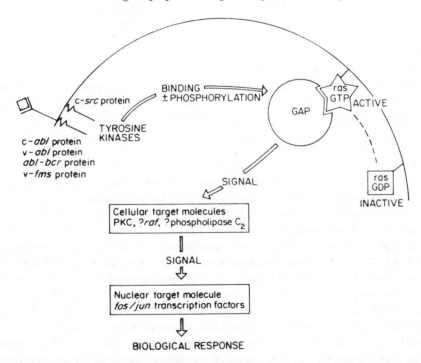

Figure 4. Schematic model for interaction of GAP with membrane-associated tyrosine kinases. Both receptor tyrosine kinases (such as v-*fms*) and non-receptor tyrosine kinases (such as c-*src*) may form complexes with GAP, in some cases phosphorylating this molecule, which reduces its ability to stimulate *ras* GTPase activity and stabilises the GAP/ras·GTP active complex. GAP may also form complexes with cytoplasmic molecules such as *raf* and phospholipase C_2

view is that in various experimental systems *ras* proteins can either increase or reduce the activity of protein kinase C, which has secondary effects on the levels of inositol phosphates in the cytoplasm. The *ras* proteins do not have direct effects on the enzymes phospholipase A_2 and phospholipase C, although the activities of both are often profoundly altered in *ras*-transformed cells. The final link in the chain of signal transduction through *ras* p21 proteins is the action of transcription factors such as AP-1 (a complex of the products of the c-*fos* and c-*jun* oncogenes), which influence the expression of a wide range of cellular genes.

SPECIFIC POINT MUTATIONS OF *ras* ONCOGENES IN HUMAN NEOPLASIA

The early studies of activated *ras* oncogenes in human and experimental tumours involved the use of biological assays for transforming activity in genomic DNA. These assays, the NIH3T3 focus induction assay and the nude mouse tumorigenicity assay, are very labour intensive but are highly sensitive and useful for validating the transforming activity of dominant oncogenes, not exclusively of the *ras* family, isolated from a range of tumour types. However, these assays have been largely supplanted by new, rapid techniques that directly identify the presence of base pair changes in the sequence of the *ras* oncogenes. These techniques all involve the use of the polymerase chain reaction with specific paired primers and a heat-stable DNA polymerase to amplify *in vitro* the sequence of interest. The most widely used (by ourselves and by many other laboratories) of the new assays is hybridisation of filter-bound amplified target DNA (from fresh tumour tissue or cryostat or paraffin sections) with batteries of sequence-specific oligonucleotide probes. The sensitivity of this approach can be tuned to an extraordinary degree by performing the hybridisation in liquid phase (as proposed by Kumar and Barbacid), and indeed it is feasible to detect a single mutant gene amongst 10^5 normal copies by this technique. Another assay, used by Perucho and colleagues, is RNAase A cleavage mismatch analysis in which the mismatched hybrid of RNA probe and amplified mutant DNA is cleaved by RNAase A and can be resolved by gel electrophoresis. Direct sequencing of double-stranded amplified DNA to detect base pair changes in sequence is becoming increasingly popular, but this method lacks the ultimate sensitivity of hybridisation and RNAase cleavage.

A wide range of human tumours has been analysed using one or more of these assays, and some interesting features have emerged. Some tumour types, such as sarcomas and carcinomas of breast, ovary, oesophagus and stomach, do not apparently possess *ras* activation. Others, such as tumours of exocrine pancreas, thyroid and colon, have a high frequency of activated *ras* oncogenes. For a more detailed catalogue of the frequencies and identities of activated *ras* alleles in human tumours, the reader should consult the references by Lemoine and by Bos (see Further Reading). I will discuss some of the more interesting examples here.

The most provocative finding has been the exceptionally high frequency of activated Ki-*ras* alleles in carcinomas of the exocrine pancreas; in series reported by Perucho and others it has been over 95% of cases. Not only is there this high frequency, but there is also some specificity of activation, with the first or second base of codon 12 of Ki-*ras* being favoured for G to A mutation. This is intriguing in view of the strong suspicion that carcinogens are involved in the aetiology of this highly malignant tumour. We are currently investigating the activation of *ras* oncogenes in experimental pancreatic tumours produced by a range of chemical carcinogens, in order to test this association.

Tumours of the thyroid gland form a useful multistage model of neoplasia which can be reproduced in experimental animals. The frequency of *ras* oncogene activation is approximately 50% in all stages from follicular adenoma through follicular carcinoma to undifferentiated carcinoma. This system was one of the first in which *ras* activation in an unequivocally benign lesion was demonstrated, and is powerful evidence that *ras* oncogene activation is associated with early stages of tumour development, such as initiation or establishment, rather than late stages, such as malignant progression, at least in some cases. Our *in vitro* reconstruction studies using retroviral introduction of activated *ras* oncogenes into primary human and rodent thyroid epithelial cultures also support this view. In contrast to the findings in fibroblast systems, our studies with this pure epithelial system suggest that expression of mutant *ras* is sufficient to rescue from senescence and partially transform primary cells without the co-operation of any other exogenous oncogene. Thyroid neoplasia is the only solid tumour type in which activation of all three members of the *ras* family has been shown to occur, but in this tumour type, as in pancreatic cancer, there is a specificity of mutation. The favoured mutation in differentiated tumours is transition (usually A to G) at codon 61 of N- or Ha-*ras*, while in undifferentiated tumours the predominant mutation is transversion at codon 12 of Ki-*ras*. It is significant that a similar specificity has been shown in the experimental model also, with carcinogen (NMU)-induced tumours invariably possessing Ha-*ras* oncogenes activated by mutation at codon 61, and radiation-induced tumours exclusively possessing activated Ki-*ras* oncogenes. Radiation exposure is a well-recognised risk factor for the development of thyroid cancer, and a range of environmental carcinogens have been shown to produce thyroid cancer in animals. It is possible that molecular analysis of activating mutations may give an insight into the possible role of such carcinogens in the aetiology of human thyroid neoplasia.

Several groups have demonstrated that activated *ras* alleles occur in approximately 40% of cancers of the colon and rectum. Vogelstein and others have shown that while large adenomas (particularly the villous type, which has a higher malignant potential) contain activated *ras* oncogenes at a similar frequency (40%), smaller adenomas are significantly less likely to contain such mutations (<20%). Hence in this multistage system too, *ras* activation is an early event occurring during the benign phase of the disease. Mutation specificity is evident here also, with most of the mutations reported being G to A transitions at the second G of Ki-*ras* codon 12.

A different mutation specificity is seen in adenocarcinomas of the lung (the frequency of *ras* mutation is 30% in this tumour type—other types of non-small cell lung cancer do not apparently contain activated *ras* genes). The favoured mutation is G to T transversion of Ki-*ras*, which has led some investigators to postulate the involvement of tobacco smoke carcinogens. However, it is of interest that epidemiological studies have in general shown that adenocarcinoma is the one subtype of non-small cell lung cancer not associated with cigarette smoking.

Ultraviolet (UV) irradiation may also be able to induce *ras* mutations. Bos has reported that in human melanomas *ras* mutations were restricted to those tumours that occurred in sun-exposed sites of the body. The majority of mutations were in the N-*ras* gene in or adjacent to dipyrimidine sites, which is a classic feature of UV-induced mutation.

Because of the relative ease of repeated sampling in patients with myeloid and lymphoid diseases, many groups have been able to analyse the incidence of *ras* activation at various stages in the evolution of these disorders. In the premalignant myeloid disorder known as myelodysplastic syndrome, *ras* mutations are found in about 30% of cases, and it appears that these patients have a higher chance of progression to AML and a worse overall prognosis. It also seems that one particular cell line is preferentially affected by *ras* mutation, since most of the reported examples are cases of AML classified as M4 (myelomonocytic) or M5 (monocytic).

As intriguing as the fact that *ras* activation occurs at high frequency in some human neoplasms is the fact that in other tumour types this oncogenic event is identified only very occasionally or not at all. For instance, only a very low frequency of *ras* activation occurs in human breast cancer, even though certain experimental models of breast cancer, such as NMU-induced rat mammary tumours, harbour mutant *ras* alleles at very high frequency. The same applies to carcinomas of the ovary, oesophagus and stomach, and also a range of sarcomas and lymphomas. It is unknown what genetic events can substitute for *ras* mutation in these tumours, but in view of the multiple links in the signal transduction pathway involving *ras* proteins there are a number of potential targets. Of course, it is likely that there are other pathways that do not involve *ras*, GAP or their associated proteins, and abnormalities of these may produce the same phenotypic effect.

ras GENES AS TUMOUR SUPPRESSOR GENES

Much interest has centred recently on tumour suppressor genes, or 'anti-oncogenes', such as the Rb gene and p53. Another candidate tumour suppressor gene is K-*rev*-1, which Noda and others have characterised in detail. This gene was originally isolated after transfecting Ki-*ras*-transformed mouse cells with a human fibroblast cDNA library and then selecting for 'flat revertants' from the transformed, tumorigenic phenotype. The K-*rev*-1 gene is identical in sequence to the *rap* 1A gene and shows much sequence homology with c-Ha-*ras* in the guanine nucleotide binding regions, in the effector domain, and at the membrane attachment motif at the C-terminus. When mutations are introduced into the sequence of K-*rev*-1 at positions analogous to those that activate c-Ha-*ras*, then very much lower levels of gene expression are required to induce reversion of transformed phenotype. The interpretation of these experiments is that this *ras*-related gene product acts as a transducer of growth inhibitory signals, or perhaps competes for the binding of GAP or other proteins involved in the effector arm of *ras* p21 signal transduction. The affinity of rap 1A·GTP binding to GAP is 100 fold higher than that of ras·GTP to GAP. The premise that *ras*-related proteins might compete for some limiting factor is supported by experiments in which expression of Ha-*ras* with an Asn 17 substitution inhibited cell proliferation, apparently by competition with the normal endogenous cellular *ras* protein.

FUTURE DIRECTIONS

The frequent involvement of activated *ras* oncogenes in common human tumour types has stimulated a search for specific anti-*ras* weapons for cancer treatment. One area that is being explored is interference with the lipid modifications that are essential for normal membrane attachment (and biological activity) of *ras* proteins, using inhibitors of mevalonate synthesis such as compactin and mevinolin. Although these compounds can inhibit cellular proliferation *in vitro,* and cells transformed with mutant *ras* may be more sensitive to this effect than those expressing only normal *ras,* the effective concentrations profoundly depress most cholesterol synthesis and hence many essential cellular functions.

Another area of interest is the use of anti-sense oligodeoxynucleotides directed specifically against the expression of mutant *ras* oncogenes. There is evidence that this approach can be effective *in vitro,* but there are many problems associated with achieving adequate dosage and stability *in vivo.* However, increasing sophistication is being achieved in the chemical modification of these compounds to protect them against serum and cellular nuclease activity.

A picture of the links in the chain of signal transduction in which *ras* proteins participate is gradually developing, and once the upstream and downstream elements are clearly identified this will undoubtedly lead to other therapeutic strategies. Already the implication of GAP as an important regulator of normal *ras* activity suggests that it may be possible to design a modified GAP molecule that could regulate mutant *ras* activity. Indeed, McCormick and colleagues report that a synthetic peptide corresponding to the potential active site of GAP (identified through sequence homologies with both the GTP-binding subunit of the stimulatory regulator of adenylate cyclase and the yeast gene *IRA*-1) is able to affect the dissociation rate of GDP from *ras* p21, causing exchange of GDP for GTP *in vitro.* GAP and other downstream elements may therefore be appropriate targets for blocking strategies in tumours expressing mutant *ras* oncogenes.

FURTHER READING

Barbacid, M. (1987) *ras* genes. *Ann. Rev. Biochem.,* **56**, 779–827.

Bos, J. L. (1989) *ras* oncogenes in human cancer: a review. *Cancer Res.,* **49**, 4682–4689.

De Vos, A. M., *et al.* (1988) Three-dimensional structure of an oncogene protein: catalytic domain of human c-Ha-*ras* p21. *Science,* **239**, 888–893.

Kitayama, H., Sugimoto, Y., Matsuzaki, T., *et al.* (1989) A *ras*-related gene with transformation suppressor activity. *Cell,* **56**, 77–84.

Lemoine, N. R. (1990) *ras* oncogenes in human cancers. In: M. Sluyser (ed.), *The Molecular Biology of Cancer Genes.* pp. 143–170. John Wiley, Chichester.

Marshall, C. J. (1988) The *ras* oncogenes. *J. Cell Sci. (Suppl.),* **10**, 157–169.

McCormick, F. (1989) *ras* GTPase activating protein: signal transmitter and signal terminator. *Cell,* **56**, 5–8.

Pai, E. F., *et al.* (1989) Structure of the guanine-nucleotide binding domain of the Ha-*ras* oncogene product p21 in the triphosphate conformation. *Nature,* **341**, 209–214.

Tong, L., Milburn, M. V., De Vos, A. M. and Kim, S.-H. (1989) Structure of *ras* protein. *Science,* **245**, 244.

3 | The *myc* Oncogene

GERARD I. EVAN

THE DISCOVERY OF THE *myc* ONCOGENE

The *myc* oncogene was first identified as the transforming gene of the avian myelocytomatosis viruses, retroviruses which cause acute myelocytic leukaemia as well as a number of other types of neoplasm in affected chickens. *In vitro,* the avian myelocytic leukaemia viruses are able to transform macrophage-like cells and bone marrow. These transformed cells bear many of the features of early macrophages and appear identical to the target cells *in vivo.* In mutants of the myelocytomatosis viruses with altered *myc* genes, the transforming potential of the virus is generally compromised or absent, demonstrating that the *myc* gene of the virus (viral or v-*myc*) is responsible for its oncogenic activity.

THE VIRAL *myc* ONCOGENE

Like almost all oncogenes found in acutely transforming retroviruses, the v-*myc* oncogene is not required for the normal life cycle of the avian myelocytomatosis viruses. Retroviruses typically contain only three genes:

1. *gag,* which encodes the virus core proteins. These polypeptides contain antigenic markers which are used to serotypically define particular groups of retrovirus, hence '*gag*' from 'group antigen'.
2. *pol,* which encodes the retrovirus DNA polymerase enzyme—reverse transcriptase.

Genes and Cancer. Edited by D. Carney and K. Sikora
©1990 John Wiley & Sons Ltd

3. *env*, which encodes the virus envelope 'spike' glycoprotein responsible for target cell specificity.

It is believed that viral oncogenes are acquired by a random mutational event. As such, they are found inserted randomly within the viral genome, the only requirement being that they can be expressed in some way, either as fusion proteins containing a hybrid of viral and oncogene protein sequence, or from separate mRNAs. Because acquisition of a viral oncogene usually occurs via the exchange of some of the virus's own sequence, such retroviruses usually lack important sequences and are thus replication defective.

Four independent isolates of avian myelocytomatosis virus have been characterised: MC29, CM II, OK10 and MH2 viruses. Each has a v-*myc* gene inserted within its genome in a unique way. In MC29 and CM II viruses, *myc* sequences are encoded by single hybrid mRNAs which contain viral *gag* (core protein) sequences at their 5' ends. In OK10 and MH2 viruses *myc* sequences are expressed both as genomic and spliced mRNAs. Each isolate of avian myelocytomatosis virus thus expresses *myc* sequence-containing polypeptides of a discrete size peculiar to that virus, because each is fused to differing amounts of other viral proteins. The fact that all viral *myc* proteins are chimaeras of *myc* and viral *gag*-encoded sequences meant that characterisation of the proteins was possible using *gag*-specific antibodies. Such early studies showed that viral *myc* proteins were largely localised to the cell nucleus, phosphorylated and had very short biological half-lives. However, the functions of these v-*myc* proteins in carcinogenesis remained elusive.

More recently, retrovirally transduced c-*myc* has been identified in isolates of feline leukaemia virus (FeLV), where it is associated with sarcomatous disease. As in the avian system, feline v-*myc* sequences are fused to viral *gag* to generate chimaeric proteins.

THE c-*myc* GENE

The viral *myc* (v-*myc*) gene, like most retrovirus oncogenes, is closely related to, and presumably derived from, a gene found in normal cells, the cellular *myc* (c-*myc*) gene. The c-*myc* gene is highly conserved throughout vertebrate evolution and has been isolated and sequenced in fish, amphibians, avians and mammals. The gene always comprises three exons, of which the first is largely non-coding. Conservation of the coding sequence of the c-*myc* gene is extensive and especially marked in certain regions, the so-called *myc* homology boxes, which may encode important functional domains of the c-*myc* protein. Although present in all species, the first exon of the c-*myc* gene is not well conserved in sequence across the vertebrate phylum. Its function, if any, is unknown, although many have proposed that it might have some role in transcriptional or translational regulation of c-*myc* expression.

c-*myc* AND CANCER

A number of independent lines of evidence have implicated the c-*myc* gene in neoplastic disease, aside from its obvious association with the v-*myc* oncogene.

The first came from a study of avian bursal lymphoma in which retroviruses were again implicated. Avian bursal lymphoma is, typically, associated with chronic infection by avian leukosis virus (ALV), a weakly pathogenic and replication-competent retrovirus lacking any obvious oncogene. Analysis showed that the c-*myc* gene locus in avian lymphoma cells had been disrupted by the nearby insertion of retrovirus promoter/enhancer sequences. Retroviruses integrate into the host genome as an obligatory part of their life cycle. Because retroviruses contain strong promoter and enhancer elements, they can, under certain circumstances, cause the inappropriate expression of neighbouring cellular genes. In the case of a cellular proto-oncogene like c-*myc*, this may have dire carcinogenic consequences. The precise mechanism by which ALV insertion activates the c-*myc* gene is unknown but in most, perhaps all, cases the ALV provirus is defective due to some mutational accident. Such defectiveness may be a requirement for c-*myc* activation.

A second, related phenomenon was identified in two B-cell lymphomatous diseases in mammals, mouse plasmacytoma and human Burkitt's lymphoma. Mouse plasmacytomas carry a characteristic chromosomal translocation involving the distal part of chromosome 15 and the distal parts of chromosome 12 or, less frequently, chromosome 6. The distal arm of chromosome 15 contains the c-*myc* gene, whilst the affected regions of mouse chromosomes 12 and 6 carry the immunoglobulin gene loci for heavy chain and *κ* light chain respectively. Thus, this translocation brings about the *de novo* juxtaposition of the c-*myc* gene with a region of the mouse genome which, in B-lineage derived cells such as plasmacytomas, is highly transcriptionally active. Aberrant expression of c-*myc* is then thought to occur, although the precise mechanisms of alteration in expression are unclear. Similar chromosomal translocations are typical of human Burkitt's lymphoma, and involve the immunoglobulin heavy chain locus on chromosome 14 (14q32) and the *κ* and λ light chain loci on chromosomes 2 (2p12) and 22 (22q11) reciprocally translocating with the c-*myc* locus on chromosome 8 (q24).

Amplification of *myc* genes has been reported in a number of diverse neoplasms, including colon carcinoma, small cell lung carcinoma, retinoblastoma, neuroblastoma, promyelocytic leukaemia and breast carcinoma. Cells exhibiting amplified *myc* genes frequently contain double minute chromosomes (DMs), C-bandless chromosomes (CMs) or homogeneously staining regions (HSRs), all visible cytogenetic abnormalities pointing to amplification of regions of the cells' DNA. *In situ* hybridization studies have shown that these regions contain multiple copies of the affected oncogene. In most cases, *myc* gene amplification is observed in cell lines derived from tumours and is not present in the primary neoplasm. This has suggested that *myc* gene amplification may solely reflect some process of habituation to growth *in vitro*. Against this argument, however, are several observations. First, in one case of promyelocytic leukaemia, and in neuroblastomas generally, *myc* gene amplification has been reported in the original primary tumours. Moreover, in the experimental mouse tumour SEWA, amplification of the c-*myc* gene is gradually lost during *in vitro* passage but regained following transplantation through a syngeneic mouse. Additionally, the degree of *myc* gene amplification observed is highly variable from tumour to tumour, ranging from one to several hundred-fold, and in neuroblastoma a greater number of copies of the N-*myc* gene correlates well with a worse prognosis (see below). Finally, amplification of *myc* genes is invariably associated with significantly greater levels of expression of *myc* proteins within the affected cells. In summary, therefore, amplification of *myc* proto-oncogenes does appear to have some role in progressive carcinogenesis.

Although both amplification and translocation can result in elevated expression of *myc* genes they seem to be mechanisms restricted to only a few types of neoplasm. Despite this, elevated expression of c-*myc* is virtually ubiquitous amongst primary tumours and its degree is frequently related to the prognosis of the disease. In the absence of obvious amplification or rearrangements, the mechanism of over-expression of *myc* genes in tumour cells is unknown. It is of note, however, that in untransformed cells steady-state levels of *myc* protein and mRNA appear to be very tightly controlled at levels much lower than those observed in tumour cells. It would thus appear that some lesion within this homeostatic regulation is a common, and perhaps obligatory, event during multi-stage carcinogenesis.

PRODUCTS OF THE c-*myc* GENE

The different isolates of avian myelocytic leukaemia viruses express *myc* mRNAs and proteins of various sizes because of the differing ways in which the *myc* gene is inserted into the various viral genomes. In man, the c-*myc* gene produces two transcripts of 2.2 and 2.4 kb in size. Both of these contain non-coding sequences from exon 1 as well as exons 2 and 3 coding sequence. The two differing transcripts arise from two promoters, both of which appear to be active in most cell types. Differential use of these promoters can occur in some tumours with translocated c-*myc* genes, but its significance, if any, is unclear. Both the 2.2 and 2.4 kb transcripts encode a protein of predicted molecular weight 49 kDa. Similar size proteins are predicted from the size of open reading frames in mouse, chicken, toad and trout. However, the apparent sizes of c-*myc* proteins on SDS polyacrylamide gels is of the order of 62 kDa. Although part of this discrepancy is due to post-translational modification, most appears to be caused by the high proportion of proline, lysine and arginine residues in c-*myc* proteins.

The c-*myc* protein has been extensively characterised and studied. However, almost all these studies have concentrated on the protein in tumour cells. This is because levels of c-*myc* protein in untransformed cells are so low as to be virtually undetectable, whereas tumour cells typically contain 10–100 times more. In human cells, the c-*myc* protein appears as a pair of closely spaced bands with molecular weights between 62 and 64 kDa on an SDS polyacrylamide gel. The higher molecular weight component is now known to be the product of a cryptic CTG initiation site for translation within the first exon, which generates a protein with an N-terminal extension of 14 amino acids. The significance of this larger protein is unknown, although some evidence suggests that it may possess functional differences from the shorter form. The transcriptional activating property of c-*myc* protein on the adenovirus E4 promoter is specific to the larger form of the protein. Both c-*myc* polypeptides are phosphorylated at serine and threonine residues, localise to the cell nucleus, bind single- and double-stranded DNA *in vitro*, and have an extremely short half-life of some 20 minutes. The rapid degradation of the c-*myc* protein is energy-dependent, and the protein is stabilised by treatment of cells with azide or deoxyglucose. High-resolution microscopic analysis of the distribution of the c-*myc* protein within the interphase cell nucleus reveals a general distribution throughout the nucleus but sparing the nucleoli. Confocal microscopy suggests a more heterogeneous pattern of distribution with some evidence of colocalisation with other known nuclear markers such as small nuclear ribonucleoproteins (snRNPs). During mitosis, c-*myc* proteins are not associated with condensed chromosomes although staining is seen throughout the rest of the cell.

OTHER *myc* GENES

The human genome contains several genes which share significant homology to the c-*myc* oncogene and can be identified using low stringency DNA hybridisation. The two best characterised of these *myc*-related genes, N-*myc* and L-*myc*, were identified and isolated on the basis of their homology to c-*myc* and because they are found to be amplified in certain types of tumour. N-*myc*, L-*myc* and c-*myc* genes all have very similar overall structures, comprising three exons of which the first is almost entirely non-coding. In addition, they share several regions of high homology and encode similar sized proteins.

The human N-*myc* gene was identified using avian v-*myc* probes at reduced stringency to analyse *myc* genes in human neuroblastoma cells. Human neuroblastoma cells, especially from more aggressive tumours, frequently show cytological evidence of gene amplification. The amplified regions of DNA were shown to contain a novel gene with substantial homology to c-*myc*, the N-*myc* gene. N-*myc* contains an open reading frame sufficient to encode a 456 amino acid polypeptide that is translated from a 2.8 kb mRNA. Antibodies raised against synthetic peptides and bacterial fusion proteins have been used to identify the N-*myc* protein in cells as a DNA-binding, nuclear phosphoprotein of about 64 kDa on SDS gels. Close inspection reveals that at least three polypeptides are present. Part of this heterogeneity is caused by differing degrees of phosphorylation and part by there being two ATG start codons used in N-*myc* protein synthesis. Thus, the N-*myc* protein possesses heterogeneity at its N-terminal end, somewhat reminiscent of the situation with the c-*myc* protein. Unlike c-*myc*, N-*myc* expression is extremely restricted in the adult. During embryogenesis N-*myc* expression is seen at high levels in many tissues, including foetal brain, kidney, retina and lung. Amplification of N-*myc* is seen in a number of tumours and tumour cell lines of neuroectodermal origin, principally neuroblastoma, Wilm's tumour, retinoblastoma and small cell lung carcinoma. In neuroblastoma, there is excellent evidence that the more serious incidences of the disease (stages III and IV) tend to have a greater degree of N-*myc* amplification than the more benign cases (stages I and II). Intriguingly, type IV-S neuroblastomas, typified by small primary tumours, extensive metastasis and frequent spontaneous remission, show low levels of N-*myc* amplification more akin to stage I and II disease. Analysis of degrees of N-*myc* amplification in neuroblastomas is thus likely to prove useful in determining strategies for therapy. However, the mechanism linking amplification of N-*myc* with more aggressive neoplasia is unknown. Studies have shown that a greater degree of N-*myc* gene amplification invariably leads to higher levels of the N-*myc* protein in cells, suggesting a role for elevated N-*myc* protein in more serious disease. However, some high-level expression of N-*myc* protein in neuroblastoma cells is not attributable to N-*myc* gene amplification. It thus seems likely that, as is the case with c-*myc*, elevated levels of N-*myc* protein in cells can occur by several mechanisms, of which amplification is but one. This implies that a high level of N-*myc* protein in neuroblastomas, whatever its cause, may prove an even better prognostic indicator than the degree of N-*myc* gene amplification.

The human L-*myc* gene was first identified as an amplified gene in a number of human small cell lung carcinoma cell lines. The L-*myc* gene comprises a three exon structure similar to c-*myc* and N-*myc*, with an open reading frame encoding a predicted polypeptide of 364 amino acids. Antibodies raised against synthetic peptide containing L-*myc* sequences identify three polypeptides of between 60 and 64 kDa in size, all probably expressed from a single 2.3 kb mRNA. The two larger L-*myc* proteins appear to be hyperphosphorylated forms of the smaller and their relative levels are raised by treatment of cells with phorbol esters—activators of protein kinase C. Some evidence also exists suggesting that L-*myc* is expressed from two mRNAs, generated by alternate splicing, and that these different mRNAs further contribute to L-*myc* protein heterogeneity. L-*myc* is expressed in many tissues throughout embryogenesis, particularly brain. Like N-*myc* however, its developmental expression is much more restricted, both temporally and spatially, than that of c-*myc*. No adult tissues have so far been identified that express appreciable levels of L-*myc* mRNA or protein.

In general, the similarities between all three characterised *myc* proteins, c-, N- and L-*myc*, far outweigh their differences. All are nuclear phosphoproteins of similar size which bind DNA *in vitro*. All have very short biological half-lives, although that of L-*myc* is notably longer (60–90 minutes; as opposed to 20–25 minutes for c- and N-*myc*). All share a number of discontinuous regions of amino acid sequence homology, regions which have also been conserved amongst *myc* genes throughout vertebrate evolution and presumably comprise important functional domains of the proteins. The major difference between *myc* gene products lies in their patterns of expression. Whereas c-*myc* is almost ubiquitously expressed in adult proliferative tissues and in embryos, N-*myc* and L-*myc* are much more restricted. Until the functions of *myc* proteins in normal cells are elucidated, it is impossible to judge the significance of these differences in expression amongst *myc* genes. It is possible that there are functional differences between the three *myc* proteins. Alternatively, they may have identical functions yet be regulated by different parameters of differentiation and proliferation.

EXPRESSION OF *myc* GENES

As with all proto-oncogenes, a distinction has to be drawn between the 'normal' functions of *myc* genes in untransformed cells and their 'pathological' functions in tumour cells. Presumably the two are related, but carcinogenic functions may only represent a subset of the normal. The c-*myc* oncogene first came to notice because of its homology to the viral oncogene v-*myc*. Subsequently, deregulated expression of c-*myc* was shown to be associated with a variety of neoplasms, but early studies showed that introduction of the c-*myc* gene into normal fibroblasts by transfection was not sufficient to transform the recipient cells. Subsequently, it was shown that c-*myc* could cause transformation of fibroblasts but only when *co-transfected* with a mutated and carcinogenic form of the *ras* oncogene. Thus, c-*myc* is only capable of transforming cells in co-operation with another oncogene. Analogous studies have since shown that both N-*myc* and L-*myc* behave similarly. Thus, all *myc* genes appear to have a transforming potential which is presumably only realised *in vivo* as part of a multi-stage carcinogenic sequence. In the absence of any known normal function for *myc* genes, the co-transfection assay described above is still the only assay available for *myc* function. However, it is important to bear in mind that it measures only one aspect of *myc* function—that associated with tumorigenesis.

c-*myc* expression in untransformed cells: relationship to the cell cycle

Untransformed cells, such as fibroblasts or lymphocytes, maintained in culture proliferate only in response to specific growth factors. In the absence of such factors, untransformed cells do not divide and are quiescent. Addition of appropriate growth factors to quiescent cells induces them to re-enter the cell cycle and subsequently proliferate. This re-entry into the cell cycle is accompanied by the rapid induction of a family of genes which presumably are involved in mediating the mitogenic process. Members of this 'early' gene family include the proto-oncogenes c-*fos* and c-*jun*, a number of other less well-defined genes, and the c-*myc* gene. Their rapid induction after mitogenesis suggested that these 'early' genes were likely to be active early in the cell cycle. However, c-*myc* differs from the majority of early mitogen response genes in a number of ways. It is induced somewhat later than the other early genes. Its expression is almost always linked with cell proliferation whereas many of the others are also induced by a wide variety of non-mitogenic stimuli. And it is frequently expressed for extended periods, whereas most early genes are expressed only transiently. Its peculiarities suggest a unique role for c-*myc* in the regulation of cell proliferation.

Careful quantitative analysis of the levels of c-*myc* protein in untransformed fibroblasts during mitogenic induction have been made. In quiescent fibroblasts, less than 300 molecules of c-*myc* protein are present. Following addition of growth factors, c-*myc* protein levels rise over about 2 hours to a maximum of some 10 000 molecules per cell. Thereafter, the level per cell falls within later G_1 to about 4000 molecules, a level which then remains constant throughout the cell cycle as long as the cells remain in log phase. At all times, the very short half-life of both c-*myc* mRNA and protein are both maintained. Thus, expression of c-*myc* in growing cells is both an active and a continuous process.

Upon removal of necessary growth factors from proliferating untransformed cells they eventually stop growing and re-enter a quiescent state, commonly referred to as G_0. However, growth arrest is not necessarily immediate and is dependent upon an individual cell's position with the cell cycle; for example, cells beyond a certain point in G_1 are committed to traversing the cell cycle irrespective of external factors. Whatever a cell's position in the cell cycle, however, removal of growth factors results in a rapid decrease in the level of both c-*myc* mRNA and protein at a rate consistent with their short biological half-lives. Thus, c-*myc* mRNA and protein appear to be sensitive and continuous indicators of growth factor stimulation, consistent with a role for c-*myc* protein in signal transduction.

Untransformed fibroblasts can also be rendered quiescent by contact inhibition. Contact inhibition is also accompanied by a fall in the level of c-*myc* protein to barely measurable levels. When confluent, i.e. contact inhibited, cells are stimulated with growth factors they will go through one cell cycle but then become quiescent again: confluent cells are unable to enter a continuous proliferative state and appear committed to a return to G_0. This is reflected in the pattern of expression of c-*myc* mRNA and protein. Although confluent cells exhibit the same rapid induction of c-*myc* as sub-confluent cells upon mitogenic stimulation, thereafter levels of c-*myc* mRNA and protein rapidly fall so that by the end of G_1 virtually no c-*myc* expression is detectable. The early disappearance of c-*myc* mRNA and protein thus correlates with commitment of confluent cells to traverse only one cell cycle. This suggests that the decision to enter quiescence in contact-inhibited cells is made in late G_1, before the onset of DNA synthesis, and may be mediated by c-*myc*.

Further evidence suggesting a role for c-*myc* in regulating entry into G_0 comes from many studies examining the role of c-*myc* expression in differentiation. Many tumour cell lines will differentiate in response to various chemical inducers and such differentiation is almost always accompanied by abrupt repression of c-*myc* expression. Similar repression of c-*myc* expression is also seen in certain untransformed cells. However, enforced expression of c-*myc* completely prevents differentiation, probably by preventing transient withdrawal of cells from the cell cycle.

The role of c-*myc* in cellular proliferation thus appears to be quite subtle. Expression of c-*myc* is dependent upon exogenous growth regulatory signals, positive and negative, irrespective of a cell's position within the cell cycle. Sustained c-*myc* expression, observed only in exponentially growing cells, requires continuous expression of the c-*myc* gene because of the short half-lives of both c-*myc* mRNA and protein. However, exponential growth is probably a rare state in tissues *in vivo* except in unusual circumstances such as embryogenesis or regeneration after wounding. In normal cells, the role of c-*myc* may thus be to determine the choice of a cell to cease or continue proliferating. In this model, transient or sustained repression of c-*myc* leads to rapid disappearance of the c-*myc* protein and acts as a signal for the cell to quiesce, whereas sustained expression of c-*myc* keeps a cell proliferating. In a multicellular organism in which unrestrained cell growth is automatically life-threatening, it makes sense to regulate the decision to continue proliferating by a short-lived signal.

Expression of c-*myc* in tumour cells

In transformed cells, c-*myc* expression is almost always at an elevated level and, moreover, is not responsive to external growth factors. Generally, tumour cells deprived of necessary growth factors show no down-regulation of c-*myc* expression and, significantly, are unable to quiesce. In unfavourable growth circumstances which would lead to sustained quiescence of untransformed cells, transformed cells continue to attempt to proliferate, with the result that many of them die.

Almost all transformed cell lines exhibit an inability to become truly quiescent.

Neither contact inhibition nor deprivation of growth factors, conditions which lead to complete and stable growth arrest in untransformed cells, causes tumour cells to become quiescent. Significantly, high levels of c-*myc* expression are also virtually ubiquitous in tumour cells, the principal exceptions being tumour cells expressing high levels of some other member of the *myc* family. The high level of c-*myc* expression in transformed cells is constitutive and entirely refractory to down-regulation by removal of growth factors. In untransformed cells, c-*myc* expression is tightly regulated to prevent excess production of c-*myc* protein. This implies that some form of lesion in c-*myc* autoregulation is responsible for the high level of c-*myc* expression in tumour cells. In some cases, such lesions are obvious as amplifications or rearrangements of the c-*myc* gene, but the cause of uncontrolled c-*myc* expression in the majority of tumour cells is unknown. Whatever the mechanism, however, the evidence does suggest that deregulation of *myc* expression is a frequent, perhaps ubiquitous, component of the multi-stage carcinogenic process.

THE FUNCTION OF *myc* PROTEINS

Elucidation of the complete function of the c-*myc* gene product remains elusive. Nonetheless, a number of diverse studies have begun to shed light on the various properties and functions of the c-*myc* protein and, thus, suggest possible roles for the protein in normal and neoplastic cells. Clues to *myc* protein function have, in the main, come from analyses of the regions of the protein required for its biological function as a transforming protein, from studies of the highly conserved domains of the protein, and from comparisons of these conserved domains with other proteins of known function.

Highly conserved regions of the c-*myc* protein

Several regions within the c-*myc* protein are highly conserved in amino acid sequence, both throughout c-*myc* gene evolution and between different members of the *myc* gene family (i.e. c-, N-, L- and v-*myc* proteins). The first regions of homology identified were the so-called 'myc boxes'—two discontinuous amino acid sequences within exon 2 and present in c-, N- and L-*myc* proteins. Subsequent analyses have shown that some seven or eight such regions of *myc* protein are highly conserved. Such conservation strongly suggests that these regions of the protein are involved in *myc* protein functions. Almost all of the conserved regions of the c-*myc* protein are now known to be associated with specific functional properties.

Regions associated with transforming potential of c-*myc*

Until recently, the only assay for c-*myc* function was the gene's oncogenic activity in a co-transformation assay. Not only is this assay slow and unwieldy, but it examines only the pathological function of the *myc* gene, usually associated with inappropriate and elevated expression. We do not understand the relationship between the normal and oncogenic functions of c-*myc*, mainly because of our ignorance of its role in normal cells. It is possible, perhaps likely, that the oncogenic properties of c-*myc* represent only a subset of its total functions in normal cells. Notwithstanding this proviso, considerable effort has gone into attempts to define regions of the c-*myc* protein responsible for its oncogenic activity. Early studies of v-*myc* identified a number of mutants with severely compromised oncogenic potential, so confirming v-*myc* as an oncogene. Unfortunately, no temperature-sensitive mutants of v-*myc* for transformation have ever been identified, a fact that has not helped elucidation of its *modus oncogensis*.

A number of attempts have been made to map regions of the c-*myc* protein necessary for oncogenic activity by site-directed mutagenesis. Mutants of the three most highly conserved domains in the second exon of human c-*myc* (corresponding to amino acid sequences 44–65, 128–144 and 185–200 in the c-*myc* protein) were constructed and examined for their oncogenic potential. Deletion of the region 185–200 made little difference to transforming activity, but loss of regions 44–65 and 128–144 severely affected the oncogenic potential of the protein. A more extensive mutagenesis study on the entire c-*myc* sequence subsequently mapped the sequences essential for cotransforming activity to two regions: amino acids 106–143 and the C-terminal 119 amino acids (residues 320–439). This later study did not find the first *myc* homology region (amino acids 44–65) to be necessary for oncogenic potential. Differences such as this probably reflect inherent shortcomings of co-transformation as an assay: it is subject to many uncontrollable variations and is difficult to score.

As well as mutational analysis, theoretical analyses of *myc* protein structure comparing sequences with other transforming proteins have also indicated possible regions responsible for transforming function.

Nuclear localisation signals

Nuclear targeting of the human c-*myc* protein is mediated by two short peptide sequences located at residues 320–328 and 364–374. Peptide 320–328 has the sequence PAAKRVKLD and is the strongest of the two signals. Attachment of this sequence to exogenous proteins causes their complete accumulation in the nucleus and deletion of the sequence results in a mutant c-*myc* protein which is distributed throughout the nuclear and cytoplasmic compartments. Interestingly, the mutant still possesses transforming activity. In contrast, sequence 364–374 (RQRRNELKRSP) induces only partial nuclear localisation but is essential for transforming function. This is probably because this region is involved in DNA binding of the c-*myc* protein (see below).

Phosphorylation of c-*myc* protein

At least three well-characterised protein kinases, casein kinase II, protein kinase A and glycogen synthase kinase 3, are known to phosphorylate c-*myc* protein. Sites of *in vivo* phosphorylation have been partially mapped to specific serine and threonine residues. The effect of phosphorylation on c-*myc* protein activity is unknown, but phosphorylation of many other DNA-binding proteins is known to modulate functions such as their degree of dimerisation and/or affinity for DNA. However, the dynamics of expression and degradation of the c-*myc* protein differ from that of most known transcriptional regulator proteins, most of which are made at specific times for specific functions and are substantially longer lived than c-*myc* protein. In contrast, the c-*myc* protein is rapidly synthesised and rapidly degraded throughout the growth phase of the cell cycle, such that cessation of synthesis results in being substantial clearance of the protein from the cell within an hour. It might thus be thought that the activity of c-*myc* protein could be adequately regulated solely by control of its synthesis. Thus, if phosphorylation of c-*myc* protein does regulate its activity, it must do so over a time scale measured in minutes or even seconds.

Oligomerisation of c-*myc* protein

The extreme C-terminus of the c-*myc* protein comprises a structural motif involved in dimerisation, the so-called 'leucine zipper'. This is an α-helical domain with a characteristic heptad repeat of leucine residues. Two such helices are able to dimerise in a parallel orientation to form a stable coiled-coil structure. All members of the *myc* protein family have leucine zippers, as do a number of transcriptional regulatory proteins such as the *fos* and *jun* oncoproteins and the GCN4 protein of yeast. Leucine zippers have even been found in some non-nuclear proteins, so it seems that the leucine zipper is an effective domain directing dimerisation which has been widely utilised throughout evolution. The leucine zipper in the c-*myc* protein is capable of directing the formation of dimeric and tetrameric structures, and an intact leucine zipper is absolutely obligatory for the transforming activity of the protein. This implies that the c-*myc* protein exerts its biological effects in an oligomeric form. Dimerisation is known to be a requirement for DNA binding by several other nuclear proteins which contain leucine zippers. Thus, the properties of the c-*myc* protein (and other *myc* proteins) is consistent with it being a DNA-binding protein.

DNA binding properties of the c-*myc* protein

Several early studies showed that the c-*myc* protein bound to single- and double-stranded DNA *in vitro* but no sequence specificity was apparent. The region of the protein responsible for this non-specific DNA binding is in the C-terminal half of the protein. It is widely presumed that the c-*myc* protein will have a DNA sequence specificity, but until this is determined it is unclear whether or not such a specificity will localise to the same region as that responsible for promiscuous DNA binding. Recently, clues as to the nature of the DNA-binding domain of the c-*myc* protein have come from comparative analysis of related DNA-binding proteins together with predictions of c-*myc* protein structure. Several proteins have been identified which share homology with the *myc* family of proteins in a region just N-terminal to the leucine zipper domain. Predictive algorithms for protein conformation suggest this region forms a helix-loop-helix structure which is likely to be involved in DNA binding. So far, this motif has been identified in several mammalian proteins, including MyoD1, *myd* protein, Myf-5 and myogenin (all involved in myoblast differentiation); the E12 and E47 immunoglobulin enhancer binding proteins; and *lyl*-1, a gene located at sites of chromosomal translocation in T-cell leukaemias. The motif has also been identified in *Drosophila* proteins: the *achaete-scute* complex proteins, involved in neural differentiation, *daughterless*, involved in sex determination and neural differentiation, and *twist*, involved in embryonic germ layer determination. All of these proteins are directly involved in the regulation of gene expression, usually in the context of differentiation.

TOWARDS AN UNDERSTANDING OF THE ROLE OF THE c-*myc* GENE

As an oncogene, c-*myc* may possess a pivotal role in the process of carcinogenesis. It appears to exert a function which is a subtle and evanescent regulator of cellular proliferation. Its precise molecular function is unknown, but it bears all the hallmarks of a multimeric DNA-binding protein, probably involved in the regulation of expression of specific genes. Further studies will doubtless elucidate targets for c-*myc* protein activity in normal and transformed cells, and reveal the function of the gene in normal and malignant growth.

FURTHER READING

Braun, H. M., Buschhausen-Denker, G., Bober, E. and Arnold, H. H. (1989) A novel human muscle factor related to, but distinct from, MyoD1 induces myogenic conversion in 10T1/2 fibroblasts. *EMBO J.*, **8**, 701–709.

De Greve, J., Battey, J., Fedorko, J., *et al.* (1988) The human L-*myc* gene encodes multiple nuclear phosphoproteins from alternatively processed mRNAs. *Mol. Cell Biol.*, **8**, 4381–4388.

DePinho, R. A., Hatton, K. S., Tesfaye, A., *et al.* (1987) The human *myc* gene family: structure and activity of L-*myc* and an L-*myc* pseudogene. *Genes Dev.*, **1**, 1311–1326.

Freytag, S. O. (1988) Enforced expression of the c-*myc* oncogene inhibits cell differentiation by precluding entry into a distinct predifferentiation state in G0/G1. *Mol. Cell. Biol.*, **8**, 1614–1624.

Luscher, B., Kuenzel, E. A., Krebs, E. G. and Eisenmann, R. N. (1989) *Myc* oncoproteins are phosphorylated by casein kinase II. *EMBO J.*, **8**, 1111–1119.

Onclercq, R., Gilardi, P., Lavenu, A. and Cremisi, C. (1988) c-*myc* products trans-activate the adenovirus E4 promoter in EC stem cells by using the same target sequence as E1A products. *J. Virol.*, **62**, 4533–4537.

Saksela, K., Makela, T. P., Evan, G. and Alitalo, K. (1989) Rapid phosphorylation of the L-*myc* protein induced by phorbol ester tumor promoters and serum. *EMBO J.*, **8**, 149–158.

Schwab, M. (1988) The *myc*-box oncogenes. In: Reddy, E., Premkumar; Skalka Anna Marie; Curran Tom, (eds.) Elsevier Science, Amsterdam, New York, Oxford, pp. 381–391.

Watt, R. A., Schatzman, A. R. and Rosenberg, M. (1985) Expression and characterization of the human c-*myc* DNA-binding protein. *Mol. Cell. Biol.*, **5**, 448–456.

4

N-*myc*—its Place as a Diagnostic and Prognostic Indicator in Neuroblastoma

JOHN T. KEMSHEAD
KALPANA PATEL

DISCOVERY OF THE N-*myc* GENE

The N-*myc* gene was first isolated by virtue of its partial sequence homology with v-*myc*. This was accomplished by using Southern blotting techniques to screen human neuroblastoma DNA with a variety of oncogene probes under conditions of reduced stringency. In particular lines, an amplified 2 kb *Eco*R1 fragment was detected with a v-*myc* probe. Cloning and sequencing of this fragment showed this to be a previously undescribed gene, which has considerable sequence homology to c-*myc*. Whilst the N-*myc* gene has not been detected in any human retroviruses, it has been shown to be capable of transforming embryonic fibroblasts *in vitro* when transfected with a mutant *ras* gene. Furthermore, it has been shown that when N-*myc* is transfected into an expression vector containing the long terminal repeat sequence of Moloney murine leukaemia virus, it can act alone in transforming fibroblasts without the co-operation of *ras*. These observations serve to strengthen the case to suggest that the N-*myc* gene is an authentic proto-oncogene.

In addition to c-*myc* and N-*myc*, other members of the *myc* gene family have been identified. The best characterized is L-*myc*, although R-*myc*, L-*myc*¥, p-*myc* and B-*myc* have been described. Whilst c-*myc* and B-*myc* expression has been noted in a relatively wide spectrum of tissues, N-*myc* and L-*myc* gene products are found in a more restricted group of tissues and tumours. Until recently it was thought that only one *myc* gene was activated in a cell at any one time, although this is now

Genes and Cancer. Edited by D. Carney and K. Sikora
©1990 John Wiley & Sons Ltd

somewhat controversial. The possible functions of the N-*myc* gene and its role in malignancy will be reviewed below

STRUCTURE AND FUNCTION OF THE N-*myc* GENE

Location

Using both *in situ* hybridization techniques and somatic cell hybrids, the N-*myc* gene has been mapped to the distal arm of chromosome 2 (2p 24). In some neuroblastomas, the gene has also been found to be associated with homogeneous staining regions and double minute chromosomes (see below). No link has been observed with the other chromosome abnormality often found in neuroblastoma and some other embryonic childhood tumours, namely deletions or rearrangements involving the short arm of chromosome 1 distal to band p32.

Structure

The *myc* family represents a group of genes that are similar in structure and share a degree of sequence homology. N-*myc*, c-*myc* and L-*myc* are rich in cytosine and guanine bases and consist of three exons interspersed by two introns. All three genes have non-coding first exons which contribute to long 5′ leader sequences. The second and third exons of the N-*myc* gene code for 255 and 201 amino acids, whereas in c-*myc* they encode 252 and 187 amino acids. Exon 2 contains two blocks of sequences where a high degree of homology between c-*myc*, N-*myc* and L-*myc* has been noted. However, the introns and 3′ untranslated regions of the three genes are totally divergent.

Transcription

Transcription of the N-*myc* gene is not completely understood although it is known that multiple mRNA species are generated. These are thought to arise from the use of both multiple initiation sites within exon 1 as well as alternative splicing. The multiple initiation sites fall into two distinct clusters, suggesting that the N-*myc* gene may have at least two promoters which are individually regulated.

Stanton and Bishop have described two N-*myc* mRNA species of approximately 3 kb, with different first exons. The mechanism underlying the generation of these two forms of N-*myc* mRNA has been elucidated. They arise as a consequence of two splice donor sites designated SD1 and SD2, present on exon 1, linking to the same acceptor site on exon 2. The choice of donor site used for splicing is controlled by where initiation begins within exon 1. Transcripts which initiate more than 150 bases 5′ of SD1 are spliced at this site, whereas those initiated close to SD1 are spliced at SD2. The significance of these and other transcriptional variations on the control of gene expression remains poorly understood. In general terms it has been suggested that these types of mechanisms may differentially influence the half-life of the mRNA species generated. The significance of this to N-*myc* mRNA remains unclear, as the half-life of the message is relatively short (approximately 20 minutes). The instability of N-*myc* mRNA is thought to be brought about by the presence of A/U-rich sequences in the 3′ untranslated regions.

Translation

The coding regions of exons 2 and 3 within the N-*myc* gene are predicted to generate a protein of 49 kDa consisting of 456 amino acids. However, Western blot analysis of the N-*myc* protein reveals that this runs as a doublet on SDS polyacrylamide gel electrophoresis with an apparent molecular weight of 63–66 kDa. In some samples of human foetal brain and neuroblastoma, we have also identified a 78–81 kDa protein doublet that may also be a N-*myc* gene product. These proteins have been identified through their binding to three different antisera raised against synthetic peptides representative of sequences present in exons 2 and 3 of the gene (see below and Chapter 15).

In comparison to N-*myc*, both the c-*myc* and L-*myc* genes code for proteins of similar sizes as determined by Western blot analysis. The c-*myc* protein consists of 439 amino acids and L-*myc* protein 362 amino acids. A high molecular weight form of the L-*myc* gene product (78–81 kDa) has also been found. However, the nature of the differences between the normally described gene product and the 'aberrant' forms of the protein have not been elucidated. It is difficult to explain the formation of high molecular weight *myc* proteins through the use of alternative reading frames. Whilst exon 1 of the N-*myc* gene is considered to be non-coding, Stanton and Bishop have pointed out that there are several open reading frames present. However, stop codons within these open reading frames suggest that a series of peptides would be generated from these sequences, rather than truncated forms of the *myc* protein. No evidence for the existence of these peptides has been found.

The half-life of all of the *myc* proteins studied to date is very short (approximately 30 minutes). The rapid turnover of the *myc* proteins suggests that they may be involved in a regulatory role within the cell, as discussed below.

Function

N-*myc*, c-*myc* and L-*myc* proteins are all found in the nucleus. The C-terminal regions of the proteins are highly charged and contain regions rich in basic amino acids. This has been suggested to indicate that one role for N-*myc* is to bind to either DNA or histones in a selective manner. Within the nucleus, immunocytochemical data suggest that the N-*myc* product is not found in the nucleolus. In normal adult tissues, the N-*myc* is not expressed in the majority of tissues studied. However, it is found in a variety of foetal tissues and tumours. In the mouse, *in situ* hybridization studies have revealed the presence of high levels of N-*myc* mRNA in foetal brain, kidney, heart and lung. Expression in the latter two organs is lost very early on in development, whilst it is maintained at low levels in brain and kidney, until birth. Far less information is available about the expression of N-*myc* in human tissues, although immunocytochemical data suggest that the gene is expressed in particular areas of foetal brain.

Studies on human neuroblastoma cell lines have shown that N-*myc* expression can be down-regulated when cells are induced to differentiate. Somewhat more controversial is the rate at which down-regulation occurs. In some studies, using the cell line SH-SY5Y and the phorbol ester 12-O-tetradecanoylphorbol-13-acetate, differentiation of cells was noted along with a gradual decrease in the level of N-*myc* mRNA. In other studies, using alternative cell lines and retinoic acid as the differentiation agent, N-*myc* levels were observed to decrease before signs of 'differentiation' were noted. The precise role of N-*myc* with respect to control of cell division and differentiation remains unclear, as several other oncogenes have been found to be both down- and up-regulated as differentiation proceeds.

A further suggestion concerning the function of the N-*myc* gene comes from studies of a rat neuroblastoma cell-line. After transfection of an N-*myc* gene into the cell line, down-modulation of major histocompatibility antigens was paralleled by an increase in both *in vivo* growth rate and metastatic ability. Down-regulation of MHC class I antigens could be reversed by treating cells with interferon without affecting the steady-state level of N-*myc* mRNA. Whilst these findings have not been repeated in a human system, the findings fit well with what is known about N-*myc* expression in neuroblastoma. In general, N-*myc* amplification has been noted to occur in advanced disease (see below). *In situ* hybridization studies have revealed higher levels of N-*myc* message in anaplastic neuroblasts as compared with their 'more differentiated' counterparts. Finally, low levels of class I antigens are often found on neuroblastoma cells. This situation can often be reversed by treatment of cells with interferon. However, the relationship with N-*myc* expression and Class I antigen remains speculative at the present time.

MECHANISMS LEADING TO OVER-EXPRESSION OF THE N-*myc* GENE

Gene amplification

Amplification of the N-*myc* gene has been noted to occur in approximately 40% of stage IV human neuroblastomas studied to date (see below). Transcription of these multiple gene copies leads to elevated levels of N-*myc* mRNA, presumably resulting in higher than normal expression of the corresponding *myc* protein. Amplification of the gene has been found to be associated with two chromosome abnormalities, namely homogeneous staining regions (HSRs) and double minute (DM) chromosomes. Where HSRs occur they apparently appear sporadically within the genotype, not necessarily at the site of the normal N-*myc* gene. At present, studies on human neuroblastoma cell lines have revealed HSRs containing amplified N-*myc* sequences associated with 18 different chromosomes. The levels of N-*myc* amplification within neuroblastomas appear almost bimodal, with tumours containing either approximtely 10–30 or 100–150 copies.

Within the homogeneous staining region, genes other than N-*myc* must often be amplified to account for the size of the HSR. *In situ* hybridization studies have revealed blocks of hybridizing sequences interspersed with non-hybridizing sequences. Whilst one might expect that sequences immediately adjacent to the N-*myc* gene on chromosome 2 to co-amplify, this is not necessarily the case. In the colon carcinoma cell line COLO320 DM, a gene designated PVT is co-amplified along with c-*myc*. PVT is found some 50 kb downstream from *myc*. Whether co-amplification of other genes along with *myc* is random or selective is not known at the present time.

Over-expression of a single gene

Far less data are available regarding the association of high levels of N-*myc* mRNA in neuroblastoma and advanced disease. This is predominantly due to difficulties in obtaining tissues in a suitable form for RNA extraction. These difficulties have been compounded in Europe by the reluctance of clinicians to biopsy tumours to make an initial diagnosis. It has been our experience that undegraded RNA is difficult to obtain from tumours which are often highly necrotic after patients have received extensive therapy. Luckily, this situation is changing now that a document unifying the staging and response criteria for neuroblastoma has been accepted by the major paediatric oncology centres in Europe, USA, Japan and Australia.

To overcome the problem of obtaining fresh tissue for mRNA studies, some groups have studied infiltrated bone marrow by *in situ* hybridization techniques. This is a simpler approach, obviously avoiding the question of the ethics of tumour biopsy. However, it is dependent on the presence of a reasonable infiltrate of neuroblasts in the marrow. In addition, few data are available on comparisons of N-*myc* levels in metastatic and primary tumours in the same patient.

The reasons why high levels of N-*myc* mRNA build up in cells in the absence of amplification of the gene are not understood. Presumably, this reflects either enhanced transcription of the gene or the generation of a more stable mRNA within the cell. Recently, the N-*myc* gene has been identified as a common proviral insertion site in murine leukaemia virus induced T-cell lymphoma. Proviral activation of N-*myc* was identified in 35% of independently induced primary tumours. The majority of the proviral insertion was found to occur within a small segment of the 3′ untranslated region of the N-*myc* gene. This resulted in an increased level of expression of a truncated N-*myc* mRNA. Unfortunately, the nature of the protein translated from the message was not discussed. The relevance of this observation to N-*myc* over-expression in neuroblastoma awaits further investigation.

DETECTION OF THE N-*myc* PROTEIN

Within the last three years, immunological approaches for studying the N-*myc* proteins have become available. Ikegaki and co-workers have generated monoclonal antibodies against a bacterially expressed LacZ fusion protein containing a portion of the N-*myc* protein sequence. Similarly, Slamon *et al.* have raised a hetero-antiserum in rabbits against a bovine growth hormone/N-*myc* fusion protein. An alternative approach to raising N-*myc* antibodies has been to use synthetic peptides as immunogens. Both our group and others have used antisera raised in this manner to detect the N-*myc* gene product using both Western blots and immunocytochemical/ immunohistochemical techniques.

A study of both human neuroblastoma cell lines and fresh tumour samples has revealed considerable heterogeneity in nuclear staining with these anti-N-*myc* reagents. Presumably, this is due to heterogeneity in the steady-state levels of the protein in the malignant population. Whether this is related to the cell cycle remains unclear. Studies on the N-*myc* protein are also complicated by the relatively short half-life of the material. This has been shown to be of the order of 30 minutes. Thus, as with studies on the N-*myc* RNA, care has to be taken to rapidly snap-freeze tumour biopsies after they have been removed from the patient. Our experience using N-*myc* antisera suggests that conventional formalin fixation and paraffin embedding of tissue destroys the antigenic characteristics of the protein. Whether this is due to the cross-linking fixative used and/or the use of high-temperature melting point waxes is not clear. Conventionally prepared histopathological samples, therefore, do not seem appropriate for the study of N-*myc* protein levels. However, whilst our studies have revealed that precipitating fixatives such as ethanol are better at preserving the epitopes on the N-*myc* protein, others have obtained antibody binding using formalin-fixed tissues.

Another problem associated with the immunological detection of the N-*myc* gene product is the relatively high amplification of the signal that has to be achieved in order to visualize antibody binding. To attempt to overcome this problem, Evans *et al*. have developed a sensitive immune assay to detect c-*myc* in tissue extracts. Whilst this technique is more sensitive than the immunocytochemical detection of *myc* proteins, it does suffer some major drawbacks. The most serious of these is that one has to be sure of the degree of tumour infiltration in the sample before beginning the assay. Using a binding assay to measure *myc* levels it is not possible to study individual cells to correlate cell phenotype wth the degree of anti-*myc* antibody binding. Evans' assay, which is of the 'sandwich type', is dependent on the capture of the *myc* protein by an antibody on a solid phase support. Binding to the primary antibody is visualized through the use of a second anti-*myc* antibody recognizing a different epitope to the primary reagent. No studies on the use of the assay to quantify N-*myc* protein levels in tumours have been reported to date.

N-*myc*: ITS ROLE IN THE DIFFERENTIAL DIAGNOSIS OF NEUROBLASTOMA

Solid tumours

In the majority of cases, establishing a diagnosis of neuroblastoma on the basis of the clinical, radiological, biochemical and routine pathological picture is relatively straightforward. However, in approximately 20% of cases diagnosis is more complex, particularly when the tumour is relatively anaplastic. Under these circumstances, it can be difficult to distinguish neuroblastoma from other small round cell tumours of childhood, namely neuroblastoma, rhabdomyosarcoma, lymphoblastic leukaemia/lymphoma and Ewing's sarcoma. In an attempt to assist the differential diagnosis of these tumour types, a variety of immunological and biochemical tests have been devised. Panels of monoclonal antibodies to both cell membrane components and intermediate filaments have proved invaluable in assisting in the characterization of certain tumours of these types. Using these reagents, it is possible to simply differentiate neuroblastoma from acute lymphoblastic leukaemia/lymphoma.

However, characterizing rhabdomyosarcoma and Ewing's sarcoma from neuro-blastoma is more difficult as few reagents are available that specifically bind to these tumour types. As N-*myc* amplification was originally thought to be strictly limited to tumours of neuroectodermal origin, the diagnostic value of this abnormality was investigated. Studies on N-*myc* amplification and over-expression of both the mRNA and protein have now revealed that this can be found in a much wider spectrum of tumours than originally thought. Within tissues of neuroectodermal origin some astrocytomas and retinoblastomas and small cell carcinomas (thought by many to be of neuroectodermal origin) have been shown to carry amplified N-*myc* sequences. The specificity of the phenomenon with respect to the neuroectoderm has also been found wanting, as two independent reports have described N-*myc* amplification in embryonal rhabdomyosarcomas. Further elevated levels of N-*myc* gene expression have been found in some Wilms' tumours, retinoblastomas and teratomas. Finally, high levels of N-*myc* protein have been identified in approximately 50% of medulloblastomas examined. Thus, the diagnostic potential of N-*myc* gene amplification and over-expression is somewhat reduced from that originally suggested, although along with other reagents, it can play a role in assisting in the differential diagnosis of the 'small round cell tumours' of childhood.

Bone marrow disease

As discussed previously, *in situ* hybridization using an N-*myc* probe has been used to detect the metastatic spread of tumour cells to bone marrow. More problematic is the use of either Southern blots or dot blots to identify N-*myc* amplification in this tissue. Here the major difficulty surrounds the sensitivity of the technique to detect amplification of the N-*myc* gene. If the bone marrow was completely replaced by tumour then, where a tumour carried 100 N-*myc* gene copies, a 100-fold amplification of the N-*myc* gene would be detected by Southern blot/dot blot hybridization. When the tumour load falls to 10% then obviously the other 90% of cells (the normal marrow component) carry a single N-*myc* gene per haploid genome. Hence analysis of this sample will reveal an approximate 10-fold gene amplification. Repeating these arguments for a 1% tumour infiltrate illustrates that only close to a single gene copy per haploid genome will be detected. This type of analysis does not fare well when compared to immunocytochemical studies on bone marrow where routinely it is possible to detect one tumour cell in approximately 1 : 1 000 normal haemopoietic progenitors.

N-*myc* AS AN INDICATOR OF PROGNOSIS

To understand the association of N-*myc* and prognosis initially requires a review of the staging systems used for neuroblastoma. Four are commonly used: the Evans system, the St Jude system, the TNM system and, recently, the Forbeck classification. The most common of these is the Evans system, which is essentially a surgical staging procedure.

Stage I defines a tumour confined to the organ of origin. Stage II indicates that the tumour extends in continuity beyond the organ of origin but does not cross the midline; regional ipsilateral lymph nodes may be involved (IIB). Stage III tumours extend beyond the midline and may involve regional lymph nodes bilaterally. Stage IV refers to large primary tumours with distant metastases involving bone, bone marrow, viscera, soft tissues or remote lymph nodes. Stage IV-s defines a group of patients (less than one year of age) with small primaries similar to Stage I or II tumours but with metastases in liver, skin or bone marrow. This clinical staging system correlates well with prognosis: thus patients with Stage I or II disease have a 75–90% chance of disease-free survival at two years, whereas Stage III and IV patients have only a 10–30% chance. Paradoxically, Stage IV-s patients have a favourable outcome in approximately 80% of cases.

Brodeur *et al.* were the first to report a correlation between N-*myc* amplification in neuroblastoma and advanced clinical stage. By Southern blotting, they detected between three- and 300-fold amplification in 38% of 63 untreated tumours. Amplification was found in none of 15 patients with Evans' Stage I or II disease, but in 24 of 48 cases (50%) with Stage III or IV. The association between N-*myc* amplification and tumour 'progression' in neuroblastoma was later confirmed in a larger study by Seeger *et al.* They observed amplification in none of eight Stage I, two of 16 Stage II, 13 of 20 Stage III and 19 of 40 Stage IV cases. Five Stage IV-s tumours had only a single copy of N-*myc* per haploid genome. Correlation of N-*myc* copy number with progression-free survival showed that those with the greatest degree of amplification had the worst prognosis. Thus, at 18 months from diagnosis, patients whose tumours had 1, 3–10 or >10 copies of N-*myc* had a 70%, 30% or 5% chance of progression-free survival, respectively. Correlation with progression-free survival was also observed within individual stages, so that of 16 Stage II tumours, two out of two with amplification metastasized, whereas only one of 14 without amplifications did so ($p=0.03$). Very similar findings have been reported more recently by Tsuda *et al.*, although in contrast to Seeger's study, amplification was noted in three out of nine Stage IV-s cases. Significantly, two of the three with amplification relapsed early and died of their disease. Tsuda concludes that 'amplification of N-*myc* is a reliable prognostic factor even in Stage IV-s and is a signal for therapeutic intervention'. N-*myc* amplification in one out of five Stage IV-s tumours has also been reported by Bartram and Berthold, but the follow-up interval (1 month) is too short for any conclusion to be drawn with regard to prognosis.

One point that is critical to establish, is whether the association of N-*myc* amplification and advanced disease is due to either an increase in the steady-state levels of the *myc* gene product or to general karyotypic abnormalities. It should be possible to deduce which of these possibilities is correct through study of patients with tumours having single copy N-*myc* genes that are activated to produce elevated levels of *myc* mRNA. If N-*myc* expression can be shown to be of prognostic importance in this group it would suggest that it is the over-expression of the gene that influences survival. Unfortunately, data on the relationship between N-*myc* expression and survival are confusing. Some groups claim that N-*myc* expression is of equal importance to N-*myc* gene amplification, with respect to prognosis. For example, Hashimoto *et al.* have undertaken a comparative study of N-*myc* amplification, detection of N-*myc* protein and survival in 13 patients with neuroblastoma and five with ganglioneuroblastoma. Whilst a correlation between N-*myc* amplification and the expression of the protein was established, this was found not to be absolute. However, high levels of N-*myc* protein were not found in tumours with single N-*myc* gene copy per haploid genome. In contrast to this finding, Garson *et al.* have detailed a tentative association between an increased risk of relapse and elevated N-*myc* protein levels in another neuroectodermal tumour, namely medulloblastoma. No N-*myc* amplification was found in any of the medulloblastomas studied ($n = 12$), whilst approximately 50% appeared to contain relatively high levels of the N-*myc* protein as determined by both immunocytochemistry and Western blot analysis. Relapses were only reported in the patients where high levels of N-*myc* protein were noted, despite the two groups of patients being well matched for age, sex, degree of tumour resection and time from their last treatment. To add to this confusing picture Nisen *et al.* have demonstrated N-*myc* over-expression of a single gene copy in all of the Stage I and II neuroblastoma tumours studied as well as 5/8 Stage IV-s malignancies. No association between survival and over-expression of the *myc* gene was reported. Thus the role of N-*myc* with respect to its use as a prognostic marker requires further evaluation. This is particularly true, as a relationship between survival and the ploidy status of neuroblastoma tumours has also been suggested.

The usefulness of studying N-*myc* amplification in neuroblastoma tumours has to be placed in context. The abnormality has only been detected in approximately 40% of Stage IV patients, the majority of whom fare poorly on conventional combination chemotherapy. Even when high-dose chemoradiotherapy is given to patients along with autologous bone marrow rescue, two-year survival rates post transplant are approximately 40%. At the present time it is not known if N-*myc* amplification predicts for relapse in this patient group. The patients where detection of N-*myc* amplification may be of most importance are those with either Stage I or II disease. Here the case for treating individuals with amplification of the N-*myc* gene along the same lines as a Stage IV patient is compelling.

One final criterion for consideration is the timing of amplification of the N-*myc* gene. All the work originally undertaken by Brodeur and Seeger was on material obtained prior to the patients receiving chemotherapy. Whether the association between survival and amplification is maintained after individuals have received extensive treatment has to be further evaluated.

OTHER PROGNOSTIC FACTORS

Many indicators of survival have been described for patients with neuroblastoma. Of these, age, and stage are considered the most important independent factors. Several serum markers have been suggested to be of prognostic importance. Serum ferritin, an iron storage protein, is one such indicator. The upper limit of normal ferritin in an age-matched group of children is 142 ng ml^{-1}. Patients with neuroblastoma having low levels of serum ferritin (< 75 ng ml^{-1}) tend to have a longer disease-free survival than those with higher levels (> 142 ng ml^{-1}). In addition, children with Stage IV-s disease tend to have normal serum ferritin levels.

Neuron specific enolase (NSE) is another serum marker thought to be of prognostic significance in patients with neuroblastoma. This is an isoenzyme of enolase found mainly in tissues of neuroectodermal origin, although it is also present in red blood cells. Lower levels of NSE have been found in the serum Stage I and II patients compared to Stage III and IV disease. The prognostic value of NSE serum levels appears to be restricted to infants under one year of age. Survival for the group of patients with NSE levels below 100 ng ml^{-1} was 100% compared to 25% for those with enzyme levels above 100 ng ml^{-1}.

Gangliosides have also been suggested as of possible diagnostic and prognostic value in neuroblastoma patients. Several monoclonal antibodies have been described as binding to gangliosides. These include A2B5 and 3F8, raised against chick retinal cells and neuroblastoma cells respectively. Monoclonal antibody 3F8 is one of a series of antibodies binding to the ganglioside GD2. Elevated levels of GD2 are found in the serum of patients with neuroblastoma. However, this abnormality has also been found in some patients with Wilms' tumours and osteogenic sarcomas. One possible confusion regarding the use of antibody 3F8 in detecting GD2 is that this antibody has also been shown to cross-react with the neural cell adhesion molecule, which in turn may also be found in elevated amounts in the serum of patients with neuroblastoma.

In addition to serum markers, the histopathological classification of Shimada has been shown to be of prognostic relevance to patients with neuroblastoma. This classification scheme includes some standard pathological observations as well as a variety of clinical parameters. The degree of stromal development within the tumour, the degree of differentiation and the mitotic-karyorrhexix index is estimated and this information is used in conjunction with the age of the patient to place the individual into a good or poor prognostic group.

Thus, in addition to N-*myc* aberrations, other chromosomal abnormalities and a variety of biochemical markers have been suggested as being of use in defining which neuroblastoma patients have a good or bad prognosis. Which of these (outside age and stage) are interrelated and which are independent variables has to be established. Nakagawara and Ikeda have reported a significant correlation between amplification of N-*myc* and decreased urinary excretion of catecholamines in children with advanced neuroblastoma. Furthermore, Tsuda *et al.* have reported that N-*myc* amplification is associated with lack of histological differentiation. Future studies will reveal the relationship of other prognostic markers for the disease. Until then the status of N-*myc* as an important factor in diagnosing and predicting the outcome of patients with neuroblastoma will remain questionable. It is of major importance to resolve which of the factors outlined above are of independent prognostic significance, as the cost and difficulty of setting up molecular techniques in a routine pathology department is considerable. However, in the future it is hoped that major advances in the treatment of patients with neuroblastoma will be made. Our greater understanding of the biology of the tumour can only help to speed up this process.

FURTHER READING

Bernards, R., Dessain, S. K. and Weinberg, R. A. (1986) N-*myc* amplification causes down modulation of MHC class 1 antigen expression in neuroblastoma. *Cell*, **47**, 667–674.

Brodeur, G. M., Seeger, R. C., Schwab, M., *et al.* (1984) Amplification of N-*myc* in untreated human neuroblastomas correlates with an advanced disease stage. *Science*, **224**, 1121–1124.

Cohen, P., Seeger, R., Triche, T. and Israel, M. (1988) Detection of N-*myc* gene expression in neuroblastoma tumours by in-situ hybridization. *American J. Path.*, **131**, 391–397.

DePinho, R., Mitsock, L., Hatton, K., *et al.* (1987) *Myc* family of cellular oncogenes. *J. Cell Biochem.*, **33**, 257–266.

Lohuizen, M. van, Breuer, M. and Berns, A. (1989) N-*myc* is frequently activated by proviral insertion in MuLV-induced T cell lymphomas. *EMBO J.*, **8**, 133–136.

Nisen, P. D., Waber, P. G., Rich, M. A., *et al.* (1988) N-*myc* oncogene RNA expression in neuroblastoma. *J. Natl. Cancer Inst.*, **20**, 1633–1637.

Schwab, M., Ellison, J., Busch, M., *et al.* (1984) Enhanced expression of human gene N-*myc* consequent to amplification of DNA may contribute to malignant progression of neuroblastoma. *Proc. Natl. Acad. Sci. USA*, **81**, 4940–4944.

Shtivelman, E. and Bishop, J. M. (1989) The PVT gene frequently amplifies with MYC in tumour cells. *Mol. and Cell. Biol.*, **9**, 1148–1154.

Stanton, L. W. and Bishop, J. M. (1987) .Alternative processing of RNA transcribed from N-*myc*. *Mol. and Cell. Biol.*, **7**, 4266–4272.

Thiele, C. J., Deutsch, L. and Israel M. (1988) The expression of multiple proto-oncogenes is differentially regulated during retinoic acid induced maturation of human neuroblastoma. *Oncogene*, **3**, 281–288.

5 | The *myb* Gene and its Regulation

E. PREMKUMAR REDDY
C. DAMODAR REDDY

INTRODUCTION

The last decade has witnessed the emergence of the field of molecular oncology as an amalgamation of four disciplines of cancer research, *viz.*, retrovirology, chemical carcinogenesis, cytogenetics and cell-growth regulation. The discovery that transforming elements (oncogenes) of acute transforming viruses are derived from normal cellular genes (proto-oncogenes), and that these genes are targets for mutation and/or rearrangements in naturally occurring human tumors and tumors induced by chemical carcinogens in animal models has provided important insights into our understanding of the role of these genes in malignancy. The discovery that oncogenes code for either growth factors or their receptors, cytoplasmic guanine nucleotide-binding proteins and protein kinases presumed to function in signal transmission, and nucleoproteins thought to regulate gene expression or initiate DNA synthesis in response to diverse external and internal signals, provided a logical connection between cell growth regulation and neoplasia.

In spite of these important breakthroughs, the precise mode of action of these gene products and the nature of the interrelationship between individual proto-oncogenes as related to cell growth and differentiation is still unclear. This is particularly true of nuclear oncogenes, which are thought to regulate gene transcription and DNA replication. Although several advances have been made in our under-standing of the function of *fos* and *jun*, the specific biochemical functions of other oncogenes and their cellular counterparts remain to be identified. In this review, we summarize the salient features of the structure, mechanisms of oncogenic

Genes and Cancer. Edited by D. Carney and K. Sikora
©1990 John Wiley & Sons Ltd

activation and transcriptional regulation of a nuclear oncogene, *myb*, which appears to play an important role in hematopoietic cell growth and differentiation.

The *myb* oncogene was first identified as the transforming gene of avian myeloblastosis virus (AMV), which causes myeloblastic leukemia in chickens and transforms myelomonocytic cells *in vitro*. AMV does not transform fibroblasts, even though it can infect these cells and produce both RNA and proteins encoded by the viral genome, suggesting that only a restricted cell population is the target of its transforming gene product. AMV has arisen by recombination between a chicken helper virus and host cellular sequences. The cell-derived sequences which constitute the v-*myb* gene are responsible for the oncogenic potential of this virus. A second virus, termed E26, also contains the *myb* oncogene in addition to a second oncogene, *ets*, and has been shown to cause erythroblastosis and a low level of concomitant myeloblastosis in chickens.

GENE STRUCTURE AND MECHANISMS OF ACTIVATION

The structure of AMV and E26 viruses is shown in Figure 1. Molecular cloning and nucleotide sequence analysis of AMV and its helper MAV proviruses revealed that the transduced cellular gene is present at the 3′ end of the viral genome, having replaced the *env* sequences of the helper virus. Complete nucleotide sequencing of the proviral genome of AMV (7141 bp) revealed that it contains the entire *gag* region as well as most of the *pol* region. The v-*myb* sequences appear to have replaced a short region of the *pol* gene (26 codons) and virtually all of the *env* gene with the exception of the last 11 codons. Analysis of the viral RNA in AMV-transformed cells showed the presence of two species of 7 kb and 2 kb. The larger, 7 kb transcript is transcribed from the entire proviral genome, whereas the smaller subgenomic RNA species is generated by a splicing event where the leader sequences from the 5′ terminus of

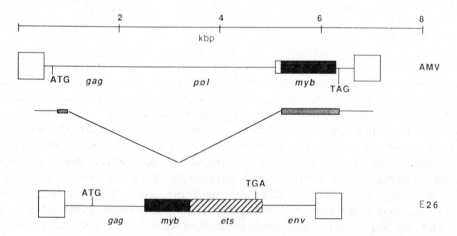

Figure 1. Structure of the AMV and E26 proviruses. Long terminal repeats are indicated in rectangles. The *myb* coding sequences are indicated by filled boxes. The structure of the subgenomic mRNA which codes for the *myb* protein is shown below the proviral genome. The coding sequences of this mRNA are indicated by dotted boxes

the provirus are spliced to the body of the v-*myb* encoded sequences. Protein synthesized by this spliced mRNA would contain six amino acids derived from the *gag* gene of helper virus followed by 371 amino acids derived from the v-*myb* region and terminating with 11 amino acids at the carboxy-terminal end derived from the *env* gene of the helper virus. Such a protein with a molecular mass of 48 kDa is readily detected in AMV-transformed cells. The E26 virus transcribes a single unspliced 5.7 kb RNA that encodes a tripartite fusion protein of 135 kDa consisting of *gag*, *myb* and *ets* sequences. Sequence analysis of the proviral genome indicates that this protein is made up of 272 amino acids derived from the viral *gag* gene, 283 amino acids from the *myb* gene and 491 amino acids from the *ets* gene.

A comparison of the sequence of the two v-*myb* sequences with that of c-*myb* revealed that the two viruses arose from the cellular gene as a result of extensive deletion at both the 5' and 3' ends of the coding region. Thus the normal c-*myb* protein was found to contain an additional stretch of 142 amino acids at the N-terminal end and 192 amino acids at the C-terminal end compared to the AMV. Comparison of c-*myb* cDNA sequences with those of v-*myb*-E26 (oncogene of E26 virus) revealed the occurrence of similar deletions in the transforming gene. Thus stretches of 150 and 272 amino acids have been deleted from the amino- and carboxy-terminals during the generation of this oncogene. The deletion of similar sequences (coding for amino- and carboxy-terminal amino acids) during the generation of two different viral isolates raises the possibility that such deletions in the coding region could be crucial for the oncogenic activation of this gene.

In addition to the avian systems, which suggest that deletions are important in the activation of *myb*, two other murine models provide support to this hypothesis. Rearrangements in the *myb* locus have been described in the ABPL tumors that arose in BALB/c mice following the injection of pristane and Abelson murine leukemia virus. These tumors do not contain the integrated proviral genome and instead undergo rearrangements in the *myb* locus, resulting in the synthesis of abnormal mRNA transcripts. Rearrangements in all ABPL tumors were due to the integration of the Mo-MuLV genome into a 1.5 kbp stretch of cellular DNA immediately upstream to the v-*myb* related sequences. This integration occurs in the intron sequences that lie between the third and fourth coding exons, resulting in the synthesis of transcripts that lack the 5' coding sequences. This results in the deletion of amino-terminal amino acids in the *myb* gene product of ABPL tumors analogous to that produced by the v-*myb* gene. A fourth example of *myb* activation is seen in some of the myeloid leukemias induced by Cas-Br MuLV in NFS mice. The nature of the *myb* rearrangements in the NFS-60 has revealed that the rearrangements are due to the integration of the proviral genome in the 3' end of the *myb* locus resulting in the premature termination of the rearranged *myb* gene transcription. The *myb* coding sequences in this aberrant mRNA terminate at a point close to the site of deletion observed in AMV and E26 viral oncogenes. Thus, in all the four model systems studied so far (Figure 2), it appears that the activation of the *myb* gene is invariably accompanied by deletions in the coding regions of the gene, which lends support to the hypothesis that these structural alterations play an important role in the oncogenic activation of the *myb* gene. The human *myb* gene is located on chromosome 6(q22→24) and abnormalities in this locus have been observed in several acute myelogenous leukemias, T-cell leukemias and colon carcinomas

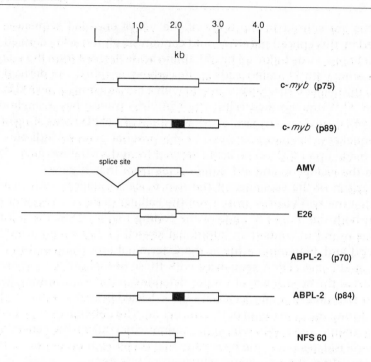

Figure 2. Structural comparison of the coding region of c-*myb* mRNA (normal) with activated forms of *myb* mRNAs in the AMV and E26 viruses and ABPL-2 and NFS-60 tumour cells. Open boxes represent *myb*-coding sequences. The blackened boxes represent sequences derived from alternatively spliced exon

as well as several melanomas. In a majority of these tumors, these abnormalities seem to be accompanied by an amplification of the *myb* gene followed by enhanced transcription. Rearrangements have not been generally observed in these tumors. However, it is possible that amplification could result in point mutations or splicing aberrations that result in the structural alterations of the protein.

TRANSCRIPTIONAL PRODUCTS AND REGULATION OF TRANSCRIPTION

The c-*myb* gene is transcriptionally active in several hematopoietic tissues of diverse species and codes for a message of 3.5–4.0 kb. In the domestic fowl, a 4 kb message has been detected in several lymphoid tissues, particularly in immature cells. These include thymus, bursa and foetal liver as well as yolk sac myeloid precursor cells. Expression of c-*myb* appears to be cell cycle dependent, as an increase in the steady-state levels of c-*myb* mRNA was observed during the late G1 and early S phase of the cell cycle in normal chicken embryo fibroblasts, in B-lymphocytes derived from the bursa as well as MSB-1 T-cell lymphoma cell line. Like its chicken counterpart, the murine c-*myb* gene is expressed as a 3.8–4.0 kb doublet in thymus, bone marrow and foetal liver but very poorly in adult spleen, liver and lymph nodes. Expression of c-*myb* undergoes a dramatic reduction during the differentiation of T-cells from immature cortical thymocytes to more mature peripheral T-lymphocytes. An interesting pattern of c-*myb* expression is also seen in the lymphoid organs of lpr/lpr mice, which exhibit an autoimmune lymphoproliferative syndrome. Peripheral lymphocytes of these mice were found to express high levels of c-*myb* and interestingly, humans with a similar disorder also exhibit similar levels of *myb* expression. Murine myeloid leukemia cell lines, such as WEHI-3, invariably exhibit high levels of *myb* expression, and GCSF-induced terminal differentiation of these cells to granulocytes seems to result in a substantial decrease in *myb* RNA levels. Friend virus-induced erythroleukemic cell lines exhibit high levels of *myb* transcription, and DMSO-induced terminal differentiation of these cells seems to result in a dramatic down-regulation of this gene transcription.

Human c-*myb* transcripts of 3.5 to 4.5 kb have been detected in several lymphoid, erythroid and myeloid cell lines. More mature cells or cells subjected to chemical induction appear to show dramatically decreased expression of the c-*myb* transcripts. Thus HL-60 cells, when treated with chemical inducers of differentiation seem to shut down *myb* synthesis. A similar rapid decrease in *myb* expression has been observed in the human myeloblastic leukemic cell line ML-1, following treatment with PMA which accompanies differentiation. Transcription of human c-*myb* gene has also been observed in breast, colon and small cell lung carcinomas and several of the cell lines derived from such tumors.

The c-*myb* locus appears to extend over a stretch of 40 kb in chicken, mouse and human species and to contain approximately 14 exons and introns. The mechanisms involved in the differential expression of *myb* gene in various hematopoietic cells have been the subject of intense study in recent years. This was first studied in two B-cell lymphomas (70Z/3B and A20.2J), where it was observed that 70Z/3B cell line (a pre-B-cell) expresses high levels of *myb* transcripts, while its more mature counterpart, A20.2J, expresses low levels of this mRNA. Recent work by various groups, essentially based on *in vitro* elongation of nascent transcripts in isolated nuclei, has revealed a very intricate pattern of transcriptional control at the c-*myb* locus. These results suggest that virtually all cells regulate *myb* RNA levels by regulating transcription elongation in the first intron of the c-*myb* gene. Thus it appears that cells which express low levels of *myb* transcripts appear to do so by prematurely terminating transcription of this gene in intron 1, whereas cells that express high levels of this mRNA overcome this transcriptional block. This developmentally regulated difference appears to be correlated to the presence of DNAase I-hypersensitive sites in this region, suggesting that the regulation of transcription elongation may be an important physiological mechanism by which *myb* expression is controlled.

To understand the molecular basis of transcriptional regulation of *myb* gene, we have recently examined the DNA–protein interactions within the first intron of c-*myb* gene and identified a 1.0 kb region which could be responsible for its transcriptional regulation. Using mobility shift assays, we showed that several nuclear factors bind to this region and the binding of these factors correlates with c-*myb* mRNA abundance in different cell types. It has also been known for some time that during the DMSO-induced differentiation of mouse erythroleukemic cells there was a dramatic decrease in c-*myb* mRNA levels, and that this reduction in the steady-state levels of mRNA is achieved in these cells by a block in transcription elongation. Our findings indicate that in the mouse erythroleukemic system, the block in transcriptional elongation is accompanied by a dramatic decrease in nuclear factors that bind to c-*myb* intron 1 sequences. These results suggest that a block to transcriptional elongation is overcome by the binding of nuclear factors to c-*myb* intron sequences and in the absence of such binding there is severe inhibition of transcriptional elongation. Characterization of the nuclear factors that bind to these intron sequences should provide us with additional insights into the mechanisms of gene regulation that operate in eukaryotic cells.

In addition to the regulation of transcription, the c-*myb* gene also appears to exhibit an intricate pattern of differential splicing which generates different proteins. Thus it is becoming apparent that most cells expressing *myb* RNA have at least two different forms of this message—a predominant form that could code for a c-*myb* protein of 75 kDa and a minor form that could code for an 89 kDa protein. The mRNA that codes for this larger protein appears to be generated by a differential splicing mechanism which results in the insertion of an additional stretch of 363 bp between exons 9 and 10. The function of this 89 kDa protein, as well as the mechanisms by which the cell regulates the balance between the two alternatively spliced mRNAs, is at present not understood. It is possible that the two mRNAs are produced using different transcriptional promoters. Alternatively, unique mechanisms may exist that regulate the differential splicing of the *myb* RNA, which results in the generation of disproportional amounts of the two species.

TRANSLATIONAL PRODUCTS OF THE c-*myb* GENE: STRUCTURAL AND FUNCTIONAL DOMAINS

Antibodies raised against synthetic peptides derived from v-*myb* DNA sequences or bacterially expressed proteins have allowed the biochemical characterization of v-*myb* and c-*myb* gene products. These studies demonstrated that the AMV v-*myb* gene codes for a protein of 48 000 Da, while the cellular *myb* gene codes for a protein product of 75 000 Da. Following the identification of alternative splicing mechanisms in c-*myb*, we developed anti-peptide antibodies specific for the alternatively spliced region of the mRNA originally observed in ABPL tumors. Immunoprecipitation analysis using these sera demonstrated the presence of two forms of c-*myb* protein— one of approximately 75 kDa and the other of 89 kDa. The function of this additional translational product is at present unclear, but it appears to be important since this alternatively spliced mRNA is observed in chicken, mouse and human species.

The structure of the two translational products of the murine c-*myb* gene and v-*myb* gene of AMV are presented in Figure 2. The murine c-*myb* protein, which is 75 kDa in size, is composed of 636 amino acids and contains several structural and functional domains (Figure 3). The first one-third of the molecule consists of an unusual structure of three direct repeats of 52 amino acids each. This region is known to mediate binding of the *myb* protein to DNA, and is highly conserved evolutionarily, being virtually identical in mouse, human and chicken, and conserved in *Drosophila*, corn *c1* gene and in two human *myb*-related genes, A-*myb* and B-*myb*. Two additional features have been noted within these tandem repeats. First, there

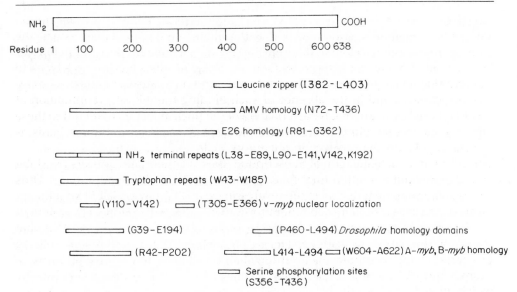

Figure 3. Structural and functional domains of mouse c-*myb* protein

is a periodic occurrence of tryptophans; each of the three repeats has three tryptophans, the first two separated by 18 or 19 residues, and the second and third by 19 amino acids. While the role of these tryptophans is unknown, it has been postulated that they could participate in DNA–protein interactions. Following the discovery of leucine zipper regions in the c-*fos* and c-*jun* proteins, which seem to play an important role in protein–protein interaction, a similar region has been identified in the c-*myb* region, though the functional significance of this region is at present unclear. This leucine zipper includes Ile 382, Leu 389, Leu 396 and Leu 403. These are conserved in mouse, human and chicken, but are absent in *Drosophila*, corn *c1* gene, A-*myb* and B-*myb*. Between Ser 401 and Phe 402, differential splicing results in the presence or absence of exon 9B, encoding 121 amino acids. Inclusion of exon 9B separates the third leucine of the leucine zipper from other leucines. Within repeat 2, a stretch of amino acids extending from Tyr 110 to Val 142 has been implicated as the nuclear localization signal; amino acid residues between Thr 305 and Glu 366 contain the second region necessary for nuclear localization. Both v-*myb* and c-*myb* proteins are mainly phosphorylated on serines. The serines phosphorylated in c-*myb* have been localized to the region between amino acids 355 and 426 of mouse c-*myb* in Figures 1 and 2 (correspsonding to amino acids 284 to 355 of v-*myb*). The role of serine phosphorylation in the biological activity of *myb* protein is at present unclear.

FUNCTION OF THE c-*myb* GENE

While it is becoming increasingly evident that the c-*myb* gene plays an important role in such diverse cellular processes as proliferation, differentiation and transformation, no specific biochemical function has been identified for the c-*myb* protein. In fact it is unclear whether its association with both growth and differentiation results from distinct functions or from a common c-*myb* function. Its short half-life, nuclear localization, DNA-binding property, conservation of DNA-binding domain and apparent cell cycle-dependent expression suggest that it may play an important role in controlling cell division and/or differentiation. It is readily induced in several T-cell lines upon treatment with IL-2 and mitogens such as PHA. Studies with anti-sense oligonucleotides demonstrate that expression of c-*myb* gene product is essential for the proliferative potential of several myeloid and T-cell lines. Exposure of human peripheral blood lymphocytes to anti-sense oligonucleotides before mitogen stimulation results in a block of T-cell proliferation but does not appear to affect the expression of early and late differentiation markers in these cells. These results suggest that c-*myb* protein deprivation does not perturb T-lymphocyte activation or early molecular events that may prepare the cell for subsequent proliferation. Rather, it appears to specifically block cells in late G1 or early S phase of the cell cycle. Studies with murine erythroleukemic cell lines and murine and human myeloid cell lines, as well as neuronal cell lines which can be induced to terminally differentiate in the presence of chemical inducers such as DMSO or growth factors such as GCSF, seem to suggest that terminal differentiation is accompanied by down-regulation of *myb* gene expression, implicating this oncogene in the process of differentiation. This concept is further strengthened by the observation that transfection of a vector carrying the c-*myb* gene under the control of an exogenous promoter that results in the constitutive expression of c-*myb*, blocks the erythropoietin-induced erythroid differentiation and partially blocks DMSO-induced terminal differentiation of mouse erythroleukemic cells.

Studies by Biedenkapp *et al.* have demonstrated that bacterially expressed v-*myb* protein binds DNA in a sequence-specific manner and the recognition sequence for this protein is PyAACG/TG. Accumulating evidence also suggests that the c-*myb* gene may act as a transcriptional transactivator. This property could be detected by co-transfection of c-*myb* cDNA expression vector into CV1 monkey kidney cells along with a reporter plasmid containing the *CAT* gene under the control of a test promoter and enhancer. Thus the two tandem repeats of SV40 enhancer were shown to mediate the c-*myb* induced activation of transcription. This notion is further supported by recent experiments of Weston and Bishop who demonstrated that fusion of v-*myb* coding sequences to the N-terminal 147 amino acids of yeast transcriptional activator GAL-4 allowed this fusion protein to activate the transcription of β-globin gene. They also present evidence that intact v-*myb* and c-*myb* function as transcriptional activators of the human β-globin gene if v-*myb* binding sequences are linked in cis to the regulatory domain of the β-globin gene.

Although the c-*myb* gene has been implicated in diverse biological functions such as cell growth and differentiation, the molecular mechanism of action of this protein is at present unclear. It is possible that these diverse functions are mediated by different translational products. The viral counterparts of this gene code for truncated proteins which lack the amino and carboxy terminal regions of the c-*myb* gene. Similarly, the NFS-60 cell line, which has undergone rearrangements in the *myb* locus as a result of retroviral integration, also produces a truncated *myb* RNA which lacks the 3' sequences. Similarly, murine retroviruses expressing truncated *myb* proteins have recently been shown to possess enhanced transforming potential. It is possible that the truncated proteins represent constitutively activated forms of *myb* which mediate cell transformation via transcriptional activation of specific cellular genes. The carboxy terminal region of the c-*myb* protein could play the role of a negative regulatory domain, and activation of this protein might require its association with a 'ligand', in the absence of which the protein could revert to an inactive state. If this model were true, it would be expected that the two translational products of c-*myb* with different carboxy terminal regions could function by association with different ligands, thus enabling the *myb* protein to accept diverse cytoplasmic signals.

Identification of cellular genes whose transcription is directly regulated by *myb* proteins should provide important clues regarding the function and mechanism of action of this nuclear protein, which appears to play a pivotal role in proliferation and differentiation of hematopoietic cells.

FURTHER READING

Bender, T. P. and Kuehl, W. M. (1986) Differential expression of c-*myb* proto-oncogene mRNA in murine B-lymphoid tumors is regulated by a block to transcription elongation. *Science,* **237,** 1473–1476.

Biedenkapp, H., Borgmeyer, U., Sippel, A. E. and Klempnauer, K-H. (1988) Viral *myb* oncogene encodes a sequence specic DNA-binding activity. *Nature,* **355,** 835–837.

Dudek, H. and Reddy, E. P. (1989) Identification of two translational products for c-*myb*. *Oncogene,* **4,** 1061–1066.

Gewirtz, A. M., Anfossi, G., Venturelli, D., *et al.* (1989) G1/S transition in normal human T-lymphocytes requires the nuclear protein encoded by c-*myb*. *Science,* **245,** 180–183.

Ramsay, R. G., Ikeda, K., Rifkind, R. A. and Marks, P. A. (1986) Changes in gene expression associated with induced differentiation of erythroleukemia: proto-oncogenes, globin genes and cell division. *Proc. Natl. Acad. Sci. USA,* **83,** 6849–6853.

Reddy, C. D. and Reddy, E. P. (1989) Differential binding of nuclear factors to intron-1 sequences containing the transcriptional pause site correlates with c-*myb* expression. *Proc. Natl. Acad. Sci. USA,* **86,** 7326–7330.

Rosson, D. and Reddy, E. P. (1987) Mechanism of activation of the *myb* oncogene in myeloid leukemias. In *Normal and Neoplastic blood Cells: From Genes to Therapy, Annals of N.Y. Acad. Sci.,* **511,** 219–231.

Thompson, C. B., Challoner, P. B., Neiman, P. E. and Groudine, M. (1986) Expression of the c-*myb* proto-oncogene during cellular proliferation. *Nature,* **319,** 374–380.

Weston, K. and Bishop, J. M. (1989) Transcriptional activation by the v-*myb* oncogene and its cellular progenitor, c-*myb*. *Cell,* **58,** 85–93.

6 Involvement of the *abl* Proto-Oncogene in Human Leukemias

RALPH B. ARLINGHAUS

Normal cellular genes capable of causing tumors in animals were first discovered as genetic elements of RNA tumor viruses. The prototype of this class of viruses, the Rous sarcoma virus, was discovered in the early 1900s by Peyton Rous, who found it had acquired a mutated form of a normal cellular gene, now called *src*. A number of other viruses that have acquired activated forms of cellular proto-oncogenes have since been discovered. These viruses are now termed retroviruses because they harbor an RNA-directed DNA polymerase (reverse transcriptase) unique to these viruses. One of these is the Abelson mouse leukemia virus; it causes pre-B-cell tumors in mice and converts lymphoid and fibroblastic cells grown in culture into tumor cells. The genetic element responsible for these tumorigenic properties is a fragment of the normal cellular gene known as the *abl* proto-oncogene. The *abl* proto-oncogene spans approximately 230 000 base pairs of DNA located on chromosome 9 in humans. The protein coding sequences are contained in two alternative 5′ exons spliced to a common set of ten exons (Figure 1), producing two major mRNA transcripts of 6 and 7 kb.

The *abl* proto-oncogene is expressed in virtually all tissues as a protein of MW 145 000 to 150 000 that places high-energy phosphate derived from ATP on tyrosine residues of proteins; it is part of an emerging group of regulatory enzymes known as tyrosine protein kinases. Tyrosine kinases play an important role in signal transduction mechanisms employed by cell surface receptors such as the insulin receptor and the epidermal growth factor receptor. The products of the normal forms of the *src* and *abl* genes are in part located at the inner side of the surface membrane

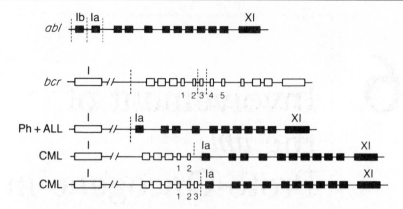

Figure 1. Molecular events in CML and related leukemias. The structure of the *abl* and *bcr* genes is indicated by filled and open boxes, respectively. The boxes refer to coding exons. The lines between exons are intervening non-coding introns. The positions of breakpoints are shown by the dashed vertical lines. Rearrangements seen in Ph[1]-positive ALL and two alternative translocations seen in CML are shown. This figure was taken from R. P. Gale in *Baillière's Clinical Haematology* **1**: 1–17, 1987

of cells, where they are believed to mediate growth signals received by ligand-activated receptors. However, in non-dividing tissues, such as brain, high levels of the *src* gene product have been detected, indicating that tyrosine kinases play important roles in terminally differentiated cells as well.

In the Abelson mouse leukemia virus genome, the cellular *abl* gene is truncated at its 5' end and becomes fused to a truncated version of the retrovirus' structural protein gene, which normally encodes four viral core proteins. Because of its fatty acid-containing amino terminal core protein, this chimeric protein localizes at the inner surface of the virus-infected cell's exterior membrane, presumably allowing specific and aberrant phosphorylation of a variety of unknown but obviously important substrates, thus converting the normal cell into a tumor cell. It is widely believed that, because of its unregulated tyrosine protein kinase activity, the viral *abl* gene product constantly sends a growth signal to the nucleus of the virus-infected cell, resulting in its unregulated growth and tumorigenic properties. Many questions remain unanswered about this process and about the role of the virus and its chimeric gene product in generating primarily pre-B-cell tumors and not other types of tumors.

THE *abl* PROTO-ONCOGENE AND THE PHILADELPHIA CHROMOSOME

The *abl* proto-oncogene has now been implicated in the cause and maintenance of certain forms of human leukemias that carry the Philadelphia chromosome (Ph[1]). The Ph[1] is present in hematopoietic cells from 95% of individuals with chronic myelogenous leukemia (CML). Approximately 5% of adults with acute myelogenous leukemia (AML), and up to 10% of children and 25% of adults with acute lymphocytic leukemia (ALL) also have the Ph[1]. In most cases the Ph[1] detected in acute leukemia is cytogenetically identical to that detected in CML.

Leukemic cells carrying the Ph[1] usually have two altered chromosomes in which a reciprocal translocation has occurred between chromosomes 9 and 22, designated t(9;22) (q34.1;q11.21), chromosome 22 being the Ph[1]. The breakpoint on chromosome 9 in CML occurs at the cytogenetic band that marks the *abl* proto-oncogene (9q34.1). Molecular cloning experiments indicate that breakpoints, which occur at variable sites over large molecular distances, usually occur 5' to *abl* exon II and typically in the long intron between the alternate first exons, termed Ia and Ib (Figure 1). The consequence of these breakpoints in most cases is that ten 3' exons of *abl* are translocated from chromosome 9 to 22 on the q arm at band q11.21; *abl* exon Ia may also be included in the translocated segment.

The positions of breakpoints near or within the *abl* gene on chromosome 9 show large variation, in contrast to the positions of the breakpoints within chromosome 22 (Figure 1). In CML breaks on chromosome 22 are restricted to a relatively small region of DNA encompassing 5–6 kbp. This restricted location was termed the *breakpoint cluster region* (bcr); it is centered within a protein-coding gene now called *bcr*. This gene (*bcr* I) and three related genes are located on the long arm of chromosome 22 in the order: *bcr* II; *bcr* IV; *bcr* I; *bcr* III. The *bcr* I gene extends over 90 kbp of DNA and is composed of at least 18 exons. The first exon is large and is located at least 30 kbp from the second exon. In Ph[1]-positive ALL, the breakpoint on chromosome 22 can occur between the first two exons of the *bcr* I gene. In CML the breakpoints usually occur in a more central location between two small exons of the *bcr* gene. The breakpoints on chromosome 9 are usually 5' to exon II, often between alternate exons Ia and Ib. The resulting mRNA transcript links the 5' three-quarters of the *bcr* I coding region to the *abl* coding region lacking the first exon (Figure 1).

The *bcr* locus is transcribed into mRNAs of 7.0, 4.5 and 4.0 kb, with smaller transcripts of 3.0, 2.5, 1.2 and 1.0 kb also being detected. The structure of the 4.5 kb *bcr* RNA has been determined by sequence analysis of molecularly cloned DNA copy: it is a single long open reading frame of 3813 nucleotides capable of encoding a protein of 1271 amino acids with a molecular mass of 142 kDa.

bcr-abl TRANSCRIPTION

CML leukemic cells and cell lines derived from patients with CML contain a novel 8.5 kb mRNA composed of about 3.3 kb of 5' *bcr* sequences and the balance as *abl* sequences. The joining of the two gene sequences occurs by splicing of the chimeric pre-mRNA. The consequence of the fusion is that the reading frames of the two segments of the pre-mRNA are joined in phase such that the chimeric mRNA is translated into authentic but altered *bcr* and *abl* proteins. It is obvious that certain critical regions of the *bcr* and *abl* polypeptides must be included within the fused protein to confer biological activity to the chimeric protein. Similar but different constraints will certainly apply to the junctions that occur in Ph[1]-positive ALL.

Alternate *abl* exons Ia and Ib are excluded from the chimeric *bcr-abl* mRNA. This can occur by two mechanisms: if the chromosomal break occurs 3' of either exon then that exon will remain on chromosome 9. However, in most cases, the break is 5' to exon Ia and 3' to exon Ib. In this case *abl* exon Ia will be included in the primary transcript. But since the *abl* exon Ia has no 5' splice acceptor site it is deleted from the spliced *bcr-abl* mRNA.

bcr-abl PROTEIN TRANSLATION

The *bcr* and *abl* genes are expressed in a wide variety of tissues. The *abl* gene product has an approximate molecular weight of 145 000 in human cells. The presence of two alternate first exons predicts the presence of at least two *abl* gene products. In the mouse, there are four alternate first exons, predicting the presence of four different but similar sized *abl* proteins with different amino termini. Regarding the products of the *bcr* genes, proteins of 190 and 160 kDa were identified initially. My recent studies have identified *bcr*-related gene products of 190, 185, 155, 135, 125 and 108 kDa in a variety of hematopoietic cells. These products shared antigenic and structural determinants consistent with their being encoded by the *bcr* gene or genes.

Proteins encoded by *bcr* are found within cytoplasmic complexes in association with a protein termed ph-p53. The identity of the latter protein is unknown. Interestingly, ph-p53 has also been found to be associated with $p210^{bcr-abl}$, sedimenting in cytoplasmic complexes ranging in size from 100 to 300 kDa. The function of these complexes and their role in cellular metabolism is not yet known.

The fused *bcr-abl* transcript is translated into a chimeric protein of about 210 kDa in CML cells. The fused protein contains either 927 or 902 amino acids encoded by *bcr*, depending on whether or not *bcr* exon 3 is included in the hybrid protein, and 1096 residues of *abl* (Figure 1). In ALL, the *bcr-abl* protein has a similar number of *abl* residues but contains only the amino acids encoded by the first exon of *bcr*. The size of the ALL-specific protein is about 185 kDa.

THE FUNCTIONAL ROLES OF THE *abl* AND *bcr* GENES IN LEUKEMIAS

The viral and cellular forms of the *abl* proto-oncogene have protein sequence patterns characteristic of protein kinases (Figure 2). In the standard assay of their enzymic activity, an immune complex containing the *abl* protein kinase bound to its antibody is incubated in a reaction mixture containing divalent cation and ATP in a suitable buffer. As with many kinases, it is important to use a site-directed antibody that attaches to the *abl* protein at a point that does not affect the protein kinase subdomain. The end result of this reaction is the covalent attachment of the gamma phosphate of ATP to tyrosine residues on either the *abl* protein itself or on an added protein substrate such as enolase.

The *abl* protein contains two structural domains characteristic of many protein kinases (Figure 2), a consensus ATP-binding site (domains I and II) and a phosphotransferase site (domains III–VII). These consensus sequences are often diagnostic of protein kinases. However, these consensus protein kinase domains encompass less than 200 amino acids of a 1200-residue protein. The remaining sequences obviously play other important roles, including sites of target protein

Domain	I	II	III	IV	V	VI	VII
Consensus	ᴸG.G..ɢ.V..(9-18)...A.K..(92-106)...ᴿDL...N..(12)..DFG..(19-25)...ᴀᴘE..(11)..D.ᴡ.G..(8-9)..ɢ..P
C-*abl* protein	[148] LG.G..ɢ.V..(12)...A.K...(90).....RDL...N..(12)..DFG.....(23)...APE..(11)..D.W.G...(9)...G..P [339]			186-216AA			
bcr protein	[163] KG.G...G.D..(16)...L.K...(103).....GPL...Q..(22)..DCG.....(3).....TPD..(11)..E.F.G...(3)...R..P [355]			191AA 192AA			

Figure 2. Comparison of consensus protein kinase domains to putative domains in the *abl* and *bcr* proto-oncogenes. The consensus protein kinase and the *abl* domains were taken from published works by Hunter and Cooper. The *bcr* sequences that resemble ATP and phosphotransferase domains were as described by Li *et al.* (Oncogene 4: 127–138, 1989). Note the discrepancies between the *bcr* pattern and the consensus pattern. The single letter code for amino acids is used. Small capital letters listed in the consensus sequence identify amino acid residues that are not strictly conserved in most protein kinases

binding, intramolecular and intermolecular sites of protein kinase regulation, and protein stability. Because of the known effects of the *gag-abl* tumor protein in which the amino terminal end of the *abl* protein is replaced by the truncated viral *gag* gene precursor protein, important sites that regulate its kinase activity are believed to reside at the amino terminus of the normal *abl* protein. Thus in both the CML- and ALL-specific *bcr-abl* proteins, it is widely believed that the substitution of some 900 amino acids from the *bcr* gene for the normal *abl* amino termini (there are two such termini stemming from the alternate first exons Ia and Ib) activates the *abl* kinase, thereby freeing it from normal regulatory control mechanisms.

However, recent studies raise the possibility that the *bcr* gene product plays more than a regulatory role in the leukemogenic activity of the *bcr-abl* protein. Gene sequence data from the 4.5 kb mRNA predicts the presence of a consensus ATP-binding site domain. Closer inspection of adjacent sequences reveals a near-consensus (see below) phosphotransferase domain (Figure 2). These data, along with the detection of an associated serine/threonine protein kinase activity, support the hypothesis that the *bcr* gene encodes a protein kinase activity. The position of the putative kinase domain is predicted to be in the first exon. The results reported by Groffen, Heisterkamp and co-workers are consistent with this prediction. They showed that the *in vitro* kinase activity associated with p160^{bcr} is neutralized by antiserum against the 5′ portion of *bcr* protein but not by antiserum against 3′ exons.

The position of the putative kinase domain in the first *bcr* exon further strengthens the proposal of an important role for this gene in Ph^1-positive leukemias since this exon is conserved in both CML-specific p210$^{bcr-abl}$ and ALL-specific p185$^{bcr-abl}$. Thus, both proteins would possess two protein kinase domains instead of the usual single domain. The joining of two protein kinases may be of great significance in the maintenance of the leukemic state. However, caution is required regarding the putative protein kinase activity of *bcr* proteins. First, the consensus kinase sequences are not strictly adhered to in *bcr* since significant differences exist between the consensus pattern and that present in *bcr* (Figure 2). Thus if *bcr* does encode a protein kinase, it has diverged from the typical structure of most kinases. Second, *bcr* proteins exist in cytoplasmic complexes and therefore one of several other proteins in the complex could account for the associated protein kinase activity originally attributed to p160^{bcr}.

Much more research needs to be done on *bcr* and *abl* gene products, and the fused forms of these proteins, to determine their roles in leukemia. Such studies will in the end lead to better health care for the cancer patient. In this regard, research is under way in a number of laboratories to develop specific compounds that will inhibit tyrosine protein kinases and new and faster methods to detect Ph^1-positive leukemia cells. Monoclonal antibodies developed in my laboratory are being used for this purpose.

FURTHER READING

Baltimore, D. (1981) Abelson murine leukemia virus-induced transformation of immature lymphoid cells. *Proc. Clin. Biol. Res.*, **45**, 297–308.

Bishop, J. M. (1983) Cellular oncogenes and retroviruses. *Ann. Rev. Biochem.*, **52**, 301–354.

Ben-Neriah, Y., Bernards, A., Paskind, M., *et al.* (1986) Alternate 5' exons in c-*abl* mRNA. *Cell*, **44**, 577–586.

Draezen, O., Canaani, E. and Gale, R. P. (1988) Molecular biology of chronic myelogenous leukemia. *Seminars in Hematology*, **25**, 35–49.

Hermans, A., Heisterkamp, N., von Lindern, M., *et al.* (1987) Unique fusion of *bcr* and c-*abl* genes in Philadelphia chromosome positive acute lymphoblastic leukemia. *Cell*, **51**, 33–40.

Hunter, T. and Cooper, J. A. (1986) Viral oncogenes and tyrosine phosphorylation. In: P. Boyer and E. G. Krebs (eds) *The Enzymes*, vol. XVII. 3rd edition, Academic Press, New York, pp. 191–245.

Li, W., Draezen, O., Kloetzer, W. S., *et al.* (1989) Characterization of *bcr* gene products in hematopoietic cells. *Oncogene*, **4**, 127–135.

Li, W., Kloetzer, W. S. and Arlinghaus, R. B. (1988) A novel 53 kDa protein complexed with P210[bcr-abl] in chronic myelogenous leukemia cells. *Oncogene*, **2**, 559–566.

Stam, K., Heisterkamp, N., Reynolds, Jr. F. H. and Groffen, J. (1987) Evidence that the Ph[1] gene encodes a 160 000-Dalton phosphoprotein with associated kinase activity. *Mol. Cell Biol.*, **7**, 1955–1960.

Whitlock, C. A. and Witte, O. N. (1985) The complexity of virus–cell interactions in Abelson virus infection of lymphoid and other hematopoietic cells. *Adv. Immunol.*, **37**, 73–98.

7 Structure and Function of *src* Family Kinases

KENTARO SEMBA

KUMAO TOYOSHIMA

To date, more than 20 retroviral oncogenes are known to have the capacity to transform cells *in vitro* and to form tumors *in vivo*. Of these retroviral oncogenes, the v-*src* gene of Rous sarcoma virus (RSV) has been studied most extensively since temperature-sensitive mutants of RSV first suggested the existence of an 'oncogene'. All retroviral oncogenes (v-*onc*) are derived from cellular counterparts (c-*onc*) in the host genome. At present, seven *src*-related cellular genes, c-*yes*, c-*fgr*, *fyn*, *lyn*, *lck*, *hck* and possibly *tkl*, as well as c-*src* have been molecularly cloned. These genes could encode tyrosine-specific protein kinases that are highly homologous with the c-*src* protein, p60^{c-src}. Thus, *src* and these other genes comprise a gene family called the *src* family.

In this review, we describe the structure of *src* family kinases and discuss the possible functions of their products.

FUNCTIONAL ANATOMY OF *src* FAMILY KINASES

The c-*src* gene and seven *src*-related genes are classified in a single gene family for the following reasons:

1. They encode 55–60 kDa protein-tyrosine kinases that lack a typical trans-membrane stretch.

2. Their products show extensive homology with each other over a contiguous stretch of approximately 460 residues towards the carboxy terminus (C-terminus).

3. So far as investigated, the positions of their exon/intron boundaries in coding regions are conserved.

Genes and Cancer. Edited by D. Carney and K. Sikora
©1990 John Wiley & Sons Ltd

The *src* family genes c-*src*, c-*yes* and c-*fgr* were identified as cellular homologues of retroviral oncogenes. The *lck* gene was identified as a proto-oncogene activated by integration of the Moloney murine leukemia virus. The other members were isolated by cross-hybridization with probes of the *src* family members at low stringency.

First, we will summarize the expression patterns of *src* family kinases, and then describe four functional regions of *src* family kinases, an amino-terminal (N-terminal) unique region, a modulatory region, a kinase domain and a C-terminal regulatory region.

Expression patterns of *src* family kinases

Although *src* family kinases are highly homologous, their expression patterns are distinct (Table 1). p60$^{c\text{-}src}$ is expressed in almost all cells, and at especially high levels in blood platelets and neurons. Expression of p60$^{c\text{-}src}$ also increases during differentiation of monocytes and neurons. In the brain, two types of c-*src* proteins have been recognized. One is identical to the regular product of the c-*src* gene expressed in other tissues, and the other is a brain-specific product that contains six additional amino acid residues at the junction of exons 3 and 4. Although c-*src*, c-*yes* and *fyn* are ubiquitously expressed, their intensities of expression vary in different tissues and organs. In contrast, the other members, c-*fgr*, *lck*, *lyn*, and *hck*,

Table 1. Molecular characaterization and expression patterns of *src* family kinases

Product	Human chromosome	Expression
c-src (533 aa)	20q13.3	Ubiquitous High in neurons and platelets Increased upon monocytic differentiation of HL-60 and U937 cells Increased in colon carcinoma
c-yes1 (543 aa)	18q21.3	Ubiquitous
fyn (537 aa)	6q21	Ubiquitous High in brain Increased in T-cells of *lpr* and *gld* mice
c-fgr (529 aa)	1p36.1	High in EBV-infected B-cells Detectable in granulocytes, macrophages and NK cells Induced upon monocytic differentiation of HL-60, U937 and THP-1 cells Induced upon granulocytic differentiation of HL-60 cells
lck (509 aa)	1p32→p35	High in T-cells Detectable in B-cells
hck (505 aa)	20q11→q12	High in granulocytes Detectable in B-cells Increased upon monocytic differentiation of ML-1 and HL-60 cells Increased upon granulocytic differentiation of HL-60 cells
lyn (512 aa)	8q13→qter	High in B-cells, platelets, monocytes and HTLV-I-infected T-cells
tkl		Detectable in spleen, brain and fibroblasts

are expressed preferentially in specific haematopoietic lineages: the c-*fgr* gene is expressed in granulocytes, monocytes and natural killer (NK) cells; the *lck* gene in resting T-lymphocytes; the *lyn* gene in B-lymphocytes, platelets and monocytes; and the *hck* gene in granulocytes and monocytes. Several lines of evidence support the idea that *src* family kinases play important roles in haematopoietic cells (see below).

Unique region

As shown in detail in Figure 1, all members of the *src* family share a common structure. In p60^{c-src} and p56^{lck}, a myristic acid is covalently attached to Gly 2 (glycine at position 2); p59^{fyn} is also myristylated. This myristylation is necessary for the binding of these proteins to the cellular plasma membrane and for the transforming ability of p60^{v-src}. Gly 2 is invariant in all members of the family. The minimum myristylation signal in p60^{v-src} is Gly 2 to Ser 6. Lys 7 is a critical residue for effective myristylation of p60^{v-src}; Lys 7 is conserved in all *src* family kinases except *lck*. These findings suggest that all members of the family are myristylated and bind to the cellular membrane. Actually, most of them have been found in the membrane fraction.

The 60–90 residues after Gly 2 are quite divergent. Since this 'unique region' is encoded by one exon in the c-*src* gene, exon shuffling may have played an important role in generation of *src* family genes with distinct functions. The unique region may contain the recognition sequences for interaction with other proteins, for example, regulatory proteins or extracellular receptors. This hypothesis was supported by

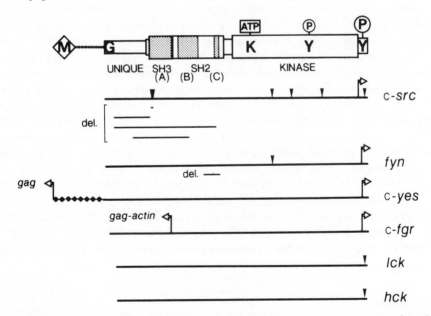

Figure 1. Schematic illustration of the structure and the oncogenic mutations of *src* family kinases. The positions of oncogenic mutations are indicated by vertical arrows for single amino acid substitutions, by thin horizontal lines preceded by 'del.' for deletions and by open arrows for recombinations with other sequences. Abbreviations: G=glycine; K=lysine; Y=tyrosine; M=myristic acid; P=phosphate; SH2 and SH3=*src* homology region 2 and 3

the recent finding that p56^{lck} interacts with the cytoplasmic regions of CD4 and CD8α through its unique region. Since the absence of amino acids 15–81 in p60^{v-src} had no effect on its transforming activity, this region is not required for the transforming activity of p60^{v-src}.

Modulatory region (SH2, SH3 region)

Residues 80 to 260 in p60^{c-src} are well conserved in all members of the family. Approximately 100 residues in this region (137–241 in p60^{c-src}) are also conserved in both the c-*fps* and c-*abl* proteins; they are designated as SH2, for *src* homology region 2 (the kinase domain is homologous region 1). The *src* family proteins and c-*abl* proteins share an additional homologous region (SH3, 86–136 in p60^{c-src}) located on the N-terminal side of SH2 (Figure 1). Surprisingly, parts of these regions have recently been shown to be shared by several other cellular proteins: phospholipase C's (PLC-γ_I, γ_{II}); the v-*crk* oncoprotein, spectrin, and GAP, the protein that stimulates the GTPase activity of p21^{ras}. These regions in p60^{c-src} are now called region A(88–137), B(148–187) and C(220–230), respectively (Figure 1). The biological significance of these regions is still unclear. One possibility is that they could interact with a common cellular protein(s). In fact, it has been suggested that the activated c-*src* protein (Tyr 527 to Phe) may interact with two phosphotyrosine-containing proteins through region B.

Deletions of SH2 and/or SH3 affect the transforming ability of p60^{v-src}. Mutant v-*src* proteins carrying deletions extending from residue 15 to 149 [del(15–149)] and del(149–169) induce comparable levels of phosphotyrosine *in vivo*, suggesting that their tyrosine kinase activity *in vivo* is similar to that of the wild-type p60^{v-src} protein. Nevertheless, the deletions attenuate, but do not abolish the transforming activity, as assayed by focus formation and anchorage-independent growth. These findings are consistent with the hypothesis that the modulatory region may help the *src* protein to recognize and to phosphorylate the cellular target(s). However, a large deletion of amino acids might influence the transforming activity by altering the whole conformation of p60^{v-src}. To avoid this possibility, the transforming ability of p60^{v-src} carrying small deletions, insertions or amino acid substitutions was characterized. Deletions or insertions of three or four amino acids within residues 155–177 included in region B abrogated the transforming activity of p60^{v-src} without significantly affecting the tyrosine kinase activity. These defective *src* proteins had significantly shorter half-lives within cells, suggesting that the region encompassing residues 155–177 may influence the stability of p60^{v-src} in the cellular membrane, possibly by interaction with cellular membrane components or substrates.

Kinase domain

Residues 260–516 in p60^{c-src} encompass the catalytic domain that exhibits tyrosine-specific protein kinase activity, called the kinase domain. The characteristic residues in the kinase domain include a glycine-rich motif, Gly-Xaa-Gly-Xaa-Xaa-Gly— residues 274–279 in p60^{c-src}—thought to form an ATP-binding pocket; Lys 295 in p60$^{c\text{-}src}$ that reacts with an ATP analogue; and Tyr 416 in p60$^{c\text{-}src}$ that can be autophosphorylated. With a few exceptions, mutations throughout the kinase domain in p60$^{v\text{-}src}$ abolished both the transforming activity and the tyrosine kinase activity, indicating that the kinase domain must be intact for both transforming and enzymic activity of p60$^{v\text{-}src}$. Mutants with insertions at residues 299 and 300 exhibit a temperature-dependent transforming phenotype, while those with insertions at residues 304 and 306 exhibit a host-dependent transforming phenotype. Thus this small region close to the ATP-binding pocket appears to be responsible for the generation of conditional mutants.

C-terminal regulatory region

Tyr 527 in p60$^{c\text{-}src}$ is conserved in members of the *src* family and is extensively phosphorylated. The following findings indicate that phosphorylation of this tyrosine residue depresses tyrosine kinase activity:

1. Spontaneous dephosphorylation of Tyr 527 occurs under some conditions of cell lysis and is correlated with augmented *in vitro* kinase activity.

2. Dephosphorylation of Tyr 527 by phosphatase treatment *in vitro* and binding of specific antibody to the region containing Tyr 527 increases the tyrosine kinase activity.

3. Avian p60$^{c\text{-}src}$ synthesized in yeast has low phosphorylation stoichiometry at Tyr 527, and is more active than the protein synthesized in mammalian fibroblast cells.

Analysis of the kinetics of substrate phosphorylation by phosphatase treatment or antibody-binding suggests that the phosphorylated C-terminus interacts with the active site, perhaps by behaving as a product analogue.

What kinase(s) can phosphorylate Tyr 527? In yeast, normal p60$^{c\text{-}src}$ is phosphorylated at Tyr 527, but kinase-inactive p60$^{c\text{-}src}$ (Lys 295 to Met) is not, indicating that p60$^{c\text{-}src}$ can phosphorylate itself at Tyr 527. When kinase-active p60$^{c\text{-}src}$ with two mutations (Tyr 416 to Phe; Tyr 527 to Phe) and kinase-inactive p60$^{c\text{-}src}$ are expressed together in yeast cells, kinase-inactive p60$^{c\text{-}src}$ is phosphorylated at Tyr 527 as extensively as normal p60$^{c\text{-}src}$ expressed alone. Thus, p60$^{c\text{-}src}$ can phosphorylate itself in an intermolecular fashion rather than in an intramolecular fashion. This autoregulation could act as a feedback regulation system in the signal transduction pathway mediated through p60$^{c\text{-}src}$.

In addition to autophosphorylation, some other factors in fibroblast cells may influence the level of phosphorylation of Tyr 527, because phosphorylation of Tyr 527 in fibroblast cells is more extensive than in yeast cells, even though the concentrations in these cells are similar. They may be, for example, other tyrosine kinases besides p60$^{c\text{-}src}$, or factors that promote phosphorylation or inhibit dephosphorylation of Tyr 527. These factors have been investigated using myristic acid-negative mutants of p60$^{c\text{-}src}$. This has demonstrated that the phosphorylation level of Tyr 527 in a mutant c-*src* protein lacking the myristylation signal is indistinguishable from that of normal p60$^{c\text{-}src}$ and that further mutational elimination of the enzymic activity of myristic acid-negative p60$^{c\text{-}src}$ does not alter the efficiency of phosphorylation at Tyr 527. These findings suggest that stable membrane association is not necessary for Tyr 527 phosphorylation and that phosphorylation at Tyr 527 may be mediated by another cellular tyrosine kinase(s) that can have access to both soluble and membrane-associated *src* proteins.

Dephosphorylation of Tyr 527 is not always required for activation of tyrosine kinase activity or for transforming ability. For example, two transforming variants activated by point mutations (Glu 378 to Gly; Ile 441 to Phe) in the kinase domain are dephosphorylated at Tyr 527, while others activated by point mutations or deletion [Tyr 90 to Phe; Tyr 92 to Phe; Arg 95 to Glu or Trp; del(92–95)] in the SH3 region are not. The N-terminal region may be required for the kinase domain to assume a conformation that can be inhibited by the phosphorylated C-terminus.

ONCOGENIC ACTIVATION OF *src* FAMILY KINASES

Mutations causing oncogenic activation

Accumulating evidence shows that the tyrosine kinase activity of *src* family kinases is usually repressed but is activated when oncogenic mutations are acquired. Figure 1 illustrates oncogenic activation of *src* family kinases schematically. Three types of mutation—substitution, recombination or deletion—can confer transforming ability on p60$^{c\text{-}src}$. Substitution of an amino acid residue in or outside the kinase domain (Tyr 90 to Phe; Tyr 92 to Phe; Arg 95 to Glu, Lys or Trp; Thr 338 to Ile; Glu 378 to Gly; Ile 441 to Phe; Tyr 527 to Phe), recombination of the C-terminus with consequent removal of Tyr 527 (S2-avian sarcoma virus), or deletion of the sequences N-terminal to the kinase domain [del(92–95), del(15–89), del(15–225), del(55–169)] or of the C-terminus [del(517–533), del(518–533), del(523–533)] are sufficient for transformation. Although the molecular mechanism of oncogenic activation has not yet been analysed in detail, these mutations are known to activate tyrosine kinase activity.

Removal of the tyrosine residue corresponding to Tyr 527 of *fyn*, *lck* and *hck* also results in oncogenicity. Comparisons of v-*yes* with human c-*yes*, and v-*fgr* with human c-*fgr*, show that each of the viral genes lacks the tyrosine residue corresponding to Tyr 527 by truncation at the C-terminus, and has an altered N-terminus owing to fusion with *gag* (v-*yes*) or *gag* and γ-actin (v-*fgr*). These N-terminal recombinations may contribute to the oncogenic activations of c-*yes* and c-*fgr*. In the case of p70$^{gag\text{-}actin\text{-}fgr}$, deletion of the C-terminal third of *gag* abolishes the transforming activity of p70$^{gag\text{-}actin\text{-}fgr}$, but deletion of γ-actin does not. Recently, three transforming retroviruses carrying the mutant *fyn* sequences were isolated by passage of the human *fyn*-containing virus through chicken embryo fibroblasts (CEF). Two of them carry deletions containing region C and the other has a substitution of Ile 338 to Thr. The tyrosine kinase activities of these mutants are enhanced *in vivo* and *in vitro*.

Correlation of *src* family kinases with human neoplasia

As described above, several types of mutations can activate the tyrosine kinase activity of *src* family kinases, and this activation causes transformation of tissue culture cells and tumor formation in experimental animals. In human tumors, however, none of these oncogenic mutations, gene amplifications or rearrangements of *src* family genes has yet been observed, except one case of gene amplification of the c-*yes* gene in a primary gastric cancer. Recently, p60$^{c\text{-}src}$ kinase activity was shown to be increased in all of 21 human colon carcinoma cell lines and all of 15 human colon carcinoma tissues examined without apparent rearrangement or amplification of the c-*src* gene. Interestingly, it has been suggested that activation of p60$^{c\text{-}src}$ in these tumor tissues is due to an apparent increase in the turnover rate of tyrosine-phosphates within the C-terminal portion (presumably, Tyr 527) of p60$^{c\text{-}src}$. This enhancement of tyrosine kinase activity at the post-transcriptional level suggests a novel mechanism of proto-oncogene activation.

The *lck* gene is expressed at high levels in thymus, at moderate levels in spleen, and at lower levels in non-lymphoid tissues. However, two of 14 colon carcinoma cell lines express similar levels of *lck* mRNA to that in T-cells. This indicates the possibility that deregulated expression of *src* family kinases may be implicated in human neoplasia. Other examples include the expression of p56^{lyn} in human T-cell leukemia virus type-I (HTLV-I)-infected T-cells and the expression of p58^{fgr} in Epstein–Barr virus (EBV)-infected B-cells (see below).

POSSIBLE SUBSTRATES OF *src* FAMILY KINASES

Analysis of phosphoamino acids of total cell proteins indicates that phosphotyrosine represents only 0.03% of the total phosphoamino acids in proteins in uninfected CEF, but that its level increases about 10 times upon transformation by RSV. The target proteins phosphorylated by p60$^{v\text{-}src}$ have been investigated by several experimental approaches, including a search for molecules associated with p60$^{v\text{-}src}$, *in vitro* phosphorylation, and immunoprecipitation with antisera specific to phosphotyrosine. The phosphotyrosine-containing proteins found so far include structural proteins (vinculin, talin, ezrin, fibronectin receptor and calpactin I), metabolic enzymes (enolase, lactate dehydrogenase and phosphoglycerate mutase), calmodulin, etc., although they may be phosphorylated by other protein kinases that are activated indirectly.

An 81–85 kDa phosphoprotein that is suggested to exhibit phosphatidylinositol (PI) kinase activity has been found to form complexes with polyoma middle T antigen and p60$^{c\text{-}src}$ in cells transformed by middle T antigen. This suggests that the 81–85 kDa protein or some related protein(s) may be a natural substrate for *src* family kinases. Transformation by p60$^{v\text{-}src}$ results in the appearance of tyrosine-phosphorylated p74$^{c\text{-}raf}$ and a five-fold increase in p74$^{c\text{-}raf}$-associated serine/threonine kinase activity, as measured in immune-complex kinase assays. GAP is also phosphorylated on tyrosine residues in rodent cells transformed by p60$^{v\text{-}src}$.

In addition to these candidates, a subset of phosphotyrosine-containing proteins has been identified as membrane-localized substrates in studies using non-myristylated v-*src* protein, which is defective in transformation activity. The myristic acid-free v-*src* protein can, however, induce proliferation of chicken neuroretina cells without morphological alteration. This finding demonstrates that there are several cellular targets of p60$^{v\text{-}src}$ and that, in contrast to the cellular targets involved in morphological transformation and anchorage independence, the targets responsible for mitogenic activity are accessible to non-myristylated *src* proteins.

BIOLOGICAL FUNCTIONS OF *src* FAMILY KINASES

src family kinases in haematopoietic cells

Despite great progress in understanding the regulation of kinase activity and in identifying possible substrates of *src* family kinases, no biological roles for any members of the *src* family, perhaps with the exception of *lck*, have yet been established. However, we may obtain some suggestions about the biological functions of *src* family kinases by analysing their expression in haematopoietic cells. In haematopoietic cells, many growth-stimulating or differentiating factors and many cell surface antigens have been identified. Accumulating information about the regulation of growth and differentiation of haematopoietic cells should be helpful in understanding the physiological and pathological functions of *src* family kinases in haematopoietic cells.

Before describing the most successful example—the biological role of p56^{lck} in T-cell activation—we will summarize the mechanism of T-cell activation. Initiation of a normal immune response occurs when T-cell receptors (TCR) on T-lymphocytes recognize molecules of the major histocompatibility complex (MHC) bound with antigen expressed on antigen-presenting cells. TCR is a multisubunit complex whose components are classified into three groups. The first group consists of antigen recognition components. On most T-cells, these components consist of α-β heterodimers, which are products of rearranged genes and are expressed in a clonally restricted manner. The second group consists of three components (CD3 complex), γ, δ, ε, which have the same sequences in all T-cells and show similarities in amino acid sequence with one another. The third group is ζ (and perhaps η) subunit, which is also invariant in all T-cells. The ζ chain exists primarily as a disulfide-linked dimer, ζ-ζ or ζ-η. The stimulation of T-lymphocytes by several agents, including antigen, mitogens or specific antibodies, is supposed to activate at least two independent protein kinases, protein kinase C and an unidentified tyrosine kinase that phosphorylates the ζ chain of TCR. CD4 and CD8 molecules are non-polymorphic surface glycoproteins expressed on T-lymphocytes, and their expression is correlated with the ability of T-lymphocytes to recognize the monomorphic regions of Class I (CD8) or Class II (CD4) MHC molecules. Several lines of evidence indicate that CD4 and CD8 potentiate the cellular responses mediated through the TCR.

An initial finding was that exposure of T-lymphocytes to a variety of agents, including mitogens and phorbol esters, causes down-regulation of *lck* mRNA and extensive modification of p56^{lck}. In several human T-cell lines and colon carcinoma cell lines, p56^{lck} was shown to be phosphorylated at serine residues within the N-terminal 18 kDa portion by 10-minute treatment with either phorbol ester or the diacylglycerol analogue, both of which activate protein kinase C. These findings raised the possibility that p56^{lck} in T-lymphocytes physiologically interacts with regulatory signal transducers and modifiers during T-cell activation. As an extension of these findings, it has been demonstrated that p56^{lck} is specifically comodulated with either CD4 or CD8 molecules by antibody-mediated cross-linking of them and that a large fraction (25–50%) of p56^{lck} proteins are associated with them. Since the cross-linking of CD4 by specific antibodies is thought to mimic the physiological interaction of CD4 with Ia$^+$ cells, the association of p56^{lck} with CD4 strongly suggests that p56^{lck} is important for the function of CD4. Furthermore, using a CD4$^+$ CD8$^-$ antigen-specific T-cell clone, C8, it has been shown that cross-linking of CD4 induces a rapid increase in the specific activity of p56^{lck} tyrosine kinase and is associated with rapid phosphorylation of tyrosine residues in the ζ chain. This finding suggests that p56^{lck} could influence the TCR-mediated signal pathway via phosphorylation of the ζ chain. However, cross-linking of the other surface molecules, CD3-ε and Thy 1, that are known to induce tyrosine phosphorylation in the ζ chain on another cell line, 2B4, did not cause any activation of p56^{lck} in C8 cells. Despite the difference in cells, this suggests that other tyrosine kinases in addition to p56^{lck} could phosphorylate the ζ chain upon stimulation of T-lymphocytes by cross-linking of CD3-ε or Thy 1.

Recently, it has been demonstrated that the expression of p56^{fyn} is elevated approximately 10-fold in CD4$^-$ CD8$^-$ (double negative) T-lymphocytes forming enlarged lymph nodes in *lpr* and *gld* mice, which are commonly used as models of autoimmune disease. Since the ζ chain is constitutively phosphorylated on its tyrosine residues in these T-lymphocytes, the abnormally expressed p59^{fyn} might be involved in deregulated expansion of double-negative T-cells through phosphorylation of the ζ chain.

Another *src* family kinase, p56^{lyn}, may be associated with HTLV-I-induced leukemogenesis. Expression of p56^{lyn} occurs in B-lymphocytes but not in T-lymphocytes or in several T-cell lines, including MT-I cells, which contain the HTLV-I provirus sequence but do not express viral proteins. However, p56^{lyn} is expressed in two HTLV-I producer T-cell lines as much as in B-cells. The proviral genome of the HTLV-I virus contains a unique gene, designated as *pX*, which encodes three proteins: p40^{tax}, p27^{rex} and p21^{x-III} . The protein p40^{tax} activates the transcription of its own genes and that of several cellular genes, including IL-2 and IL-2 receptor genes, so it is a candidate for a transcriptional activator of the *lyn* gene. Deregulated expression of p56^{lyn} may perturb normal proliferation of T-lymphocytes.

As in the similar case of p56^{lyn}, p58^{c-fgr} may be associated with EBV-induced B-cell immortalization. Granulocytes, monocytes and NK cells express p58^{c-fgr}, but not B-lymphocytes. However, six EBV-positive B-cell lines examined expressed c-*fgr* mRNA while seven of eight EBV-negative B-cell lines did not; moreover, infection with EBV induced c-*fgr* mRNA. This suggests that transcriptional activation of the c-*fgr* gene may be involved in EBV-induced B-cell immortalization. In further studies, the gene(s) of EBV responsible for induction of the c-*fgr* gene must be identified.

Regulation of p60^{c-src} by maturation promoting factor (MPF) and PDGF

Besides possible regulators of the level of phosphorylation of Tyr 527, some other factors have recently been shown to influence the tyrosine kinase activity of p60^{c-src} via phosphorylation of this molecule. p60^{c-src} is phosphorylated at Thr and Ser residues and has enhanced kinase activity without apparent change in the phosphorylation levels of Tyr 416 and Tyr 527 during mitosis. This novel mitotic phosphorylation occurs at Thr 34, Thr 46 and Ser 72. Further, p34^{cdc2}, a catalytic component of the maturation promoting factor (MPF), phosphorylates p60^{c-src} at these sites *in vitro*. MPF is a protein kinase complex that plays a central role in regulation of entry of cells into mitosis in many species. Since p60^{c-src} is well positioned to mediate the dramatic cytoskeletal rearrangements that occur during mitosis, MPF may induce these effects via phosphorylation and subsequent activation of p60$^{c\text{-}src}$.

Phosphorylation of p60$^{c\text{-}src}$ at Ser 12 and Ser 48 (only in chicken p60$^{c\text{-}src}$) occurs rapidly and stoichiometrically when cells are treated with tumor promoters, mitogens and hormones that activate protein kinase C. The same sites can be phosphorylated by purified protein kinase C *in vitro*. Thus, p60$^{c\text{-}src}$ is a *bone fide* physiological substrate of protein kinase C. Phosphorylation by protein kinase C has no effect on the *in vitro* tyrosine kinase activity of p60$^{c\text{-}src}$ as measured by immune-complex kinase assay. However, this does not exclude the possibility that protein kinase C may change the physiological state of p60$^{c\text{-}src}$ *in vivo*; for example, its specific activity *in vivo*, substrate specificity, or subcellular localization. In contrast to other protein kinase C activators, platelet-derived growth factor (PDGF) treatment induces phosphorylation of one or two additional serine residues and one tyrosine residue within the N-terminal 16 kDa region, in addition to phosphorylation of Ser 12, and causes the two- to three-fold increase in tyrosine kinase activity. This implies that tyrosine kinase(s) and another serine/threonine kinase(s) in addition to protein kinase C are activated by PDGF treatment.

Activation of transcription factors by p60$^{v\text{-}src}$

There is considerable evidence that tyrosine phosphorylation is crucially important in the signal transduction pathway from the plasma membrane to the nucleus and that subversion of this phosphorylation leads to cellular transformation. How then do tyrosine kinases transduce signals to the nucleus? One hypothesis is that tyrosine kinases directly or indirectly activate transcriptional regulators and subsequently modulate the transcription rates of several genes. As described above, p74$^{c\text{-}raf}$ may be involved in the signal transduction pathway mediated by p60$^{v\text{-}src}$. Consistent with this hypothesis, activated c-*raf* and A-*raf* proteins as well as p60$^{v\text{-}src}$ can increase the activity of a transcription factor, AP1. p60$^{v\text{-}src}$ can also enhance CAT activity from HTLV-I long terminal repeat (LTR), human immunodeficiency virus LTR, *fos* promoter, etc. It will be helpful to identify the signal transduction pathway from p60$^{v\text{-}src}$ to the nucleus to determine the transcriptional factors affected by p60$^{v\text{-}src}$.

CONCLUSION

The recent finding of the association of p56^{lck} with CD4 and CD8 has confirmed the hypothesis that *src* family kinases are functionally associated with some receptor molecules that receive extracellular signals and transduce them to the nucleus. In addition to extracellular signals, MPF, an intracellular signal of mitosis, may also utilize p60$^{c\text{-}src}$ for the purpose of changing the cellular architecture during mitosis. These findings suggest that a variety of signals may induce biological phenomena through change in the tyrosine kinase activity of *src* family kinases. For determination of the functions of *src* family kinases, studies are required on what signals can influence the tyrosine kinase activity of *src* family kinases, what molecules are associated with them, and what effects they have on second messenger cascades and on transcriptional regulators.

FURTHER READING

Cooper, J. A. (1989) The *src*-family of protein-tyrosine kinases. In: Kemp, B. and Alewood, P.F. (eds.), *Peptides and Protein Phosphorylation*. CRC Press, Boca Raton (in press).

DeClue, J. E. and Martin G. S. (1989) *J. Virol.*, **63**, 542.

Ellis, C., *et al.* (1990) *Nature*, **343**, 377.

Fujii, M., *et al.* (1989) *Mol. Cell Biol.*, **9**, 2493.

Gould, K. L. and Hunter, T. (1988) *Mol. Cell Biol.*, **8**, 3345.

Katagiri, T., *et al.* (1989) *Proc. Natl Acad. Sci. USA*, **86**, 10064.

Morrison, D. K., *et al.* (1988) *Proc. Natl. Acad. Sci. USA*, **85**, 8855.

Shaw, A. S., *et al.* (1989) *Cell*, **59**, 627.

Shenoy, S., *et al.* (1989) *Cell*, **57**, 763.

Turner, J. M., *et al.* (1990) *Cell*, **60**, 755.

Veillette, A., *et al.* (1989) *Nature*, **338**, 257.

Wang, H-C. R. and Parsons, J. T. (1989) *J. Virol.*, **63**, 291.

Wasylyk, C., *et al.* (1989) *Mol. Cell Biol.*, **9**, 2247.

Yamanashi, Y., *et al.* (1989) *Proc. Natl Acad. Sci. USA*, **86**, 6538.

8 The Role of Oncogenes in Metastasis

SUZANNE A. ECCLES

The genetic and/or epigenetic mechanisms underlying the evolution of a localized focus of 'transformed' cells to an invasive, metastatic cancer are of considerable interest. This propensity of neoplastic cells for 'progression' provides significant challenges in both clinical oncology—since disseminated disease is responsible for most treatment failures—and in cellular and molecular biology, where we seek to explain the normal social interactions of cells in order to understand their aberrations. While the involvement of oncogenes in the aetiology of certain cancers now seems likely, their role(s) in tumour progression and metastasis remain controversial. Many of the conflicting data relate to difficulties in accurately assaying the activity of oncogenes and their products, and in quantitating the 'metastatic potential' of tumours. In this review I will attempt to summarize the available evidence while drawing attention to some of the technical difficulties inherent in such studies.

'THE METASTATIC PHENOTYPE'— PROBLEMS OF DEFINITION AND MEASUREMENT

The literature abounds with references to 'the metastatic phenotype' which may mislead the uninitiated into believing that there is a definable blueprint associated with cells which metastasize, which distinguishes them from others which fail to metastasize. In practice, such distinctions are far from clear. The metastatic capacity as measured for experimental tumours is a relative value which depends upon a multitude of factors. For example NIH/3T3 fibroblasts have been shown to produce tumours in the footpads of *nu/nu* mice that metastasized to lung, whereas the same cells injected s.c. in the supraclavicular region did not. The former site is more

Genes and Cancer. Edited by D. Carney and K. Sikora
©1990 John Wiley & Sons Ltd

permissive of metastasis than the latter, due to mechanical pressures; but should this particular cell line be defined as 'metastatic' or 'non-metastatic'? Immuno-compromised hosts may allow expression of the 'metastatic phenotype' which would be obscured if the cells expressed antigens recognized by immunocompetent hosts, and this is generally true within a species; however *xenogeneic* tumours rarely metastasize as readily as in the autochthonous or syngeneic host. 'Spontaneous' metastasis assays of short duration are less sensitive than those extended by extirpation of the primary tumours, and definition of a particular cell line as '*non-metastatic*' is not necessarily justified. When transfection of an oncogene is claimed to 'induce the metastatic phenotype', therefore, one must be satisfied that it has not merely accelerated a pre-existing tendency. Similarly, the least demanding 'metastasis' assay involves the direct inoculation of cells into the venous circulation. This lung colonization capacity may or may not correlate with the ability to metastasize from a primary site and cannot be assumed unless tested.

Clinically, evidence of the malignancy of different types or stages of tumours are usually based on population statistics and retrospective analyses. Occasionally, both primary and secondary lesions are available for study, but frequently assays are performed on fixed or cryopreserved material. Analyses of cell lines derived from human tumours suffer from the problem that changes in genotype and/or phenotype may occur during or subsequent to their establishment in culture (e.g. N-*ras* activation or over-expression in human breast and teratocarcinoma cell lines) and hence cannot be correlated definitively with their natural history. The final problems, common to both human and experimental tumours, relate to the phenotypic heterogeneity and instability of tumour cell populations and the complex nature of the metastatic process.

ONCOGENES—WHAT ARE THEY AND HOW DO WE TEST FOR THEIR ROLE(S) IN METASTASIS?

Oncogenes were first defined as the 'transforming' elements in acutely transforming retroviruses (v-*onc*). Subsequently, work has shown them to have been transduced from normal mammalian DNA (cellular proto-oncogenes, c-*onc*). By and large they encode proteins involved in regulation of cell proliferation and differentiation. When these genes are abnormally expressed or 'activated', cells may fail to respond to normal growth and differentiation controls and exhibit features of malignancy. Not all c-*onc* genes have a v-*onc* counterpart, for example N-*ras*, although this is closely related to Ha-*ras* and Ki-*ras*, the transforming genes of the Harvey and Kirsten sarcoma viruses respectively. Similarly, it has been suggested that cellular genes not classically regarded as 'oncogenes' nevertheless could be considered as such, based on a degree of sequence homology with known v-*onc* genes, and the fact that they code for growth factors or their receptors. Examples include homologies between the product of v-*erb*A and the glucocorticoid and oestrogen receptors, and the polyomavirus middle T protein and gastrin. The present discussion will focus on established oncogenes, but it seems timely to consider also their interactions with other cellular control elements such as steroid and peptide hormones.

The assays available for measurement of c-*onc* activity continue to improve, but some early work suffered from the inability to distinguish the 'normal' and 'activated' forms of a gene (e.g. *ras*), and from the lack of accurate quantitation. Cellular DNA can be examined for the presence of an oncogene, its amplification, translocation and methylation status. However, it is increasingly evident that *expression* is of greater significance. Transcription (mRNA levels) may or may not relate to gene amplification, and problems with the instability of RNA and variability of the 'dot blot' assay render this technique somewhat unreliable. Measurement of the protein product and, ideally, assays of its functional integrity, can be performed using antibodies raised against critical peptide sequences and the appropriate ligands or substrates. These assays are perhaps the most pertinent since the presence of the gene, and its levels of transcription are not necessarily reflected in the quantity or quality of gene product. Using such techniques (ideally in combination) it is possible to probe for oncogene expression in tumours, and enquire whether correlations exist with their metastatic capabilities. In human cancers this has been attempted either by comparing multiple samples of normal, benign (premalignant) and malignant tissues, or, more rarely, by comparison of primary and secondary tumours from the same patients. In addition to studies probing for specific oncogenes, two other, related, types of investigation have been attempted. For example, benign and metastatic colon cancers have been compared by screening cDNA libraries for differential gene expression; the results showed that both increases and decreases in abundance of several mRNAs occurred, suggesting subtle alterations in multiple genetic loci. A gene with no homologous sequence to known oncogenes was found to be more abundant in liver metastases than primary tumours; its significance as a marker of colon carcinoma metastasis remains to be evaluated. Further evidence for the existence of genes controlling invasion and metastasis in human cells has been inferred from somatic cell fusion studies. Non-invasive mouse lymphoma cells were fused with invasive human T-cells; invasive hybrids retaining only human chromosome 7 were isolated. In this instance the 'metastatic capacity' of the hybrids was assayed by direct intravenous inoculation but there is no a priori reason to presume that the invasive and migratory properties of normally circulating cells are dependent upon the same genetic machinery as in malignant carcinomas or sarcomas. Nevertheless, identification of the gene or genes involved could focus attention on their expression in metastases to address this question. In experimental models, similar comparisons of oncogene expression in 'metastatic variant' and 'parental' cell lines have been undertaken. In addition, the effects of transfecting oncogenes into cells with no or limited capacity for tumorigenicity and/or metastasis have been examined.

ASSOCIATIONS BETWEEN ONCOGENE ACTIVITY AND METASTASIS

Human cancers

Table 1 illustrates some of the studies in which associations between oncogene amplification, over-expression or activation, and tumour progression have been examined. It must be noted that in many cases the authors have referred only to tumour grade or stage, or to patient prognosis. Nevertheless, since advanced cancer is associated with the development of regional or distant metastasis, which ultimately

Table 1. Examples of associations between oncogene expression and malignancy in human cancers

Tumour material	Oncogene/product assayed	Observations
Breast—normal, benign, malignant, metastases	pan-*ras* p21 immunocytochemistry	No correlation with malignancy; normal cells in stroma also positive
Breast—benign, malignant	pan-*ras* p21 immunohistochemistry	Enhanced p21 expression in invasive carcinoma versus carcinoma *in situ*; heterogeneity in 1° and 2° tumours; 2° higher or lower than 1°
Breast—primary tumours	pan-*ras* p21 immunocytochemistry	19/20 'node positive' cases expressed p21 versus 10/21 'node negative' cases
Breast 189 1° cancers	*erb*B2 gene amplification	2–20-fold amplification. Positive correlation with nodal status, prognosis and survival
86×1° and 12×2° cancers	*erb*B2 gene amplification and protein expression	17% 1° and 25% 2° cancers showed gene amplification; more common in 'node positive' patients
Breast—108 1° cancers	EGF^R-radioligand assay; immunohistochemistry	Inverse correlation with oestrogen receptor, no correlation with nodal status; association with large tumour size and poor prognosis
Breast—121 1° cancers	c-*myc* gene amplification	32% c-*myc* amplified—no correlation with disease status
Gastric carcinoma—171 cases	pan-*ras* p21	Early carcinoma 11% positive; advanced—44%; associated with prognosis. p21 immuno-reactivity increased with depth of invasion
Gastric carcinoma—156 cases	EGF/EGF^R immunohistochemistry	No EGF in early carcinoma; positive in 29% advanced—high levels in 2° tumours. Correlation with depth of invasion

Table 1. (*continued*)

Tumour material	Oncogene/product assayed	Observations
Colorectal carcinoma—1° and 2° and benign	pan-*ras* p21	1. p21 decreased in metastases from colorectal carcinoma; expressed in lung metastases of other carcinomas. 2. High levels in deeply invasive carcinomas, low in benign/normal; metastases—heterogeneous expression
Bladder carcinoma—31×1°	EGF[R] and immunohistochemistry	Correlation between EGF[R] levels and stage and grade of tumours; normal structure. Amplification in 1 advanced case
Neuroblastomas	N-*myc* gene/mRNA	Amplification and expression correlate with stage and survival. Gene copy number predicts prognosis
Small cell lung cancer	N-*myc* gene	Amplification correlates with stage. No difference between 1° and 2° lesions

determines survival in most cases, it seems reasonable to assume that these parameters reflect 'metastatic capacity' for the purposes of this discussion. I have omitted references to established cell lines derived from human tumours for reasons discussed above.

The data illustrate a good deal of heterogeneity, both between different tumours and their metastases, and between different studies ostensibly measuring the same end-point, presumably reflecting differences in the specificity and/or sensitivity of the assays employed. Nevertheless, a few tentative generalities can be proposed: gene amplification, and/or over-expression are far more common than mutation/ rearrangement. Heterogeneity *within* a tumour suggests that highest oncogene activity may occur in association with the invasive edge; heterogeneity *between* metastases suggests that maintenance of a lesion does not depend on continued expression of the oncogene(s) that may have facilitated its initiation. The fact that different oncogenes appear to be 'active' in different cancers suggests that cellular susceptibility varies and may depend on lineage, differentiation status or environmental influences. Although *ras* seems to be one of the most frequently expressed families of oncogenes in human cancer, the most consistent associations between oncogene activity and prognosis appear to involve the *erb*B genes encoding related EGF^R-like molecules.

Experimental studies

Table 2 illustrates examples of oncogene expression in rodent tumours of varying 'metastatic capacity' and also changes in malignancy induced by the transfection of oncogenes and/or DNA from malignant cells into 'normal' or tumorigenic acceptor cells. Much of the early work compared endogenous c-*onc* expression in long-established cell lines from which metastatic 'variants' had been derived. In view of the frequent instability of the metastatic phenotype and the propensity for 'non-metastatic' cells spontaneously to acquire malignant characteristics, these studies would have been better controlled if metastatic capacity had been accurately and contemporaneously quantitated. Ki-*ras* and Ha-*ras* appear to be expressed in several independent studies using mainly murine lymphomas and sarcomas, but in rat mammary carcinomas expression was either not detected, or appeared to be associated with tumour initiation induced by MNU, rather than with the (rare) metastases observed.

In transfection experiments, the bulk of studies have investigated the influence of Ha-*ras* on murine 3T3 'immortal' fibroblasts. In most cases, evidence that this gene could induce the metastatic phenotype was offered, but the degree of enhancement of metastasis over various control cells varied enormously. There is some suggestion that the genotype of the recipient cell influences the action of the *ras* oncogene; metastatic capacity has been induced in rodent fibroblasts, but not mammary carcinoma cells. However, other studies have shown that similar cells can respond to transfection with c-Ha-*ras*-1 by an increased incidence and rate of development of metastases. Taken together, these reports strongly suggest that activated c-Ha-*ras*, possibly c-Ki-*ras* but apparently not N-*ras* (although this is less extensively investigated) can influence spontaneous metastasis of several cell types either directly or indirectly, with the magnitude of the observed effects probably being modulated by the environment of the recipient cell and/or its host. In most instances enhanced expression of the normal Ha-*ras* proto-oncogene did not induce metastasis beyond that seen with other control transfections, suggesting that the mutant p21 is required to exert maximum influence. Our own studies indicated that the 'activating' mutation in c-Ha-*ras*-1 of both Gly→Val or →Ser at codon 12 were equally capable of dramatically enhancing widespread spontaneous metastasis in mouse mammary carcinoma cells. Such data, however, cannot be taken as conclusive proof that the activity of an incorporated oncogene *per se* is permissive of metastasis, since it is clear that the manipulations involved in transfection and subsequent *in vitro* selection procedures may themselves introduce genomic instability and phenotypic changes in the recipient cells. Isolated examples of the transfection of other oncogenes apparently influencing metastasis (e.g. v-*fos* and those encoding kinases) are interesting, but require confirmation and further analysis before their significance becomes clear.

Possible mechanisms by which activated oncogenes may influence tumour invasion, dissemination and metastasis

If we accept the circumstantial evidence that activation of certain 'oncogenes' in certain tumours may be associated with their progression to a more malignant phenotype, determination of the underlying molecular mechanisms will be critical to our better understanding of, and ultimately therapeutic control of metastatic disease. However, it must be recognized that tumour cell populations may employ different strategies to achieve the same end. Analogies with the phenomenon of drug resistance, where multiple mechanisms appear to operate, caution against over-extrapolation of results from one experimental system to another. Many researchers have sought to determine the phenotypic traits which distinguish metastatic cells, yet no single characteristic has been unequivocally recognized as being constitutively required by all cells capable of metastasis.

It is often difficult to determine whether oncogene expression is a primary (i.e. causal) or secondary (i.e. induced) event in malignant cells, since many oncogenes are active during normal growth and development. It is possible, therefore, that oncogenes simply confer greater growth potential on cells already possessing the genetic elements required for metastasis. On the other hand, insertion or activation of an oncogene in the host DNA may trigger a 'pre-programmed' cascade of events normally undertaken by migrating cells during embryogenesis or wound healing. Either or both of these mechanisms could account for the paradox that a single gene (Ha-*ras*) can apparently influence a complex multi-step sequence of events such as invasion and metastasis. In some cases failure of cells to generate metastases may be due to host defence mechanisms, and oncogene expression has been linked with changes in tumour cell susceptibility which may influence the survival of such cells in the circulation or at secondary sites. In some systems, co-regulation in the expression of MHC glycoproteins and p21^{ras} has been observed, which may have a bearing not only on cellular recognition in immune reactions, but on other cell–cell interactions concerned with regulation and stabilization of developmental processes.

There is also circumstantial evidence to support the proposal that oncogene activity may also influence *specific* sequences of the metastatic process. Firstly, as already

Table 2. Endogenous or transfected oncogene activity and metastasis in experimental models

A. Endogenous oncogenes

Cell line/type		Observations
Murine lymphomas	Probed for v-erbA and B, Ki- and Ha-ras, myc, abl, fes, fms, fos, myb, sis, rel, raf, yes	'Metastatic variants'‡ compared with 'parental' tumours. Increased expression of Ki-ras, myb and raf
Murine mammary carcinoma		30-fold Ha-ras amplification, but no increase in p21 in metastasis-derived cell line
Murine lymphoma, fibrosarcoma	c-Ki-ras gene	Expressed in 'metastatic variant'‡, not parental cells
Murine B16 melanoma and UV-induced sarcomas	c-Ki-ras mRNA and p21, and 10 other oncogenes assayed	Major oncogene expressed—Ki-ras; no correlation between amount, expression and metastasis‡
1° or passaged NMU-induced rat mammary carcinoma	Endogenous Ha-ras mutated by NMU	1° tumour 10-fold higher Ha-ras DNA than 2° tumours; 10 individual metastases* higher or lower than 1°
Spontaneous rat mammary carcinoma clones	myc, N-ras, Ha-ras and fos mRNA assayed	fos expression higher in metastatic clones*; myc and N-ras no correlation; Ha-ras not expressed

B. Transfected Oncogenes

Cell line/type		Observations
Murine NIH/3T3 fibroblasts	T24 activated c-Ha-ras-1	Transfection accelerated formation of metastasis*; evident in controls in 'sensitive' assays
NIH/3T3 and 10T½	T24 c-Ha-ras-1	Direct relationship between ras expression and metastasis*; amplification of H-ras in metastases; pre-induction of p21 increased metastasis
NIH/3T3	Human DNA containing Ha-ras or N-ras	Both oncogenes induced capacity for lung colonization† (i.v.); only Ha-ras induced spontaneous metastases (nu/nu)
NIH/3T3	Ha-ras+DNA from metastatic human tumour	Ha-ras alone—no effect; other (non-myc or ras) sequences from 'metastatic DNA' required
NIH/3T3 or rat embryo fibroblasts (REF)	c-Ha-ras±v-myc or E1a ras proto-oncogene or c-mos	c-Ha-ras±v-myc transfectants metastatic*; c-Ha-ras +E1a non-metastatic, similarly c-mos and c-ras
NIH/3T3	v-Ki-ras (replication-deficient)	v-Ki-ras gene amplified and over-expressed in tumours; 2/5 lung colonies or metastases from footpad tumours—rearranged Ki-ras; not in micrometastases from s.c. site

B. Transfected Oncogenes

Cell line/type	Transfected Oncogenes	Observations
NIH/3T3	c-Ha-ras, v-mos, v-raf, v-src, v-fes, v-fms, v-myc, c-myc, p53	Lung colonization assay[†]. All oncogenes encoding serine/threonine kinases (ras, mos, raf, src, fes, fms) induced 'metastasis'; myc and p53 induced tumorigenesis only
NIH/3T3, REF and murine C127 mammary cell line	H-ras proto-oncogene or v-Ha-ras, T24 c-Ha-ras-1	c-ras proto-oncogene inactive; ras oncogenes induced 'metastatic phenotype'[†] in 3T3 cells and REF[†][*] but not in C127 cells
REF and Chinese hamster lung fibroblasts	c-myc and Ha-ras-1 (T24 and normal); 9 endogenous proto-oncogenes assayed	Lung and lymph node metastases* induced from both cell lines by T24 Ha-ras (~30%) and myc (8%). Proto-oncogene induced nodal metastases in 13% mice: c-abl and c-fos strongly expressed in all transfectants
REF passage 2	T24 c-Ha-ras-1 ± E1a	ras alone induced metastatic* and lung colonization[†] potential; plus E1a this activity suppressed
Rous sarcoma virus transformed rat fibroblasts	v-fos	Higher number of lung metastases* from i.m. tumour developing from transfectants than control cells; also enhanced lung colonization potential[†]
REF low passage	Polyoma large T or middle T, v-myc, c-Ha-ras-1	Transfectants had increased growth rate; ras and myc produced invasive metastatic* tumours, but control cells showed high spontaneous rates of progression to metastasis competence
Mouse mammary carcinoma MT1	c-Ha-ras-1 proto-oncogene or activated T24 gene	Parental cell lines 10% incidence of metastasis*; control transfectants 23–67%; those containing activated oncogene 82–100% and increased organ distribution. Lung colonization[†] unaffected
Mouse mammary carcinoma SP1	c-Ha-ras-1 proto-oncogene or activated oncogene	$CaPO_4$ transfection technique alone induced metastatic capacity (6–18%); increased further by activated oncogene (26–31%) short-term assay

*'Spontaneous' metastasis assayed; i.e. development of distant secondary (2°) tumours disseminated from primary (1°) site.
[†]'Metastasis' (i.e. lung colonization) assayed by direct intravenous inoculation of cells.
[‡]Metastatic capacity not assayed during study, but based on previous experience of 'variants'' behaviour.
Most assays were performed in nu/nu mice.

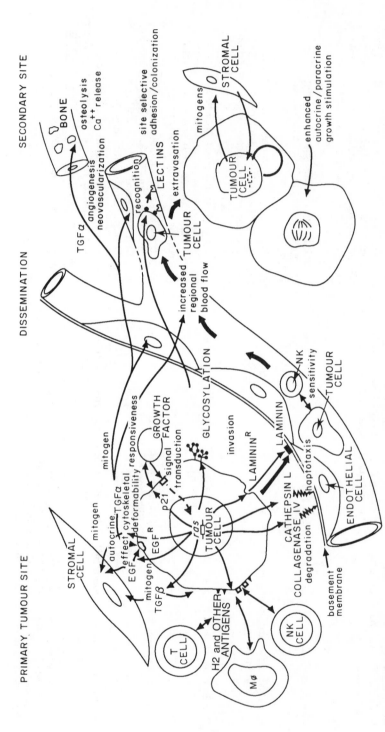

Figure 1. Possible mechanisms by which oncogenes (exemplified by *ras*) may influence discrete portions of the metastatic process

1. Increased production of TGF α-mitogenic for epithelia and stromal cells, and endothelia (1° and/or 2° sites). May be involved in osteolysis (? bone metastases). Increased blood flow (? aids dissemination).
2. Increased production of TGF β-mitogenic for stromal cells. Modifies cellular adhesion (? increased release of cells).
3. Major excreted protein of *ras* transfected cells is capthespin L. This and collagenase type IV involved in degradation of basement membranes (bm). Increased laminin[R] enhance interaction with bm and haptotaxis. Cytoskeletal deformability <(invasion).
4. Altered expression of antigens influences cellular interactions, and sensitivity to immune effectors (tumour cell survival in circulation).
5. Increased responsiveness to growth factors–stimulates growth (2° sites?).
6. Altered glycosylation (increased branching) decreases cell contact/communication; enhances extravasation (? lectin interactions influence organ colonisation patterns).

mentioned, the fact that many secondary tumours show heterogeneity of expression of oncogenes (often less than is observed in primary tumours) suggests that their role may be in the initiation, rather than the maintenance of metastases. $p21^{ras}$ and EGF^R have been shown to occur predominantly at the 'invasive edge' in gastric, colorectal, and possibly bladder cancers (Table 1), and to stimulate invasive capacity of tumour cells assayed *in vitro*. Our own experiments with c-Ha-*ras*-1 transfected mouse mammary carcinoma cells suggested that the oncogene was enhancing escape of cells from the primary tumour rather than later events in dissemination and organ colonization. Some possible mechanisms by which oncogenes may influence discrete portions of the metastatic processes are schematically represented in Figure 1. Although direct causal links between the phenotypic modifications observed and metastasis remain to be established, they nevertheless provide a starting point from which to define the targets for future therapy at the molecular level.

Although most of the work involving dissection of the sequelae of oncogene activation or transfection has been performed with fibroblasts, of greater interest, complexity and clinical relevance are studies utilizing epithelial cells, from which most solid tumours arise. In these cells additional features such as cell lineage, differentiation status, and production of and response to endocrine growth factors may be involved in their progression towards autonomy and metastasis. Intriguing parallels and interactions are emerging between the action of steroid hormones and oncogene activity in breast carcinoma; for example, both exposure to oestrogen and transfection with Ha-*ras* induced increased expression of c-*myc*, laminin receptors, collagenase type IV production, invasive capacity and metastasis and growth factor secretion. It appears therefore that in defined examples the malignant phenotype is under hormonal control, but that this can be bypassed by Ha-*ras* transfection, and that an increase in growth factor secretion may contribute to escape from oestrogen dependence and increased malignancy via common pathways. Preliminary evidence suggests that higher levels of TGF-α may be present in those 1° human breast tumours expressing elevated $p21^{ras}$, but correlation with oestrogen receptor levels are generally poor. A further possibility is that tumour progression, or stimulation of proliferation at secondary sites, may be facilitated by paracrine stimulation of endothelial or stromal elements by growth factors produced by tumour cells.

CODA

Circumstantial evidence has implicated the activity of certain known, and perhaps as yet unidentified 'oncogenes' in tumour progression and metastasis. The data are compelling, but as yet not definitive. It is certain, however, that future developments in molecular biology will clarify the role of such genes in both normal cellular growth and development, and in neoplasia. Only with such knowledge will opportunities arise for new therapeutic strategies based on more refined discrimination than those obtained with current cytotoxic modalities.

FURTHER READING

Albini, A. *et al.* (1986) *Proc. Natl. Acad. Sci. USA*, **83**, 8182.
Alon, Y. *et al.* (1987) *Cancer Res.*, **47**, 2553.
Collard, J. G. *et al.* (1987) *Cancer Res.*, **47**, 6666.
Dickson, R. B. *et al.* (1987) *Proc. Natl. Acad. Sci. USA*, **84**, 837.
Egan, S. E. *et al.* (1987) *Molec. Cell Biol.*, **7**, 830.
Elvin, P. *et al.* (1988) *Br. J. Cancer*, **57**, 36.
Greenberg, A. H. *et al.* (1987) *Cancer Res.*, **47**, 4801.
Greig, R. G., *et al.* (1986) *Proc. Natl Acad. Sci.*, **82**, 3698.
Kahn, P. and Graf, T. (eds) (1986) *Oncogenes and Growth Control.* Springer-Verlag.
Kendal, W. S. and Frost, P. (1986) *Pathol. Immunopathol. Res.*, **5**, 455.
Mareel, M., *et al.* (1986) *Anticancer Res.*, **6**, 419.
Muschel, R. J. *et al.* (1985) *Am. J. Pathol.*, **121**, 1.
Nicolson, G. L. (1987) *Cancer Res.*, **47**, 1473.
Perroteau, I. *et al.* (1986) *Breast Cancer Res. Treat.*, **7**, 201.
Price, J. *et al.* (1986) *Eur. J. Cancer Clin. Oncol.*, **22**, 349.
Salomon, D. S. (1986) *Cancer Invest.*, **4**, 43.
Shafie, S. M. (1980) *Cancer Letters*, **11**, 81.
Sluyser, M. (ed.) (1987) *Growth Factors in Breast Cancer.* Ellis Horwood.
Stacey, D. W. *et al.* (1987) *Exp. Cell. Res.*, **171**, 232.
Van Roy, F. M., *et al.* (1986) *Cancer Res.*, **46**, 4787.
Vousden, K., *et al.* (1986) *Int. J. Cancer*, **37**, 425.

PART

B

Gene Control

9 Inherited Cancer Syndromes

B. A. J. PONDER

Inherited predisposition may be a significant factor in the aetiology not just of rare inherited cancer syndromes, but of the common cancers as well. Identification of the genes involved and of their mechanisms of action has potentially important implications for cancer control. The genes may have biological interest as representatives of new classes of genes involved in normal growth and differentiation.

THE RECOGNITION OF INHERITED PREDISPOSITION

The recognition of inherited predisposition is the starting point of any search for the predisposing genes and for the clinical management of families, but it can be a surprisingly difficult problem. Predisposition is most easily recognised in the so-called 'inherited cancer syndromes' (Table 1). In these syndromes, which account for perhaps 1–2% of cancer incidence, predisposition is often strong enough to result in striking family pedigrees (Figure 1). Often, however, it is not the pedigree which identifies a particular cancer as a heritable type, but the association with one of a variety of characteristic phenotypic abnormalities. Thus, for example, if a colonic cancer is associated with multiple intestinal polyps, irrespective of the family history this is a strong indication of a genetic predisposition. Similarly, a melanoma occurring in the context of multiple atypical naevi should alert one to the 'dysplastic naevus syndrome', in which an autosomal dominant gene confers a lifetime risk of melanoma which may exceed 50% in carriers.

Many of the common cancers—e.g. breast cancer and ovarian cancer—tend to occur in families; but extensive pedigrees which would argue strongly for a hereditary cause are rare. Furthermore, there is usually no distinguishing phenotype. With

Genes and Cancer. Edited by D. Carney and K. Sikora
©1990 John Wiley & Sons Ltd

Table 1. Examples of inherited cancer syndromes

Syndrome	Principal cancers	Associated features	Chromosomal locus
Familial adenomatous polyps (FAP) and Gardner's syndrome variant	Colonic, rectal	Diffuse proliferative abnormality of gut epithelium, multiple g-i polyps Congenital hypertrophy of retinal pigment epithelium, osteomas of jaw, fibroblastic 'desmoid' tumours, occasional tumours at other sites	5q
Multiple endocrine neoplasia (MEN) type 2	Thyroid 'C' cells. Adrenal medulla (usually benign)	Hyperplasia of 'C' cells and adrenal medulla, parathyroid hyperplasia; disorganised autonomic ganglion plexuses, neuromas of somatic nerves, skeletal abnormalities (MEN 2b variant)	10
von Hippel-Lindau syndrome	Kidney. Adrenal medulla (usually benign)	Angiomatous malformations and proliferation in retina, central nervous sytem; cysts of internal organs	3p
Dysplastic naevus syndrome	Melanoma	Clinically and histologically atypical naevi	?1p

these cancers, therefore, it is much more difficult to decide whether the cluster is due to chance, environment or genes. Averaged across the whole population, familial clustering of the common cancers does not seem to be very strong: in general, siblings of a cancer patient have a two-to-three-fold increased risk of the same cancer. Within this average figure, however, are concealed some families in which predisposition is probably as strong as in any inherited cancer syndrome (see below). The practical guidelines which should be used in deciding whether a cancer is likely to be of a heritable type include: family history of the same or related cancers—examples of 'related' cancers would be breast, ovarian, uterine and colorectal, which occur in the cancer family syndrome, or known syndrome associations, such as anterior pituitary and pancreatic islet cell tumours in multiple endocrine neoplasia (MEN) type 1, or renal carcinoma and phaeochromocytoma in von Hippel-Lindau syndrome; concurrence in the family of rare cancers; young age at diagnosis; multiple or bilateral primaries in one individual; and phenotypic associations (for example, neurofibromatosis associated with glioma, the characteristic facies of MEN type 2b). A careful and extensive family history and physical examination will recognise many cases of inherited predisposition that are currently missed: but often, for example, in the case of two siblings who develop breast cancer in their forties, it will only be possible to say that there is a certain probability that a given family cluster *may* reflect inherited predisposition.

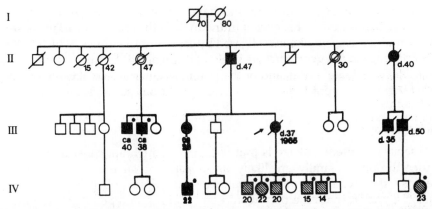

Figure 1. An inherited cancer syndrome: FAP. The pattern of inheritance is consistent with a single autosomal dominant gene and susceptibility in this family is restricted to colorectal cancer. The diagnosis of FAP in this family was not recognised until 1965, when III-10 (arrowed) presented with colonic cancer metastatic to liver and was found to have multiple colonic polyps (the phenotypic marker indicating that this was not 'ordinary' colonic cancer). The family were subsequently screened by endoscopic examination of the colon, and the individuals marked * were found to have polyps (or carcinoma: III 5,6) and underwent prophylactic colectomy at the ages shown. Key:■ ● =confirmed colonic cancer; d 50=died of cancer; ▨ ◍ =multiple polyps;□ ○ =probable colonic cancer (by history)

Although inherited predisposition can be recognised clinically by the features listed above, it is important to appreciate that, from a population or public health standpoint, the most significant contribution of inherited risk to total cancer incidence may occur without causing obvious familial clustering at all. The argument is well set out by Peto (1980) (see Further Reading). To take one example, consider a dominant gene with frequency 0.1, which confers a 100-fold increased risk of a specific cancer from 1 in 1000 to 1 in 10. The Hardy–Weinberg law predicts that such a gene would result in 95% of the cancer incidence being concentrated in the 19% of the population who carry the gene; but the relative risk of the cancer in siblings of cancer patients, compared to the whole population, would only be 2.87. By similar calculations, it can be shown that, for example, a common recessive gene which conferred a 50-fold increase in susceptibility could result in 97% of the incidence of a particular cancer being confined to 25% of the population. The implications for cancer control by screening are clearly enormous. If, as seems plausible in at least some cases, susceptibility is the result of altered metabolic interactions with environmental carcinogens, identification of the genetic mechanism of susceptibility might lead to identification of the carcinogen, and thence to rational strategies for prevention.

THE SEARCH FOR THE PREDISPOSING GENES

When a cancer is inherited through a family the predisposing gene can be sought by the classical methods of genetic linkage analysis. This has the important advantage that it requires no prior knowledge of the gene at all. The methods of genetic linkage and the implications of the results are explained briefly below. When there is no evident family clustering, on the other hand, these methods cannot be applied. Genetic predisposition at the level of individuals within the population, postulated above, can therefore only be investigated by case-control studies, which must start with knowledge of the genes that are likely to be involved. Because so little is known of possible 'candidate' genes and of the potential environmental carcinogens with which they could interact, progress in this group has so far been slow.

Genetic linkage

The essence of genetic linkage is that two genes which are consistently inherited together through a family are likely to be adjacent on the same chromosome. Otherwise, they would become separated by crossing-over between chromosomes at meiosis, and in that case they would be inherited independently (Figure 2). If one of the genes is responsible for predisposition to cancer, its chromosomal location can be found by systematic screening of a panel of other 'marker' genes whose location is already known, until one is found to have a pattern of inheritance through the cancer family which precisely corresponds to that of the cancer. The marker gene must of course exist in at least two distinguishable allelic forms (just as the cancer gene has a wild-type and mutant allele), so that the co-inheritance of one allele with the cancer gene can be tested. These allelic markers are now generally provided by restriction fragment length polymorphisms (RFLPs) in DNA. For a detailed account of the method, see White (1985).

The very rapid development of the human gene map in the past five years has increased enormously the number of genetic markers which can be tested. As a result, between 1986 and 1988 the genes for no fewer than six of the inherited cancer syndromes have been mapped (polyposis coli, neurofibromatosis types 1 and 2, von Hippel-Lindau syndrome and multiple endocrine neoplasia types 1 and 2).

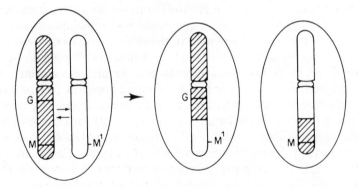

Figure 2. Crossing-over and genetic linkage. At the left is a diploid germ cell about to undergo meiosis with the production of haploid gametes. One chromosome in the diploid cell is paternal in origin, the other maternal. The gametes will each contain one copy of the chromosome, which as a result of crossing-over between paternal and maternal homologues in meiosis will contain segments derived from each chromosome of the parental chromosome pair. Two genes (e.g. the disease gene G and the 'marker' gene M) which lie close together on the chromosome will tend to be inherited together: if they lie far apart they will tend to be separated by crossing-over and to be inherited separately. The extent to which the marker is co-inherited through a family with the disease gene is a measure of how far apart they are on the chromosome

In principle, familial clusters of the commoner cancers, such as breast or ovarian cancer, can be analysed in the same way. There are, however, several problems. Linkage analysis relies on establishing a correlation between the inheritance of alleles at two genetic loci. In the case of the locus for the cancer gene, 'affected' status is taken to indicate the presence of the cancer-causing allele, and 'unaffected' the wild-type. In the inherited cancer syndromes, for the most part, the presence of the cancer gene can be reliably inferred from the characteristic phenotype of the syndrome— polyps in familial polyposis, retinal angiomas in von Hippel-Lindau syndrome— and family members who lack the phenotype by a certain age can reliably be scored as having the wild-type allele. The linkage analysis can thus use most of the members of the family with only a small risk of misclassification—which would destroy the correlation that is being sought. In familial breast cancer, by contrast, there is no marker phenotype, and examination of pedigrees suggests that many individuals who must have carried the presumed gene, including of course many males, developed cancer only at a late age or not at all. 'Unaffected' status is thus not a reliable indication that the individual does not carry the gene. Conversely, because breast cancer is common, not all 'affected' individuals will necessarily be gene carriers. This threatens to weaken considerably the correlation upon which linkage analysis depends. To achieve significant results, it becomes necessary to combine data from several different families, and this brings a second problem, that of genetic heterogeneity. It is reasonable to think that familial polyposis is caused by only one or a very few genes, but there could easily be several genes that predispose to breast cancer, and different genes might be involved in different families.

These difficulties would be somewhat eased if there were a clue to the location of the predisposing gene or genes. The statistical power of linkage is much greater if the marker and disease genes are close together, so a clue might allow a significant result to be obtained with smaller family material. (Also, of course, it would cut down the labour of searching through all 22 chromosomes.) In some of the inherited cancer syndromes listed above—e.g. retinoblastoma and polyposis—such a clue was in fact available in the form of a constitutional chromosomal deletion, visible in the lymphocytes of rare individuals with the syndrome. In each case, these individuals had additional abnormalities such as mental retardation, presumably reflecting the loss of several genes in the deleted chromosomal segment. A search for similar abnormalities in young individuals with the common cancers, especially those with a family history or with other features associated with chromosomal abnormality such as mental retardation or multiple miscarriages, would probably be worthwhile.

Another clue to the chromosomal location of predisposing genes may come from the patterns of so-called 'allele losses' in tumours (Figure 3). In many of the inherited cancer syndromes, the genetic mechanism of tumour development involves loss of both alleles at the locus of the predisposing gene. The first loss is inherited in the germline. The second occurs in the somatic cell, which as a result develops into the tumour. The second, somatic, event often involves loss of a large segment of chromosome. Compared to the first mutation, this larger second event is relatively easily detected by an analysis in which DNA extracted from tumour is compared with DNA from a normal tissue such as blood. A positive result is indicated by a consistent loss, in DNA from tumour samples, of one allele of a polymorphic DNA marker which maps to a particular chromosomal region. Such losses may indicate

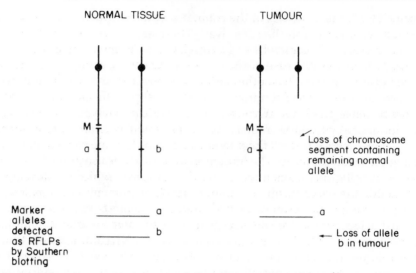

Figure 3. Allele loss in tumours. A pair of chromosomes is shown in normal tissue and in tumour from the same individual. In this example, the individual has inherited a gene loss mutation (M) on one chromosome which predisposes to cancer: loss of the remaining normal allele by mutation in a somatic cell leads to formation of the tumour. a, b are alleles at an arbitrary marker locus some distance from the inherited mutation, revealed by restriction fragment length polymorphisms (RFLPs). The somatic mutational event which leads to loss of the normal allele for the inherited gene will sometimes involve quite extensive loss of chromosomal material, leading to loss of the marker allele b

that a corresponding germline mutation, and hence a genetic locus for inherited susceptibility to the tumour, lies in the same region. 'Allele loss' studies of most of the common tumours are now in progress. It is important to realise, however, that not all allele losses found in tumours will correspond to the loci of germline mutations; for further discussion see Ponder (1988).

IMPLICATIONS FOR THE BIOLOGY OF NORMAL AND TUMOUR TISSUES

Several features of the inherited cancer syndromes suggest that the genes which are involved have important functions in the control of normal growth and development. Thus:

1. The development of the cancer is often preceded by multiple areas of abnormality in the target tissue: for example, the multiple polyps or the dysplastic naevi which were described above. Some of these abnormalities are focal, which might suggest the need for a second clonal (or at least local) event to be superimposed on the germline mutation which is present in every cell. However, others are more general to the tissue and may reflect the direct phenotypic expression of the inherited mutation. In familial polyposis, for example, there is a generalised proliferative disturbance of the intestinal epithelium which precedes polyp formation. The normal role of the polyposis gene is therefore presumably concerned with regulation of

the balance between proliferation and differentiation in the epithelium of the intestinal crypt.

2. There may be abnormalities of growth and development in tissues other than those in which the cancer develops: for example, hypertrophy of the retinal pigment epithelium in affected individuals in most families with polyposis, and jaw cysts and extra dentition in some individuals with the Gardner's syndrome variant of familial polyposis. While in some cases these may reflect the involvement of additional nearby genes in the same chromosomal deletion or rearrangement which has given rise to the cancer syndrome, probably more often they are the result of pleiotropic effects of the mutation in the same 'cancer gene', suggesting the wide-ranging involvement of many of these genes in normal development.

3. Finally, the mechanism of tumour development in retinoblastoma (and probably some others of the inherited cancer syndromes) requires loss of both alleles at the locus of the predisposing gene, as noted above (Figure 3). This implies that the mutations which lead to the cancer are recessive at the level of the cell. It is envisaged that the normal (not mutated) gene has a regulatory or 'tumour suppressor' function, perhaps by interacting with and controlling some other gene or gene product which, unopposed, would drive the cell towards malignancy. With the cloning of the retinoblastoma gene and identification of the *Rb* gene product, these interactions are beginning to be elucidated (see Chapter 8). Study of the inherited cancer syndromes has led in this way to the uncovering of a new class of cellular regulatory genes.

CLINICAL IMPLICATIONS

Families with inherited susceptibility to cancer are a population at high risk, who may benefit from screening, provided always that early diagnosis is possible and will lead to better treatment. This is probably the case in several of the inherited cancer syndromes such as familial polyposis, multiple endocrine neoplasia type 2 (MEN 2), dysplastic naevus syndrome, and in von Hippel-Lindau syndrome where death from renal carcinoma in middle age is common. In all of these syndromes, the family members at risk can be identified by the phenotypes associated with the cancer gene. Often, however, the screening procedures—for example, colonoscopy for familial polyposis or stimulated calcitonin measurement for MEN 2—are unpleasant, worrying for the families and expensive in resources. As a result, family screening is generally far from complete. Even before the genes themselves are identified, linked genetic markers can be used to predict which members of a family are at risk, and which can be excluded from risk. The accuracy of the prediction is determined by the closeness of the DNA markers to the cancer gene: for example, if there is on average one genetic crossing-over between them in 50 matings this will under the best conditions give an error of 2%. It is likely that such predictions will improve the management of families by concentrating screening on those who need it most. The clinical use that is made of a particular prediction will however remain a matter of judgement, taking into account the likely accuracy and the circumstances. It is, for example, arguable to what level the risk of carrying the gene for familial polyposis should be excluded before colonoscopic screening is deemed no longer to be necessary.

In the long term, identification of the predisposing genes and consequent understanding of the mechanisms of predisposition may turn out to be more important than diagnosis using genetic markers. Current indications are that the sequence of genetic events which leads from a normal cell to a cancer cell in a given tissue is the same, whether the cancer is familial or not. The successive steps in carcinogenesis may be analogous to hurdles in a race in which individuals who are genetically predisposed have a head start because one of the hurdles has already been jumped in the germline. In that case, understanding the mechanisms of genetic predisposition in familial cancers may tell us about the processes of carcinogenesis not just in these cancers, but in many non-familial cancers as well.

FURTHER READING

Hansen, M. F. and Cavenee, W. K. (1988) *Trends in Genetics*, **4**, 125–128.

Harnden, D., Morten, J. and Featherstone, T. (1984) *Adv. Cancer Res.*, **41**, 185–255.

Mulvihill, J. J., Miller, R. W. and Fraumeni, J. F. (eds.) (1977) *Genetics of Human Cancer. Progress in Cancer Research and Therapy*, Vol 3. Raven Press, New York.

Omenn, G. S. and Gelboin, H. V. (eds.) (1984) Genetic variability in responses to chemical exposure. *Banbury Report*, **16**. Cold Spring Harbor, New York.

Peto, J. (1980) Genetic predisposition to cancer. In: Cairns, J., Lyon, J. L. and Skolnick, M. (eds.), *Cancer Incidence in Defined Populations. Banbury Report*, **4**, pp. 203–213. Cold Spring Harbor, New York.

Ponder, B. A. J. (1988) *Nature*, **335**, 400–402.

Schwartz, A. G., *et al.* (1985) *JNCI*, **75**, 665–668.

Vogelstein, B., *et al.* (1989) *Science*, **244**, 207–211.

White, R.L. (1985) *Trends in Genetics*, **1**, 177–180.

Wolf, C. R. (1986) *Trends in Genetics*, **2**, 209–214.

10 An Introduction to Transcription

MATTHEW ELLIS

The synthesis of mRNA is a critical control point in gene regulation during development and in response to hormones, growth factors and other cellular signals. Advances in our understanding of how genes are switched on and off by transcriptional mechanisms has depended on techniques to identify regulatory information within the nucleotide sequence of responding genes and to investigate the structure and function of proteins that translate sequence information into differential patterns of transcription. This chapter is intended as an introduction to experimental techniques; the next chapter will focus on the disturbances in transcriptional regulation that occur in malignant cells and demonstrate that transformation may result from the mutation of genes involved in the transcriptional response to hormones and growth factors.

ENHANCERS AND PROMOTERS

Early studies on gene regulation defined two types of sequence involved in regulating transcription, *promoters* and *enhancers*. Current evidence indicates that rather than being functionally single entities, these sequences consist of elements, 7 to 20 nucleotides long that form binding sites for sequence-specific DNA-binding proteins (transcription factors). The term 'promoter' refers to a group of such elements clustered around the transcriptional start site. At least one of these elements operates to fix the site of initiation. A highly conserved sequence centred around −28, the TATA box, serves this function in many genes, although in genes lacking a TATA box, sequences around the start site itself help to place the first nucleotide of the message (designated nucleotide +1; negative numbers indicate 5′ untranscribed

Genes and Cancer. Edited by D. Carney and K. Sikora
©1990 John Wiley & Sons Ltd

nucleotides). Upstream, in the region spanning -30 to -110 are multiple binding sites for proteins that function to regulate the rate of mRNA initiation and elongation.

Enhancers appear quite different to promoters through their ability to stimulate transcription at a distance (hundreds to thousands of base pairs away from the initiation site) and their insensitivity to experimental changes in orientation and position. Even when located within introns, or downstream of the transcription unit, they can activate mRNA synthesis, although always depending on the presence of position-fixing promoter elements. In these terms, enhancers and promoters are operationally quite different. However, three types of observation argue against the idea that the two classes of sequence function through separate families of transcription factors. First are examples of binding sites for a number of transcription factors appearing in both promoters and enhancers. Second is the fact that sequences with enhancer-like properties can be generated by multimerisation of promoter elements. Third, some elements, although situated close to the start site in the natural situation, are capable of operating as enhancers if artificially separated. Interactions over long distances probably occur by looping out of the intervening DNA so that protein molecules widely separated on the DNA are brought into contact. Through this mechanism, transcription factors could work both at a distance or in close proximity to the transcriptional start depending on the organisation of each gene (Figure 1).

Table 1 summarises information on a few representative transcription factors that mediate constitutive, inducible and tissue-specific gene expression and their cognate binding sites. Many of the earliest examples of promoter elements came from the investigation of the SV40 DNA tumour virus early promoter/enhancer that drives the transcription of genes required early in the virus life cycle. This it achieves by containing binding sites for a number of cellular transcription factors. One of these, the sequence TGAGTCA binds the phorbol ester-inducible transcription factor

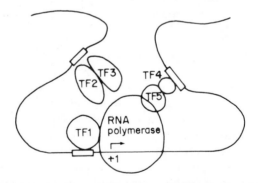

Figure 1. Transcription factors (TFs) are a class of regulatory molecules that target RNA polymerase molecules to active genes. In the model depicted here a number of potential mechanisms are illustrated whereby DNA, transcription factors and RNA polymerase are brought together to form an active transcription complex. TF1 binds close to the transcriptional start and interacts with RNA polymerase directly. TF2 and 3 bind DNA as a heterodimer to a sequence distant from the start. The intervening DNA loops out to accommodate the interaction. TF4 interacts with polymerase via a second protein TF5 that itself does not itself bind DNA

Table 1. Typical transcription factors and their binding sites

Transcription factor	Consensus binding site	Features
Sp1	GGGCGG	Identified through investigation of the SV40 early promoter, Sp1 is involved in constitutive expression from many promoters. Three zinc fingers in DNA binding domain
Glucocorticoid receptor	GGTACAN₃TGTTCT	A member of a super-family that includes steroid, thyroid hormone and retinoic acid receptors. Ligand binding leads to nuclear translocation and transcriptional activation
Serum response factor	GATGTCCATATTAGGACATC	Mediates transcriptional activation by serum, epidermal growth factor, TPA and insulin. Similar, if not identical, protein involved in muscle-specific transcription. No sequence homology with other TFs.
CREB and ATF	TGACGTCA	Binding site confers cAMP response and sensitivity to the viral transactivator, E1A. Several genes encoding CRE-binding proteins recently cloned, that have leucine zippers and DNA binding domains with homology to c-*jun*
c-JUN	TGAGTCA	One of a number of TFs that bind AP1 sites, to confer TPA inducibility. Forms heterodimer with c-Fos via leucine zipper domain
OCT-1	ATTTGCAT	Ubiquitous distribution; same binding specificity as OCT-2 but mediates constitutive activity in many cell types
OCT-2	ATTTGCAT	Expressed mainly in T- and B-lymphocytes; activates immunoglobin genes with octomer binding sites

AP1 that subsequently was found to be encoded by the oncogene v-*jun*. A second sequence within this enhancer, the 'octamer' ATTTGCAT, exemplifies the complexity of transcription factor DNA interactions, as this sequence binds a family of transcription factors, two of which are now cloned: one appears to be ubiquitous and involved in transcription from a number of genes; one is B-cell-specific, involved in immunoglobulin gene transcription. Others appear to be active in early embryogenesis. Increasingly it is recognised that multiple factors can interact with the same consensus sequence, and indeed competition between factors for binding to the same sequence may be an important feature of transcriptional regulation. In addition to positive regulatory elements, the promoters of tightly regulated genes (such as those involved in inflammation, growth control and endocrine homeostasis) show evidence of negative regulation, demonstrated by promoter mutants that show increased transcriptional activity relative to the wild-type gene. These mutants are thought to affect the binding of factors that repress transcription. Clearly, just as in prokaryotic gene expression, negative- as well as positive-acting proteins play important roles in regulation.

PROMOTER MUTATION

Consideration of the way sequences that regulate transcription are analysed is important, as the information provided by these techniques is fundamental to our understanding of how promoters and enhancers function. *In vitro* mutagenesis techniques are used to generate multiple promoter mutants. Comparison of the transcriptional activity of these mutants with each other and with the wild-type gene allows the position and sequence composition of each regulatory element to be mapped (Figure 2). This comparison depends on DNA-mediated gene transfer, and a variety of techniques that allow the quantification of the message in question amongst the millions present in cellular extracts.

Details of how recombinant DNA technology allows purification, cutting, joining and mutation of specific sequences is inappropriate here and many reviews are available on the subject (see Further Reading). Deletions through the promoter sequence, either from the 5' or 3' end, are usually the initial approach, followed by internal deletions and point mutations to further clarify where exactly the key regulatory nucleotides lie. Automated oligonucleotide synthesis now allows the construction of any desired sequence, and this has greatly aided the production of informative mutants.

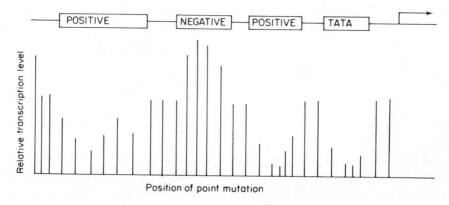

Figure 2. The effect of point mutations in the promoter sequence on the expression of a hypothetical gene containing both positive and negative regulatory elements. Negative elements are most often detected in inducible genes, where point mutations produce increases in basal expression in the absence of the inducing signal

DNA-MEDIATED GENE TRANSFER

There are a variety of ways in which cells can be made to take up and express exogenous DNA, a process termed *transfection*. The commonest technique is to co-precipitate plasmid DNA containing the test gene with calcium phosphate. In this form cells take up DNA, and expression can be detected within 48 hours. Detectable transcription from the exogenous gene is slowly extinguished during subsequent growth of the recipient cell line in culture. For this reason analysis of mutant promoters using this technique is said to be based on *transient gene expression*. A number of alternatives have been developed, as calcium phosphate precipitates are taken up inefficiently and cell to cell expression is heterogeneous because some cells take up and express DNA more efficiently than others. Finer precipitates with high molecular weight substances, such as DEAE dextran and polybrene, are taken up more readily and evenly. *Electroporation* achieves high-efficiency DNA uptake through permeabilising the cells to high molecular weight molecules by subjecting them to an intense electric field. *Protoplast fusion* involves removing the cell walls of bacteria containing the plasmid, then fusing them to cells, using polyethylene glycol.

Analysis of gene expression by transient expression has the advantage that data can be assimilated rapidly. However, since cells receive multiple copies of the test gene that are not organised into a normal chromatin structure, questions are often raised as to how accurately these experiments reflect normal regulatory events. These objections can in part be addressed by the observation that a tiny proportion of the DNA introduced by calcium phosphate transfection integrates randomly into the host cells' chromosomes, where the activity of test genes can still be detected (*stable gene expression*). Recombination between the transfected gene and the recipient cells' chromosomes can be selected for by linking the test gene to a second gene that codes for resistance to a cell poison, G418 for example—an antibiotic related to the aminoglycosides, toxic to eukaryotic cells, resistance to which is coded by the bacterial *neo* gene. Unfortunately, expression of the integrated test gene is affected by transcriptional activity in the surrounding host chromatin and this leads to marked differences in gene expression between individual clones. This can hamper data interpretation and requires analysis of large pools of transformants, to 'average out' the effect of different integration sites.

A third technique, which overcomes this problem, involves linking the test gene to a vector that replicates independently outside the host cell chromosomes to provide a stable platform to analyse transcription. These vectors were developed from the observation that infection with number of DNA viruses can result in persistence of the viral DNA in host cells as *episomes* (i.e. circles of double-stranded DNA, replicating extrachromosomally). Examples of viruses that behave in this way include bovine papillomavirus and Epstein–Barr virus. Various vectors have been made by fusing genes from these viruses responsible for the maintenance of DNA episomally, to bacterial sequences that enable the vector to behave as a plasmid in bacteria so that test genes can be introduced using standard techniques. Genes cloned into these episomes or 'artificial chromosomes' are stably maintained within the host nucleus at a known copy number in a defined genetic background and outside the influence of host cell sequences. The principal disadvantage of this technique is the limited host range of the episomal vectors described so far.

ANALYSIS OF PROMOTER ACTIVITY

The activity of a promoter can be measured in a variety of ways, the choice depending on the type and accuracy of the data required since each assay has its limitations (Figure 3).

Nuclease protection analysis is a technique frequently used to directly quantify the amount of a particular mRNA in a cellular pool. Radioactive anti-sense probes, either

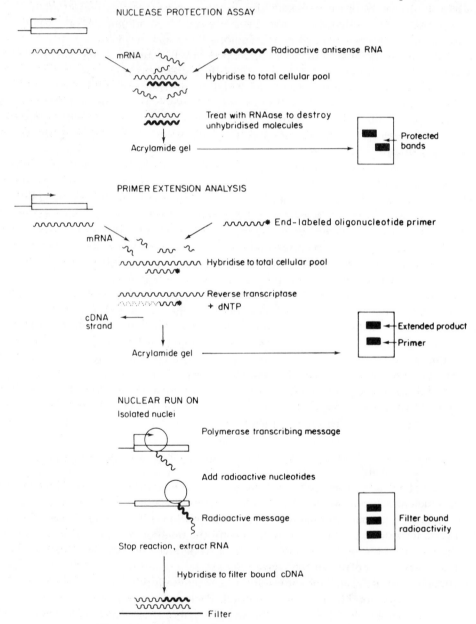

Figure 3. Assays used to measure promoter activity

DNA or RNA, are hybridised to total cellular RNA containing the mRNA in question (sense RNA). The sample is then subjected to nuclease digestion (S1 nuclease for RNA/DNA hybrids and RNAase T1 and A for RNA/RNA hybrids). This destroys all single-stranded molecules, including unhybridised probe. Hybridised probe is protected from digestion since it is present as a double-stranded molecule. It is then visualised by denaturing acrylamide gel electrophoresis and autoradiography.

An alternative is *primer extension analysis*. A primer complementary to the sequence of interest is synthesised, radiolabelled and hybridised to RNA. Treatment with reverse transcriptase generates a cDNA strand that forms in the 3' to 5' direction terminating at the beginning of the message. The resulting end-labelled product is then run on an acrylamide gel as before.

Both these techniques have the limitation that they measure the accumulation of stable specific RNA after transfection, a result of both the rates of synthesis, processing and degradation of the message, rather than just the specific rate of transcript initiation. If it is suspected that there are differences in mRNA stability or processing between mutants, the rate of RNA synthesis can be directly measured by the *nuclear run-on assay*. Nuclei are purified and incubated with labelled precursor nucleotides. RNA polymerases engaged in transcription will add radioactive nucleotides to any nascent RNA chain. The amount of radioactive RNA, specific to the gene of interest, is quantified by hybridisation to complementary DNA immobilised on a filter. The amount of bound radioactivity gives an estimate of the number of polymerase molecules engaged in transcribing the transfected promoter.

Direct analysis of RNA is time consuming, particularly when large numbers of promoter mutants are involved. An alternative is to isolate the promoter and fuse it to a gene that codes for an enzyme that has an easily assayable activity in cytoplasmic extracts (a *reporter* gene). The principal advantage of this system is rapid analysis of multiple promoter mutants based on the assumption that the amount of the translated enzyme is directly proportional to the level of transcription (an assumption that limits the value of this technique). The most common example of a reporter gene is that coding for chloramphenicol acetyl transferase (CAT), the activity of which is measured by acetylation of [^{14}C]chloramphenicol, followed by thin-layer chromatography and autoradiography. A recent alternative, firefly luciferase, is sensitive and easy to assay and may take the place of CAT in some circumstances: cytoplasmic extract, firefly luciferin and ATP are mixed in a luminometer and the amount of enzyme present is proportional to the peak light emission. If information is required on the activity of a promoter in a particular cell type or tissue, for example in studies of development, the promoter can be fused to the *E. coli* gene *lacZ*, that codes for the enzyme β-galactosidase. Cells that have an active promoter, and are therefore expressing this enzyme, stain blue in the presence of a chromogenic substrate, X-gal.

ANALYSIS OF PROTEIN–DNA INTERACTIONS

Promoter mutation and transfection studies have led to the definition of a large number of regulatory sequences that direct transcription. The question now being addressed by many laboratories is how exactly does the cell translate information contained in the sequence of enhancers and promoters into changes in the rate of transcription in response to cellular signals? These investigations depend on the identification of proteins that interact with DNA in a sequence-specific manner and of proteins that influence the formation of an active transcription complex indirectly by protein–protein interactions. Methods of analysing protein-DNA complexes to detect sequence-specific, high-affinity, DNA-binding proteins in crude nuclear extracts have been crucial to progress and are generally based on one of two approaches, bandshift analysis or DNA footprinting (Figure 4).

Bandshift analysis

The *bandshift* or *gel retardation assay* involves the incubation of nuclear proteins with radiolabelled promoter (either as synthetic oligonucleotides, or restriction enzyme fragments). Under these conditions DNA-protein complexes form in solution. The binding reaction is then analysed by native polyacrylamide gel electrophoresis. DNA-protein complexes migrate through the gel more slowly than protein-free DNA and appear as retarded or shifted bands. The specificity of the protein–DNA interaction can be increased by adding non-specific competitor DNA to the binding reaction. Furthermore, mutant promoter elements can be used as cold (non-radioactive) competitor, or as radioactive probe to further characterise the precise contribution of particular nucleotides to protein binding. One of the principal advantages of this technique is that it allows analysis of stable multicomponent complexes.

Footprinting assay

The footprinting assay provides information on the localisation of protein-DNA contacts within a promoter. This assay is based on the ability of a DNA-bound protein to modulate, at or near the protein-binding site, chemical modifications produced by the footprinting agent. *DNAase I footprinting* employs a nuclease that can digest double-stranded DNA into its constituent nucleotides. By limiting the digestion, conditions can be defined to cut promoter DNA fragments (radiolabelled at one end) on average once within each molecule at random positions. Gel electrophoresis results in a ladder of bands, each 'rung' or band representing a nucleotide position within the promoter. To localise the position of protein binding, the end-radiolabelled promoter is incubated with nuclear extract before digestion with DNAase I. Nucleotides 'buried' within a DNA-protein complex are protected from nuclease cleavage and after electrophoresis can be identified as bands missing from the ladder. Often, nucleotides at the edge of protein-binding sites show enhanced sensitivity to nuclease and show up as accentuated bands, referred to as *hypersensitive sites*. By radiolabelling either strand, contacts on either side of the helix can be identified. One of the problems of this type of analysis is that unlike bandshifts, it gives no information on the components of the protein complexes binding DNA. In addition, since the DNA–protein interaction is analysed in solution rather than in a gel, where there is a strict requirement for stable interaction, the footprints observed may not represent functionally relevent high-affinity interactions. However, a combination of the two techniques, by isolating proteins from a bandshift gel and then using

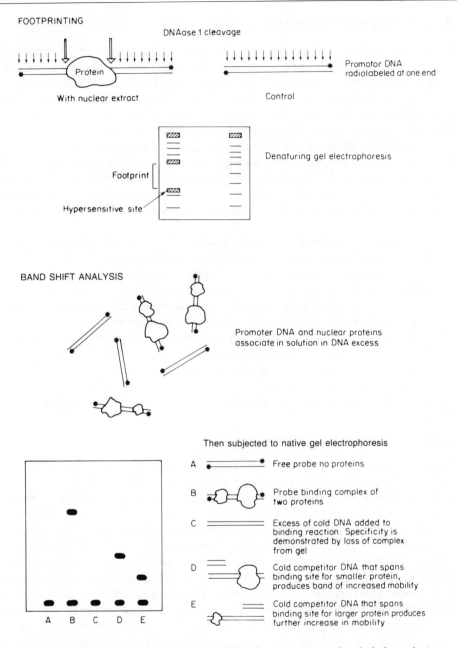

Figure 4. Schematic representations of DNA footprinting and gel shift analysis

this purified protein to produce footprints, can be very informative. A number of alternatives to DNAase I footprinting have been developed, using low-molecular weight reagents such as dimethyl sulphate (DMS). One of the advantages of DMS footprinting is that it is possible to map protein/DNA contacts in intact cells.

CLONING TRANSCRIPTION FACTORS

The DNA-binding assays have led to the detection and characterisation of numerous sequence-specific DNA-binding proteins. The isolation of recombinant clones encoding such proteins is essential for further genetic and biochemical analysis of their structure and functional properties. Only a brief description of the various cloning strategies that have been developed for cloning such rare regulatory molecules is possible here. The most fruitful approach has been the purification of these proteins on DNA affinity columns containing recognition site sequences, to obtain enough purified protein for limited amino acid sequence analysis. From this information, a series of oligonucleotide probes are synthesised to screen cDNA libraries for complementary sequences. Alternatively amino acid sequence data can be used to generate antibodies by peptide immunisation for expression library screening.

These approaches depend on the availability of substantial amounts of protein for amino acid sequencing. The requirement for large amounts of starting material, either tissue or cells, makes purification on this scale difficult. An alternative to protein purification is direct screening of expression cDNA libraries (usually phage lambda gt II) with a recognition site probe in an analogous fashion to screening with antibodies. Proteins are lifted from the phage plaques onto nitrocellulose filters and exposed to radioactive probes that contain sequences that bind the transcription factor in question. Radioactive hotspots indicate the presence of DNA-binding activity, and phages from positive plaques are rescreened several times, each time enriching for the clone responsible for probe binding. Finally, protein from positive plaques is analysed using band shifts to demonstrate sequence specific binding.

Investigating cloned transcription factors

Cloned transcription factors are subjected to an experimental strategy aimed at elucidating the structural requirements for sequence-specific DNA binding and protein interactions within the transcription complex. Initially, computer programs are used to scan the amino acid sequence for homologies with previously identified proteins and to make secondary structure predictions. In order to localise functional regions within the protein, mutants are constructed, deleting or altering the coding sequence. On translation these constructs generate proteins that are tested for DNA binding and transactivation using bandshift, footprinting and transfection assays as described. The existence of hypothetical DNA- and protein-binding structures predicted by these techniques can be further investigated using X-ray crystallography.

Results of such investigations on transcription factors cloned so far allow a number of generalisations to be made. First, transcription factors have a modular structure with usually quite separable DNA-binding and transactivation domains. Second, whilst a surprising variety of different structures have evolved to achieve sequence-specific DNA binding, these structures are highly conserved, perhaps most graphically illustrated by the observation that some mammalian transcription factors have secondary structures reminiscent of bacterial transcriptional regulators. Furthermore, conservation of basic transcriptional mechanisms between species can be demonstrated by fusion of a DNA-binding domain to a transactivation domain cloned from another, phylogenetically quite different organism. The resulting chimaeric proteins demonstrate that, for example, a yeast DNA-binding domain can recognise its cognate binding site in a mammalian cell and activate transcription if fused to an appropriate transactivation domain. The third generalisation is that transactivation domains have less rigid structural requirements than DNA-binding domains, with mutant studies demonstrating that, at least for some examples studied, all that is required for transactivation is excess of negative charge, presumably resulting in electrostatic interactions with neighbouring proteins.

Whilst the reader should consult the reading list for more detailed explanation, three still largely hypothetical structures implicated in sequence-specific DNA binding have recently been defined by these techniques. X-ray crystallographic analysis of several prokaryotic regulatory proteins such as lambda repressor and *Cro* has demonstrated a *helix-turn-helix* 'motif' (a peptide sequence shared between proteins) which appears to bind DNA by alignment of each of the two helices of the motif within and alongside the grooves of the DNA helix. The *homeobox* is a strongly conserved DNA-binding motif identified by comparing a family of transcription factors involved in development. Analysis of the amino acid sequence suggests that it could form a helix-turn-helix structure similar to that defined for prokaryotic proteins.

A second DNA-binding structure, the *zinc finger*, consists either of a pair of histidines and a pair of cysteines or two pairs of cysteines that act together to coordinate a zinc ion. The amino acids in between loop out to form the finger. Sequence specificity probably resides in the amino acid residues at the base rather than the tip of each finger. This structure has been found in a number of transcription factors, including steroid receptors and developmentally expressed genes, such as *kruppel* and *hunchback* (identified during studies of *Drosophila* development).

Finally, dimer formation between some DNA-binding proteins is necessary for transcriptional activation and has been shown to involve another conserved structure, the *leucine zipper*. This motif consists of a periodic array of leucine residues, at every seventh position, along an alpha helix. Similar motifs on different proteins then interdigitate, to facilitate dimerisation. The motif is of particular interest as it appears to underlie the interactions between two oncogenes, *fos* and *jun*, and is also present in all the *myc* family of proteins, where it appears to be necessary for *myc* tetramerisation and transformation.

CONCLUSION

The aim of this chapter has been to introduce and stimulate interest in a rapidly expanding and complex field. Investigations in the immediate future will concentrate on efforts to clone all the components of transcription complexes so that the molecular interactions underlying the transcriptional regulation of genes can be worked out in detail. In addition to the techniques mentioned, *in vitro* systems will play an important role, as will transgenic mouse experimentation, and site-directed mutation of the mouse genome in particular.

FURTHER READING

Darnell, J., Lodish, H. and Baltimore, D. (1986) *Molecular Cell Biology*. Scientific American Books, New York.

Dynan, W. S. (1989) Modularity in promoters and enhancers. *Cell*, **58**, 1–4.

Jones, N. C., Rigby, P. W. J. and Ziff, E. B. (1988) *Trans* acting protein factors and the regulation of eukaryotic transcription: Lessons from studies on DNA tumor viruses. *Genes and Development*, **2**, 267–281.

Maniatis, T., Fritsch, E. F. and Sambrook, J. (1989) *Molecular Cloning, A Laboratory Manual*. Cold Spring Harbor Laboratory.

Maniatis, T., Goodbourn, S. and Fischer, J. A. (1987) Regulation of inducible and tissue specific gene expression. *Science*, **236**, 1237–1245.

Mitchell, P. J. and Tjian, R. (1989) Transcriptional regulation in mammalian cells by sequence specific DNA binding proteins. *Science*, **245**, 371–375.

Old, R. W. and Primrose, S. B. (1985) *Principles of Gene Manipulation—an Introduction to Genetic Engineering* 3rd edn. Blackwell Scientific Publications, Oxford.

Ptashne, M. (1986) *A Genetic Switch*. Cell and Blackwell Scientific Press, Cambridge and Palo Alto.

Ptashne, M. (1988) How eukaryotic transcriptional activators work. *Nature*, **335**, 683–689.

11 Modulation of Transcription Factors by Oncogenes

YOSHIAKI ITO
KATSUYA SHIGESADA
MASANOBU SATAKE

Growth of cells in tissue is usually controlled by a variety of mechanisms, including growth stimulatory or inhibitory factors which exert their effects through binding to specific receptors on the cell surface. Recent studies of oncogenes have shown clearly how the abnormalities in the structure of growth factors or their receptors could result in the uncontrolled growth of cells.

The control mechanism of mammalian chromosomal DNA replication is unknown. When serum growth factors are added to serum-starved, quiescent rodent fibroblast cells, cellular DNA synthesis starts only after some 8–10 hours. During this long latency, a variety of events occur, which ultimately lead to the initiation of DNA replication. Among the very early events is transient induction of the synthesis of proto-oncogene c-*fos*. The c-*fos* gene is a cellular homologue of a transforming gene, v-*fos*, present in the genome of a transforming retrovirus, FBJ or FBR murine sarcoma virus. Therefore, the regulation of the expression of c-*fos* gene and the possible function of its product have been attracting much interest in recent years.

More recently, a 55 kDa c-*fos* protein was found to be associated with the product of another oncogene, c-*jun*, and to form a DNA-binding complex. Furthermore, this complex was found to be transcription activator protein, AP-1. It became evident, therefore, that transcriptional abnormalities caused by the Jun-Fos complex could lead to cell transformation.

One of the most characteristic properties of AP-1 is that its function is enhanced by a tumor-promoting phorbolester, 12-*O*-tetradecanoylphorbol-13-acetate (TPA). Since TPA is the activator of protein kinase C (PKC) and mimics the effect of some growth factors,

Genes and Cancer. Edited by D. Carney and K. Sikora
©1990 John Wiley & Sons Ltd

transcriptional regulatory proteins interacting directly with DNA have been considered as the end-receivers of the signals initiated by growth factors. Considering that many oncogene products are located in various parts of a complex network of signal transduction pathways, it is not surprising that some oncogene products modulate the function of transcription factors.

We have been studying modulation, mainly by the products of the Ha-*ras* oncogene, of transcription factors that bind to the polyomavirus (Py) enhancer. The Py enhancer contains the consensus sequence for AP-1 binding. Because only a few regulatory factors bind to the Py enhancer probe that we use, we have been examining the effect of the Ha-*ras* gene on transcription factors through a very narrow slit; however, we believe we have been observing an important part of the events, as we discuss later.

This chapter summarizes the recent findings about c-*fos* and c-*jun* and the findings we obtained with our system, and discusses the possible implication of our results in the carcinogenic process.

THE NATURE OF THE AP-1 TRANSCRIPTION FACTOR

Enhancers are segments of DNA required in *cis* configuration for the stimulation of transcription from the promoters transcribed by RNA polymerase II. They act from a distance in an orientation-independent fashion. Enhancers are composed of multiple sequence motifs to which various transcription factors bind. Some enhancer elements function to maintain a certain basal level of gene expression, while others respond specifically to outside stimuli to activate transcription. Tissue-specific gene expression is largely attributed to the inducible nature of enhancer elements of the latter type. Therefore, transcription factors interacting with inducible elements must be receivers of signals initiated by a particular tissue-specific growth factor.

AP-1 was originally identified as a transcription activation factor that binds selectively to promoter and enhancer sequences of the human metallothionein IIA gene and SV40. As noted above, similar enhancer elements have since been detected in various other genes, including human collagenase, c-*fos* and the polyomavirus enhancer. From comparison of these binding sites, the consensus sequence for AP-1 is deduced to be C/GTGACTC/AAG. Purified AP-1 contained a group of polypeptides ranging in size from 40 to 47 kDa, representing multiple protein complexes; their constituents are encoded by the oncogenes *jun*, *fos* and related genes. c-*jun*, a cellular homologue of the oncogene, v-*jun*, was isolated and was shown to code for a 39 kDa protein (340 aa) with sequence-specific DNA-binding properties identical to AP-1. Concurrently, two other c-*jun*-related genes were identified (*jun*B and *jun*D) whose encoded proteins also have the same sequence-specific DNA-binding activities as AP-1. The additional intriguing connection of AP-1 to another oncogene, *fos*, was discovered from the finding that Fos and the antigenically related protein, Fra-1, tended to form non-covalent complexes with several other cellular proteins, one of which was identified as the c-*jun*-coded protein p39. Furthermore, both Fos and Jun were noted as sharing a characteristic structural motif that consisted of a heptad repeat of leucine residues (the 'leucine zipper') preceded by clustered basic amino acids. Protein–protein and protein–DNA interactions involving Jun and Fos have been investigated extensively and the results are summarized as follows.

The three *jun* homologues, c-*jun*, *jun*B and *jun*D, are all capable of binding to the AP-1 site. These *jun* proteins can form dimers, either homologously or heterologously, and bind to DNA in the dimeric state. Fos and Fra-1 proteins can neither form dimers nor bind to DNA by themselves; however, Fos and Fra-1 form heterodimers with Jun proteins, and the resulting complexes exhibit highly increased affinities for the AP-1 site. Thus, a unified model for DNA binding of the Jun-Jun and Fos-Jun dimers is proposed, based on mutagenesis analysis in which pairing of two protein subunits by their leucine zippers allows the adjacent basic segments to form a composite DNA-binding domain with each subunit coming into contact with a half site of the palindromic recognition sequence.

POLYOMAVIRUS ENHANCER AS A PROBE

To study the modulation of the function of transcription factors by growth signals we have been using the Py enhancer as a probe. There are three reasons for using the Py enhancer:

1. The Py enhancer does not function in embryonal carcinoma (EC) cells, such as F9 and PCC4 cells. EC cells share many properties with the cells in the inner cell mass in the blastocyst and are often used as an *in vitro* model of undifferentiated embryonic cells. When the cells are induced to differentiate, the Py enhancer becomes active. Therefore, the Py enhancer is useful in studying the mechanism of tissue-specific functioning of enhancers.

2. As will be discussed below in detail, the function of the Py enhancer can be activated or repressed by a variety of oncogenes. Furthermore, this modulation appears to correlate well with the transforming activity of oncogenes. An important aspect of the transformation process could be studied.

3. Although enhancers are initially described as a *cis*-acting element to enhance transcription, the Py enhancer is also required for Py DNA replication. The observation of enhancer-dependent DNA replication has now been extended to other viral DNA replications. It is now generally believed that the initiation of eukaryotic DNA replication is probably controlled by enhancer function. Studies on the role of Py enhancer in Py DNA replication may serve as a model to explore the control of the initiation of chromosomal DNA replication.

FACTORS INTERACTING WITH Py ENHANCER A ELEMENT

The Py enhancer is usually represented by a 244 bp fragment from the *Bcl*I site (nt5021) to the *Pvu*II site (nt5265) shown diagrammatically in Figure 1. The entire enhancer region is divided into BP and PP fragments by the *Pvu*II site in the middle (nt5130). The origin of DNA replication and the promoter for the early gene transcription are located immediately adjacent to the right-hand side of the diagram. The promoter for the late genes is present within the BP fragment, and the late transcripts extend toward the left of this diagram.

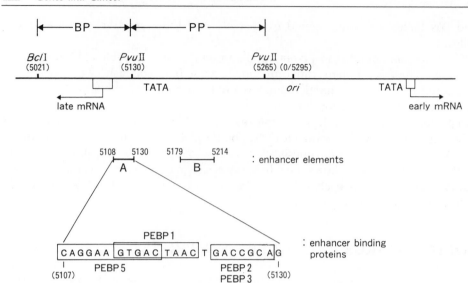

Figure 1. Structure of the polyomavirus enhancer and nuclear factors interacting with the A element

There are two cores important for the enhancer function, termed A and B, or α and β. They are conveniently located within the BP or PP fragment, respectively. We will concentrate our discussion mainly on the 24 bp A core element, since the target of the oncogene effect that we describe is the A element. Three sequence motifs can be recognized within the A element, to which regulatory protein factors are found to bind. The factors were originally termed PEA1, PEA2, PEB1, and so on by the group in the Pasteur Institute. However, we would like to use the terms polyomavirus enhancer binding proteins (PEBP) 1, 2, 3, and so on for reasons described elsewhere (Yamaguchi *et al.*, 1989; see Further Reading).

The binding site of PEBP1 (PEA1) belongs to the consensus sequence for AP-1 binding. PEBP1 shares many properties with AP-1 and is considered to be a member of an AP-1 family. PEBP2 (PEA2) and PEBP3 recognize the same sequence motif. It is currently believed that PEBP2 and PEBP3 share the DNA-binding domain and that PEBP2 is composed of PEBP3 plus an additional subunit. The sequence recognized by PEBP5 is homologous to the core of the enhancer of adenovirus type 5 *Ela* gene, called element I. The binding sites of PEBP1 and PEBP5 partly overlap as indicated in Figure 1.

It has been shown that the A element does not function in undifferentiated F9 cells but becomes active in F9 cells induced to differentiate by retinoic acid (dF9). Concomitantly PEBP1, PEBP2 and PEBP5 are not detectable in F9 cells but become detectable in dF9 cells (Table 1). The expression of these factors is, therefore, developmentally regulated. PEBP1 and PEBP5, and possibly PEBP2 also, are positive factors on transcription and the reason why the A element does not function in F9 cells is, at least partly, due to the low levels of positive factors in these cells.

Table 1. Expression of polyomavirus enhancer binding proteins in cells

	F9 cells	dF9 cells	NIH3T3 cells	COP5 cells*	Ha-*ras*/NIH3T3 cells
PEBP1	−	+	+	+	−
PEBP2	−	+	+	+	−
PEBP3	−	−	−	−	+
PEBP5	±	+	+	+	N.D.[†]

*COP5 cells are mouse fibroblasts expressing polyomavirus large, middle and small T antigens.
[†]N.D. = not done.

EFFECTS OF TPA AND TRANSIENTLY EXPRESSED Ha-*ras* ONCOGENE ON PEBP1 AND PEBP5

When the function of enhancers is tested, they are often linked in *cis* to the bacterial chloramphenicol acetyl transferase (CAT) gene driven by a given promoter, and CAT enzyme activities expressed in the cells from a transfected gene are measured. Using such an assay as well as other methods, the Py enhancer was found to be activated by TPA, resulting in the enhancement of transcription. Since 4α-phorbol 12,13-didecanoate (4α-PDD), a phorbol ester lacking tumor-promoting activity, does not show such activity, TPA stimulation of Py enhancer function seems to be closely related to the ability of TPA as a tumor promoter. The target of TPA stimulation was identified as being contained in the A element. Since the AP-1 binding site was known to be a TPA-responsive element (TRE), it was expected, and subsequently confirmed, that the PEBP1 binding site would respond to TPA. In addition, the PEBP5 binding site was also found to be responsive to TPA independently. Therefore, the Py enhancer contains two overlapping sequence motifs which are independently the targets of stimulation by TPA.

The next question is whether PEBP1 and PEBP5, which are identified as factors binding to these sequence motifs *in vitro*, are in fact responsible for TPA stimulation of transcription. Binding of AP-1 to TRE has been shown to be enhanced by treating cells with TPA. Similar enhancement of binding was also observed for PEBP1. These results suggest that AP-1 and PEBP1 receive growth signals and acquire higher binding ability to TRE, and this increased DNA binding is directly related to the enhancement of transcription. How does TPA increase PEBP1 binding to DNA? The fact that TPA is an activator of protein kinase C (PKC) immediately implies that protein phosphorylation by PKC would play a primary role. In the case of AP-1, it has been suggested that PKC phosphorylates a yet unknown target protein resulting in the stimulation of heterodimer formation between Fos and Jun proteins. However, post-translational modification, such as phosphorylation of PEBP1, may not be the only explanation of the TPA effect. Both the function of PEBP1 binding site and PEBP1 binding activity to DNA cannot be fully increased by TPA, if protein synthesis inhibitors are present. Thus, *de novo* synthesis of protein factors may also be involved in the process of activation by TPA.

A proto-Harvey *ras* oncogene (c-Ha-*ras*) acquires the ability to malignantly transform NIH3T3 cells when a point mutation is introduced into one of several places within the coding region. When activated c-Ha-*ras* gene is co-transfected into cells and expressed transiently, Py enhancer activity is stimulated in such cells. This stimulation is not observed if a non-activated c-Ha-*ras* gene is used. Therefore, in this case, too, the stimulation seems to be closely related to the transforming ability of the Ha-*ras* gene. The targets of this stimulation were found to be identical to those of TPA stimulation, namely the binding sites of PEBP1 and PEBP5. This suggests that activation of the PEBP1 and PEBP5 binding sites by the Ha-*ras* gene involves the pathway of PKC.

More recently, some other oncogenes or serum have been shown to have similar effects on Py enhancer function. They include v-*mos*, v-*src* and Py middle T antigen. However, c-*myc*, Py large T antigen and adenovirus *E1a* gene do not stimulate Py enhancer function.

It is interesting to note that an oncogene, c-Ha-*ras*, activates the function of the complex of the products of two proto-oncogenes, *AP*-1. Cell transformation by the Ha-*ras* gene may, therefore, involve the alteration of the function of the c-*jun* product towards a hyperactive state. Indeed recent reports indicate that the level of c-*jun* mRNA is constitutively high in several transformed cells. DNA binding activity of PEBP1 is also shown to be elevated in NIH3T3 cells transformed by the SV40 large T gene. Thus, constitutive activation of AP1/Jun/PEBP1 may be an underlying mechanism of cell transformation by several oncogenes. However, when we examined transformed cells more closely, we also encountered a paradoxical phenomenon, which is discussed below.

PEBP1 AND PEBP2 IN CELLS STABLY TRANSFORMED BY Ha-*ras* ONCOGENE

When PEBP1 binding activity was tested for the extract obtained from transformed cells, unexpected observations were made. In about half of the randomly collected NIH3T3 cell clones transformed by *ras* family genes (Ha-*ras*, Ki-*ras* and N-*ras*), PEBP1 was detected in greatly reduced amounts (Table 1). The other half contained PEBP1 at levels comparable to those in untransformed parental NIH3T3 cells. Although the biological significance of the above observation is not yet clear, we note that the cells with a morphologically fully transformed phenotype tend to have reduced PEBP1 binding activity. Therefore, a possibility emerges that such cells represent cells at a more advanced state of transformation, or cells with a higher degree of progression.

The biochemical basis for reduced binding activity of PEBP1 in transformed cells was also studied. Dephosphorylated PEBP1 (by phosphatase treatment) was found to have lost its DNA-binding ability. Furthermore, untransformed cells incubated in the presence of protein kinase inhibitors resulted in the loss of PEBP1-binding activity in their extract. These results suggest that the level of phosphorylation of PEBP1 is lower within the transformed cells, possibly due to down-regulation of PKC.

When PEBP1 is not detected in Ha-*ras*-transformed cells, it is expected that the PEBP1 binding site would not respond to TPA or serum growth factors. Indeed, experimentally this has been shown to be the case. This loss of responsiveness of PEBP1 to TPA or serum growth factors after transformation seems to be analogous to the state of cells which express a defective epidermal growth factor (EGF) receptor, such as *erb*B1, and thereby are not responsive to EGF. Activation of phospholipase C through the platelet-derived growth factor (PDGF) receptor was reported to be uncoupled in *ras*-transformed cells, leaving PKC to be non-responsive to PDGF. Apparent down-regulation of the protein kinase system in transformed cells might represent a new type of mechanism to explain the non-responsiveness of transformed cells to external growth stimuli.

In Ha-*ras* transformed NIH3T3 cells, another dramatic change has also been observed. In such cells, PEBP2 is present in a very small amount whereas, another factor, PEBP3, can be detected in a large amount (Table 1). These two factors have the same recognition sequences as shown in Figure 1. Proper phosphorylation of PEBP2 is necessary for its integrity, and apparent PEBP2 to PEBP3 conversion seems to be due to down-regulation of the protein kinase system as in the case of PEBP1. The biological significance of these observations has not been elucidated.

PERSPECTIVE

We have summarized the current concept that the main target of growth signals is a class of transcription factors interacting with DNA and involved directly in the regulation of gene expression (Figure 2).

One of the most interesting observations is that an AP-1 related factor, PEBP1, is frequently undetectable in cells stably transformed by the Ha-*ras* oncogene in spite of the fact that it is strongly stimulated by the same gene when it is expressed only transiently. This phenomenon appears to be related to the state of protein kinase(s), including PKC. Since not all transformants show the same pattern, it could be argued that it reflects different degrees of 'malignancy' or 'state of progression' of cell transformation. This system might offer a unique tool to uncover one aspect of carcinogenesis.

It is not clear how transcriptional activation of some genes by AP-1, Fos or PEBPs would lead to uncontrolled DNA replication. In this context, one must be reminded

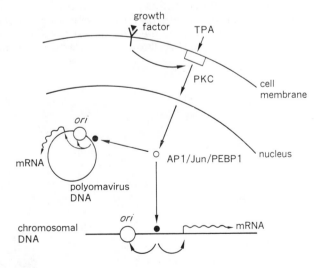

Figure 2. Model of regulation of transcription and DNA replication by AP1/Jun/PEBP1

that Py enhancer is required not only for its gene expression but also for its DNA replication. Eukaryotic chromosomal DNA replication may also be controlled by enhancers. TPA treatment and microinjected *ras* protein have been shown to induce DNA synthesis in quiescent cells. We have shown that TPA and Ha-*ras* gene activate the transcriptional enhancement function of the Py enhancer. The obvious and testable question is whether TPA or Ha-*ras* gene stimulate Py DNA replication via activation of the function of PEBP1 or PEBP5. In fact, several transcription factors are already known to be involved in the control of both transcription and replication. The Py enhancer may serve as a unique model to study the role, if any, of enhancer-binding proteins on the regulation of chromosomal DNA replication.

FURTHER READING

Bishop, J. M. (1987) The molecular genetics of cancer. *Science*, **235**, 305–311.

Curran, T., Rausher, III, F. J., Cohen, D. R. and Franza, Jr., B. R. (1988) Beyond the second messenger: oncogenes and transcription factors. *Cold Spring Harbor Symposia on Quantitative Biology*, **53**, 769–777.

Imler, J. L., Schatz, C., Wasylyk, C., *et al.* (1988) A Harvey-*ras* responsive transcription element is also responsive to a tumor-promoter and to serum. *Nature*, **332**, 275–278.

Kryszke, M.-H., Piette, J. and Yaniv, M. (1987) Induction of a factor that binds to the polyoma virus A enhancer on differentiation of embryonal carcinoma cells. *Nature*, **328**, 254–256.

Satake, M., Ibaraki, T. and Ito, Y. (1988) Modulation of polyomavirus enhancer binding proteins by Ha-*ras* oncogene. *Oncogene*, **3**, 69–78.

Veldman, G. M., Lupton, S. and Kamen, R. (1985) Polyomavirus enhancer contains multiple redundant sequence elements that activate both DNA replication and gene expression. *Mol. Cell. Biol.*, **5**, 649–659.

Vogt, P. K. and Tjian, R. (1988) Jun: a transcriptional regulator turned oncogenic. *Oncogene*, **3**, 3–7.

Wasylyk, C., Imler, J. L., Perez-Mutul, J. and Wasylyk, B. (1987) The c-Ha-*ras* oncogene and a tumor promoter activate the polyoma virus enhancer. *Cell*, **48**, 525–534.

Wasylyk, C., Imler, J. L. and Wasylyk, B. (1988) Transforming but not immortalizing oncogenes activate the transcription factor PEA1. *EMBO J.*, **7**, 2475–2483.

Yamaguchi, Y., Satake, M. and Ito, Y. (1989) Two overlapping sequence motifs within the polyomavirus enhancer are independently the targets of stimulation by both the tumor promoter 12-*O*-tetradecanoylphorbol-13-acetate and the Ha-*ras* oncogene. *J. Virol.*, **63**, 1040–1048.

12 Mitochondria in Cancer Cells

LAN BO CHEN
ELISSA N. RIVERS

THE STRUCTURE AND FUNCTION OF MITOCHONDRIA

Mitochondria are the organelles within aerobic cells that specialize in the rapid oxidation of a limited number of substrates (particularly NADH, fatty acids and succinate), with conservation of the resulting free energy in the form of ATP. The mitochondria are enveloped by two separate lipid bilayer membranes. The outer membrane is pierced by pores that allow free passage of charged and uncharged solutes up to 5000 Da in size. The inner membrane involves energy transduction by a proton current. The surface area of the inner membrane is greatly increased by infoldings called cristae, which bear components of the respiratory chain and the FoF1ATPase respiratory assemblies. Substrates are generated within the mitochondrial matrix by the Krebs cycle and by the enzymes of fatty acid oxidation. Electrons removed during oxidation of these substrates are passed along the respiratory chain and ultimately transferred to oxygen. The free energy released by electron transport is then coupled to phosphorylation of ADP to form ATP (see review by Harold, 1986, under Further Reading).

Mitochondrial electron transport and ATP synthesis are tightly coupled processes. The most widely held theory explaining this energy coupling was formulated in the early 1960s by Mitchell. He proposed that the respiratory chain pumps protons across the inner membrane, thereby generating an electrochemical gradient which has two components: a membrane potential (protons are positively charged) and a pH gradient (protons determine acidity). The interior of the membrane is negative and alkaline. Free energy released by the passage of electrons along the respiratory chain is thus transduced into the electrochemical potential of protons. Return of protons through the FoF1ATPase assemblies releases this energy, which is used to drive ATP synthesis. It is believed that mammalian mitochondria express this electrochemical

Genes and Cancer. Edited by D. Carney and K. Sikora
©1990 John Wiley & Sons Ltd

gradient mostly as a membrane potential of about 180 mV, and to a lesser extent as a pH gradient equivalent to about 60 mV (the total energy yielded would be approximately 240 mV). However, whether mitochondria in all cells express the proton gradient in this manner is still unknown. Conceivably the magnitude of the proton gradient and its expression either as the pH gradient or the membrane potential may differ among cell types and change to meet the special needs (differentiation, changes in function, transformation) of individual cells. Regulation of the proton gradient may play a fundamental role in cellular programming, since each of its components also affects the transport of metabolites, ions, precursor enzymes, mitochondrial protein synthesis, etc. Even less is known about whether mitochondria in diseased cells, such as cancer cells, alter the expression of this gradient, either in its overall magnitude or relative proportions between the pH gradient and the membrane potential.

EXPERIMENTAL STUDIES OF MITOCHONDRIA

Although a vast amount of work has been done with mitochondria, either isolated or in fixed cells, we do not know how relevant these studies are to mitochondria in intact, living cells. Mitochondria interact with cytoplasm, and very little is known about the non-substrate factors that influence mitochondrial respiration and proton gradients *in vivo*. Recently, fluorescent dyes have been employed as optical probes to assess mitochondrial bioenergetics in living cells. The advantages of such probes include their non-invasive nature, the availability of thousands of fluorescent dyes, the development of a highly sensitive detection system, and changes in fluorescence in response to environmental changes. Of particular interest to us have been the lipophilic, cationic rhodamine and cyanine dyes, which are selectively taken up by mitochondria in living cells. Of these fluorescent dyes, rhodamine 123 (Rh123) has become the dye of choice for routine studies of mitochondria in living cells because of its specificity and generally low toxicity (Figure 1). Although Rh123 can be toxic if cells are exposed to high concentrations over long periods of time, the standard procedure, using up to $10 \, \mu g \, ml^{-1}$ Rh123 for 10 minutes at 37°C, produces no obvious effect on cellular function or mitochondrial morphology.

The specificity of Rh123 uptake and retention by mitochondria apparently correlates with the plasma and mitochondrial membrane potentials. Lipophilic cationic compounds carry a delocalized positive charge (at physiological pH) throughout the entire molecule, which allows them to equilibrate across biological membranes according to the Nernst equation. Because mitochondria are located intracellularly, the amount of Rh123 accumulated by the mitochondria at equilibrium depends not only upon the mitochondrial membrane potential, but also upon the plasma membrane potential. The plasma membrane potential, which is negative inside, serves to pre-concentrate the cationic dye in the cytoplasm relative to the medium. Indeed, in the presence of high extracellular potassium ion (137 mM), which dissipates the plasma membrane potential, mitochondrial uptake of Rh123 is reduced. To confirm that the mitochondrial accumulation of Rh123 in intact cells is related to the mitochondrial membrane potential, a variety of agents that disrupt the metabolism of mitochondria have been tested for their effects on the uptake

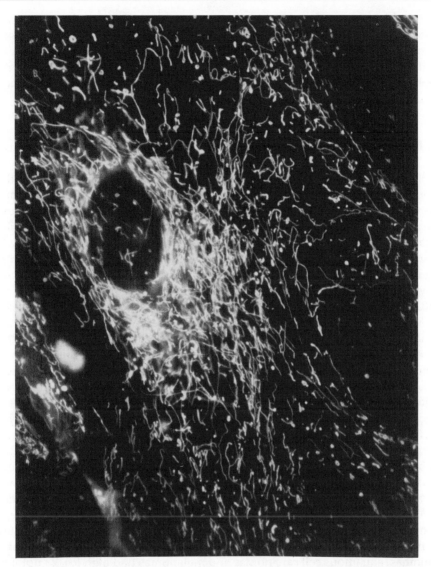

Figure 1. Fluorescent micrograph of mitochondria in a human fibroblast selectively stained with rhodamine 123 and 10 μg ml^{-1} for 10 min

of Rh123. The potassium ionophore valinomycin and the proton ionophores FCCP (*p*-trifluoromethoxyphenylhydrazone) and DNP (dinitrophenol), all of which dissipate the mitochondrial membrane potential, markedly decrease mitochondrial uptake and retention of Rh123. Electron transport inhibitors (rotenone, antimycin A, cyanide, azide), in conjunction with an inhibitor of FoF1ATPase (oligomycin), completely eliminate Rh123 uptake by all cells. The most compelling evidence comes from pretreating cells with the ionophore nigericin. During continuous respiration nigericin induces an electrically neutral exchange of protons for potassium ions, which eliminates the pH gradient across the mitochondrial membrane but increases the mitochondrial membrane potential (because nigericin also hyperpolarizes the plasma membrane, it is necessary to include ouabain in the medium). Indeed, nigericin dramatically enhances the accumulation of Rh123 by mitochondria. Inhibitors of mitochondrial protein synthesis (chloramphenicol), cellular protein synthesis (cycloheximide), and RNA synthesis (actinomycin D) have no effect on Rh123 uptake in living cells.

MITOCHONDRIAL CHANGES IN TUMOUR CELLS

The 50-year-old debate initiated by Otto Warburg over whether mitochondria in tumour cells differ from those in normal cells remains unsolved. For the past 25 years or so, the prevailing opinion has held that the mitochondria of tumour and normal cells do not differ. This position, however, has been based largely on *in vitro* studies with isolated mitochondria. Observations discussed below show that oncogenic transformation affects mitochondria, but not in a consistent manner.

Bladder epithelial cells have low mitochondrial membrane potentials, which lead to low uptake and short retention of Rh123. In contrast, dimethylbenz(a)anthracene (DMBA)- or butyl nitrosamine (BBN)-transformed mouse bladder epithelial cell lines (MB48, MB49, BBN6), a benzo(a)pyrene-transformed rabbit bladder epithelial cell line (RBC), and human bladder carcinoma-derived cell lines (EJ, RT4, RT112) have been shown to have significantly higher Rh123 uptake and retention. These initial results encouraged further comparisons of Rh123 uptake and retention between normal epithelial and carcinoma-derived cells. For instance, while CV-1 cells (normal monkey kidney epithelium) lost Rh123 in a few hours, mitochondrial fluorescence in MCF-7 cells (human breast carcinoma) could still be observed days after dye was removed from the medium. The increased accumulation and retention of Rh123 by cultured carcinoma cell lines was paralleled by our studies on primary explants from patients at this institute. Most, but not all, explanted carcinomas exhibited the phenotype of increased accumulation and long retention of Rh123. The results of a six-year study overwhelmingly indicated that all normal epithelial cells tested had low mitochondrial membrane potentials and, hence, low Rh123 uptake and retention. In contrast, screenings of 200 transformed cell lines/types and more than 100 surgical specimens showed that a great majority of adenocarcinomas, transitional cell carcinomas, squamous cell carcinomas and melanomas had high Rh123 uptake and retention. Examples of the difference in Rh123 retention between primary explant cultures of normal human colonic epithelium and differentiated human colon adenocarcinoma are shown in Figures 2 and 3. Both cultures were stained with Rh123 ($10 \, \mu g \, ml^{-1}$ for 10 min) and left in dye-free medium for 24 hours. Whereas the normal cells lost almost all of the Rh123 fluorescence, the carcinoma cells still retained a significant level of Rh123 fluorescence. The difference in mitochondrial membrane potential between normal epithelial cells and carcinoma cells was at least 60 mV. The most significant exceptions were human oat cell and large cell carcinomas of the lung, and poorly differentiated carcinoma of the colon. High Rh123 uptake and retention were not detected in leukemias, lymphomas, neuroblastomas or osteosarcomas.

Rh123 experiments involving heterokaryons suggest that mitochondrial membrane potential in living cells is influenced by slowly diffusing, as yet unidentified,

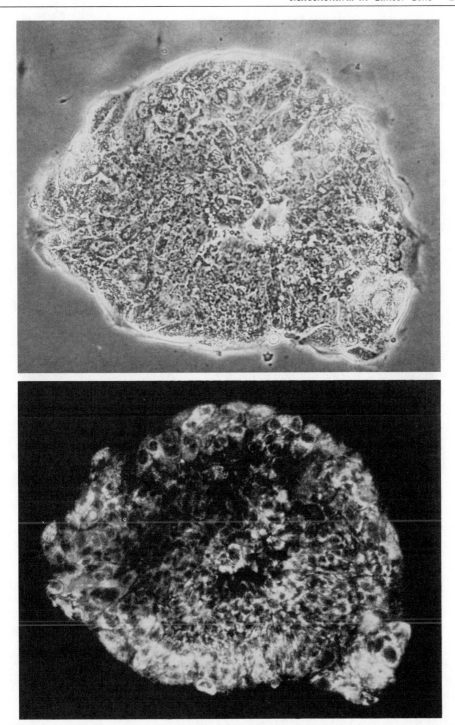

Figure 2. Prolonged rhodamine 123 retention by primary explant culture of differentiated human colon adenocarcinoma. Cells were stained with rhodamine 123 at $10\,\mu g\,ml^{-1}$ for 10 min and left in dye-free medium for 24 hours. Top: phase-contrast; bottom: fluorescence

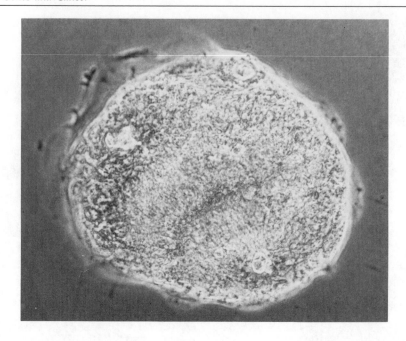

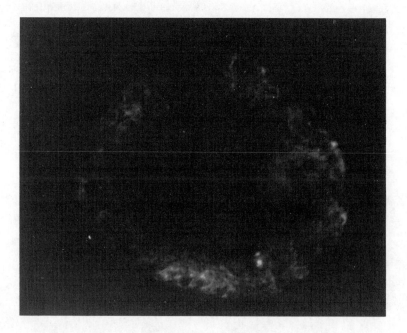

Figure 3. Lack of rhodamine 123 retention by primary explant culture of normal human colonic epithelium. Cells were stained with rhodamine 123 at 10 μg ml^{-1} for 10 min and left in dye-free medium for 24 hours. Top: phase-contrast; bottom: fluorescence

cytoplasmic factors. Heterokaryons have been obtained by fusing cells having high mitochondrial membrane potentials (MCF-7, human breast carcinoma) with cells having low mitochondrial membrane potentials (PtK2, normal kangaroo rat kidney epithelium). During the first 6 hours following exposure to Rh123, differential uptake of the dye by the two mitochondrial populations within the heterokaryons is maintained. Within 18 hours, however, all the mitochondria in the heterokaryons have taken up an equal amount of Rh123. The level of uptake by these mitochondria is intermediate between that of unfused MCF-7 and PtK2 cells.

Recently, v-*fos* oncogene-transformed fibroblasts have been shown to have higher Rh123 uptake and retention than their normal counterparts. Mink fibroblasts, which normally have a high mitochondrial membrane potential and low pH gradient, change the expression of their mitochondrial proton gradient to a very low mitochondrial membrane potential and very high pH gradient following transformation by the v-*fos* oncogene. Other oncogenes (*src*, *myc*, *ras*, *mos*, *E1A*, middle T) seem to have no effect on mitochondrial membrane potential (see review by Chen, 1988).

Therapeutic potential of differential dye uptake

The increased accumulation and retention of Rh123 by carcinoma cells prolongs exposure of their mitochondria to the cationic dye. It was expected, therefore, that any toxicity due to Rh123 would be more acute in carcinoma cells than in normal cells. The possibility of selective killing of carcinoma cells based on differential uptake and retention of lipophilic cationic dyes was encouraging. Subsequently, it was shown that Rh123 is selectively toxic to carcinoma cells *in vitro*. The concentration of Rh123 required for the inhibition of clonal growth of various carcinoma cell lines was much lower than that needed for the same response in corresponding untransformed cells. Standard chemotherapeutic agents such as Ara-C and methotrexate displayed no such selectivity. In addition, prolonged treatment (more than 24 hours) of cells with Rh123 ($10 \mu g \, ml^{-1}$) showed a selective inhibition of colony-forming ability in carcinoma cells but not in normal epithelial cells.

Potential anticarcinoma activity of Rh123 was also demonstrated *in vivo*. Rh123 was found to prolong the lives of mice implanted intraperitoneally with Ehrlich ascites or MB49 mouse bladder carcinoma cells, both of which exhibit long retention of Rh123 *in vitro*. Control mice implanted with Ehrlich ascites carcinoma cells had a median survival time of 19 days. Tumour-bearing mice treated with a non-toxic dose of Rh123 had a median survival time of 50 days, with treated/control (T/C) = 260%. Treatment with 2-deoxyglucose only, an inhibitor of glycolysis, did not prolong survival. Combined treatments of 2-deoxyglucose and Rh123, however, markedly prolonged survival (T/C = 420%). Approximately 40% of mice were cured (no evidence of tumours after 90 days). Rh123 has also been shown to be a sensitizer for the killing of tumour cells by hyperthermia and by photodynamic therapy.

Possible mechanism of dye selective toxicity

The specific mechanism of selective toxicity during prolonged exposure to Rh123 is not completely understood. The highest subcellular concentration of Rh123 is in the mitochondria, making these organelles the most attractive target for dye toxicity. Gross morphological changes occur in mitochondria of Rh123-treated cells. *In vitro* studies using isolated mitochondria have shed more light on the problem. In energized, tightly coupled mitochondria, low concentrations of Rh123 ($5 \, \mu g \, ml^{-1}$) inhibit FoF1ATPase synthesis of ATP by 90%. Slightly higher levels of Rh123 also inhibit the reverse reaction (FoF1ATPase uncoupling activity). Assays of Rh123 effects on segments of the respiratory chain using freeze-thawed (membrane-disrupted) mitochondria have eliminated several enzyme complexes as possible targets. The above results suggest that FoF1ATPase assemblies could be the primary target for Rh123 toxicity. Additional evidence supports this notion. FoF1ATPase assemblies reconstituted in phospholipid vesicles can also be directly inhibited by Rh123. It is evident that certain carcinoma cells *in vitro*, when compared to normal epithelial cells, take up and retain more Rh123 in their mitochondria. The higher dye concentration coupled with increased sensitivity of FoF1ATPase to the dye contribute to the selective toxicity of Rh123 for carcinoma cells.

Rh123 exhibits other activities which may contribute to its cytotoxic effects. Prolonged exposure of cells to Rh123 has been shown to inhibit the synthesis, transport and processing of enzymes by mitochondria. Moreover, it inhibits mitochondrial protein synthesis, bacterial DNA and RNA polymerases (enzymes which share some similarities with those of mitochondria), and the activities of protein kinase C and calmodulin. It may actually be the combined effects of several inhibitory activities that lead to the cytotoxicity observed when cells with high mitochondrial membrane potentials are exposed to Rh123 for longer than 24 hours.

Future developments

Further exploitation of mitochondrial membrane potential for cancer therapy should be given serious consideration. We propose a model whereby the mitochondria of carcinoma cells would serve as accumulating reservoirs of lipophilic cationic dye. According to the Nernst equation, if the plasma membrane potential is 60 mV and the mitochondrial membrane potential is 180 mV, then the concentration of lipophilic cations inside mitochondria at equilibrium could be 10 000-fold greater than in the medium. Since mitochondria occupy a significant portion of the cell volume, the total amount of lipophilic cations accumulated by mitochondria would be substantial. Once the extracellular dye concentration drops, dye accumulated within mitochondria would be released gradually into the cytoplasm and extracellular medium because of the dye concentration gradient. Membrane potential, however, would oppose dye diffusion; high mitochondrial and plasma membrane potentials favour the intracellular retention of lipophilic cations. Thus, mitochondria could serve first as an intracellular depot for dye accumulation and then as slow-releasing devices for the dye. It should be possible to design dye compounds that exert regulatory or cytotoxic effects for use in this model.

Dequalinium, a topical antimicrobial lipophilic cation which also exhibits significant anticarcinoma activity, is an example of the potential usefulness of lipophilic cations for cancer therapy. Doubly positively charged, dequalinium is accumulated by mitochondria, where it can inhibit mitochondrial electron transport. Upon release from mitochondria it can intercalate into DNA, and it can also inhibit the activities of calmodulin and protein kinase C. When cultured cells were exposed to dequalinium for 3 hours, the drug was 125-fold more toxic to carcinoma (MCF-7) cells than to normal epithelial (CV-1) cells. Dequalinium was also effective *in vivo* against MB49 (DMBA-transformed mouse bladder carcinoma) cells planted intraperitoneally, with T/C=250% under the best condition. The most significant anticarcinoma activity was observed against mammary tumours induced *in situ* by the carcinogen DMBA. In this case, which avoided transplantation, dequalinium inhibited growth and led to regression of tumours.

Lipophilic cations may also be used as vehicles to deliver other drugs whose uptake by tumour cells is not driven by membrane potentials. By exploiting the membrane potential, these cations may be moved across lipid bilayers electrophoretically. A 60 mV potential across a 5 nm plasma membrane would be equivalent to 120 000 V across 1 cm. Numerous drugs that have low membrane permeabilities or depend on membrane transport systems could be complexed with lipophilic cations. Thus facilitating their entry into cells via an electrical field.

FURTHER READING

Chen, L. B. (1988) Mitochondrial membrane potential in living cells. *Ann. Rev. Cell Biol.*, **4**, 155–181.

Chen, L. B., Summerhayes, I., Johnson, L., *et al.* (1982) Probing mitochondria in living cells with rhodamine 123. *Cold Spring Harbor Symposia on Quantitative Biology*, vol. XLVI, pp. 141–155.

Davis, S., Weiss, M., Wong, J., Lampidis, T. and Chen, L. B. (1985) Mitochondrial and plasma membrane potentials cause unusual accumulation and retention of rhodamine 123 by human breast adenocarcinoma-derived MCF-7 cells. *J. Biol. Chem.*, **260**, 13844–13850.

Harold, R. (1986) *The Vital Force: A Study of Bioenergetics*. W. H. Freeman, New York.

Johnson, L., Walsh, M. and Chen, L. B. (1980) Localization of mitochondria in living cells with rhodamine 123. *Proc. Nat. Acad. Sci. USA*, **77**, 990–994.

Mitchell, P. (1961) Coupling of phosphorylation to electron and hydrogen transfer by a chemiosmotic type of mechanism. *Nature* (London), **191**, 144–148.

Modica-Napolitano, J. and Aprille, J. (1987) Basis for the selective cytotoxicity of rhodamine 123. *Cancer Res.*, **47**, 4361–4365.

Nadakavukaren, K., Nadakavukaren, J. and Chen, L. B. (1985) Increased rhodamine 123 uptake by carcinoma cells. *Cancer Res.*, **45**, 6093–6099.

Summerhayes, I., Lampidis, T., Bernal, S., *et al.* (1982) Unusual retention of rhodamine 123 by mitochondria in muscle and carcinoma cells. *Proc. Nat. Acad. Sci. USA*, **79**, 5292–5296.

Weiss, M., Wong, J., Ha, C., *et al.* (1987) Dequalinium, a topical antimicrobial agent, displays anticarcinoma activity based on selective mitochondrial accumulation. *Proc. Nat. Acad. Sci. USA*, **84**, 5444–5448.

13 Viral *Trans*-Activating Genes

ALEXANDER C. BLACK
JOSEPH D. ROSENBLATT
IRVIN S. Y. CHEN

Viral *trans*-activating genes encode proteins that can affect expression from multiple non-contiguous viral and cellular genes. These viral proteins regulate the viral life cycle and can interact with a variety of cellular genetic elements involved in cellular growth control. Many viruses encode two or more *trans*-acting viral proteins: one *trans*-activates transcription from viral promoter/enhancer elements; the other mediates the temporal sequence of viral gene expression. The mechanisms for regulation are complex, and occur on both transcriptional and post-transcriptional levels, usually requiring interaction with host cell factors involved in cellular gene expression. Further elucidation of these interactions should in turn help explain on a molecular level how productive viral infection and occasional malignant transformation of virally infected cells may occur.

This chapter focuses on several well-characterized DNA and RNA viruses that possess *trans*-activating viral genes, and that have been associated with *in vitro* transformation or with clinically significant human disease. The DNA virus genes discussed below are adenovirus E1A, SV40 T-antigen and herpes simplex virus 1 VP16; the RNA virus genes considered are *tat* and *rev* of human immunodeficiency virus type 1 (HIV-1), and *tax* and *rex* of human T-cell leukemia virus types I (HTLV-I) and II (HTLV-II). Despite marked differences both in the organization of the viral genomes and the nucleotide sequences of the respective *trans*-activating viral genes,

Genes and Cancer. Edited by D. Carney and K. Sikora
©1990 John Wiley & Sons Ltd

the proteins encoded by these genes share fundamental functional characteristics. To explore these characteristics further, each viral gene will be described separately, followed by a summary of the underlying features. For a more detailed account, the reader is directed to the reviews listed under Further Reading.

ADENOVIRUS

E1A Gene

Adenovirus, a common cause of upper and lower respiratory infections in man, encodes the earliest described and most completely characterized group of *trans*-activating viral proteins, the E1A proteins. They are the first viral proteins expressed after adenoviral infection, and play a critical role in the adenoviral life cycle by stimulating efficient transcription from all early adenoviral promoters and also from the major late promoter. Despite the lack of clinically recognized human malignancy associated with adenovirus infection, the E1A proteins are also active transforming agents *in vitro*.

Adenovirus has a genome of approximately 36 kb encoding a variety of proteins involved in viral DNA replication and packaging, virion structure and host regulation. The major late promoter, which is active within one hour following viral infection, initiates two classes of viral mRNA transcripts: the L1 family, before viral DNA replication; and transcripts encoding most adenoviral structural proteins after viral replication. Experiments in HeLa cells involving transient transfections with mutant E1A-expressing plasmids or infections with mutant E1A-containing Ad5 viruses demonstrate that an intact E1A region stimulates a many-fold higher rate of transcription through the major late promoter. In addition to E1A, accurate transcription for the major late promoter requires at least five cellular transcription factors.

The E1A region yields three differentially spliced mRNAs encoding three proteins, two of which, p289 and p243, are active throughout the viral life cycle; the third is expressed only in late phase. No viral proteins other than E1A proteins are required for *trans*-activation of the early viral promoters, and recent mutational analysis of E1A restricts the *trans*-activation function to p289 only. Both p289 and p243 are located in the nuclei of infected cells, and both appear to form complexes with several cellular proteins.

Promoter mutagenesis studies and biochemical analysis of infected cell extracts demonstrate that the same host cell transcription factors bind to adenovirus promoters whether or not the cells are expressing E1A proteins. Since no additional sequence-specific binding proteins are required for E1A *trans*-activation, E1A presumably interacts with these cellular factors to augment transcription. The cellular factor that appears to be responsible for the increased transcription as determined both by testing of phosphocellulose column infected cell extracts and template commitment assays, is TF-III-C, a sequence-specific DNA-binding transcription factor.

E1A proteins also stimulate transcription from a variety of non-adenoviral promoters, including those for globin, HSV1 glycoprotein D and several different thymidine kinase genes. However, in infected cells, total polyadenylated heterologous nuclear RNA is not altered during the early phase of viral infection, despite the strong stimulation to viral gene transcription by E1A proteins, suggesting a preferential activation of viral promoters.

In addition to stimulating transcription from many types of promoters, the E1A proteins have been shown to immortalize cells in tissue culture and to transform cells *in vitro* in concert with other viral *trans*-activating factors such as adenovirus protein E1B and polyoma middle T antigen, and oncogene products such as the Ha-*ras* protein. Mutational analysis of E1A by several investigators has demonstrated that different areas of E1A are involved in *trans*-activation and transformation. Using radio-immunoprecipitation assays (RIPA) of extracts of HeLa cells infected with adenovirus containing different E1A deletion mutants, Whyte and co-workers established that the E1A proteins interact with three cellular proteins, a 300 kDa species, a 170 kDa species and a 105 kDa species, corresponding to the retinoblastoma gene product. The E1A deletion mutants were also tested for *in vitro* transforming activity by quantifying the number of mutant colonies resulting from co-transfection of plasmids expressing E1A mutants and plasmids expressing T24 Ha-*ras* into primary baby rat kidney cells. Efficient transformation required intact binding sites in the E1A proteins for all three cellular factors, suggesting that E1A proteins interact with specific cellular proteins to induce transformation of infected cells. Of particular interest is the interaction with the retinoblastoma gene product, a putative growth inhibition factor or anti-oncogene, since it suggests that inactivation of the anti-oncogene may lead to malignant transformation. Retinoblastoma occurs in patients when both alleles have been mutated, either through inheritance of one defective gene with spontaneous somatic mutation of the remaining normal gene or by spontaneous mutations in both genes.

SV40 T-ANTIGEN

Although not implicated in human malignancy, SV40 (simian virus 40) has a well-characterized *trans*-acting and transforming viral gene which encodes the SV40 T-antigen. SV40 is a small, 5 kb double-stranded DNA virus that contains two transcription units, early and late, defined by the period of peak activity after infection of susceptible cells. During the early phase, the SV40 DNA is replicated and the host cell is primed to manufacture more viral DNA; during the late phase, viral coat proteins are produced and new virions formed. The switch from early to late phase viral gene transcription is mediated by the SV40 large T-antigen, which is translated from early viral mRNA. SV40 T-antigen is essential to the viral life cycle since SV40 virions with defective T-antigen genes do not produce significant amounts of viral DNA.

SV40 T-antigen forms a tetramer that binds several *cis*-responsive sequences. At initial low levels of SV40 T-antigen, the tetramer preferentially binds to site I, the furthest downstream in the early transcription unit. But in higher concentration it also binds to sites II and III, immediately downstream and upstream, respectively, of the early transcription unit cap site and TATA box. At higher concentrations, T-antigen stops or markedly diminishes transcription from the early transcription unit by impeding RNA polymerase II initiation of RNA synthesis. By diminishing transcription of SV40 early mRNA, which encodes the T-antigen, SV40 T-antigen also appears to have an autoregulatory function by down-regulating its own expression.

In addition to its essential role in the viral life cycle, SV40 T-antigen has been implicated in the process of transformation. In non-permissive cells, the induction of S-phase by SV40 T-antigen does not lead to viral DNA replication or the switch to late phase viral gene expression. If intact early gene sequences of SV40 DNA become permanently integrated into the non-permissive host cell genome, the cell becomes transformed. This integration event is not site-specific, but rather, transformation may involve constitutive expression of the early viral gene products which prevent entry by the host cell into the resting G_0 phase.

To explore further the role of SV40 T-antigen in this process of transformation, several investigators have tested SV40 T-antigen mutants in transformation assays, and have mapped *trans*-activating and transforming functions to different regions of the T-antigen protein. The amino terminal, approximately 130 residues, has readily measurable transforming and immortalizing activity which, in particular, depends upon amino acids (aa) 105–114. However, the 105–114 aa region of SV40 T-antigen is not required for SV40 origin of replication binding, DNA replication initiation, or nuclear localization of the protein. This 105–114 aa region also has primary sequence and predicted secondary structure homology to domain 2 of the adenovirus E1A gene products, which is essential for the Ha-*ras* and E1B co-transforming activity of E1A. The 105–118 aa region of T-antigen can functionally substitute for domain 2 of E1A in a chimeric protein, as tested in *in vitro* transformation assays.

As with the E1A proteins of adenovirus, the SV40 T-antigen appears to interact with the retinoblastoma gene product. Several investigators have found in radio-immunoprecipitation experiments that the SV40 T-antigen forms a specific complex with the retinoblastoma gene product, and that complex formation requires an intact 105–114 aa T-antigen region. Thus, it has been postulated that binding of the retinoblastoma gene product by either E1A or SV40 T-antigen may neutralize its growth-suppressing function and help induce host cell transformation.

HERPES SIMPLEX VIRUS 1 (HSV-1), VP16 AND ICP27 PROTEINS

HSV-1 causes several clinically important human diseases, including transient mucocutaneous ulcers, corneal scarring, meningoencephalitis and, occasionally, inflammation of other visceral organs. HSV-1 often remains latent in sensory ganglia nerve cell bodies with potential, both *in vivo* and *in vitro*, to reactivate and produce infectious virus. Despite the high frequency of latent infection, there is no report of association between HSV-1 and human malignancy.

HSV-1 is a linear double-stranded DNA virus of 153 kb with three *cis*-acting origins of replication and more than 70 open reading frames. As with other large complex DNA viruses, the HSV-1 genome can be divided into three categories based on requirements for gene expression; alpha—immediate early genes that do not require prior viral protein synthesis; beta—delayed early genes that require some alpha gene products but not viral DNA replication, and that usually encode proteins involved in viral DNA replication; and gamma—late genes that require both viral protein synthesis and viral DNA replication for expression, and that generally encode viral structural proteins. *Trans*-acting HSV-1 proteins control the appropriate temporal expression of viral genes during lytic infection.

The HSV-1 alpha genes are specifically induced by a *trans*-activating protein that is a component of the infecting virion, VP16. VP16 is a 65 kDa protein that has been shown by several laboratories to prime transcription from five alpha genes through *cis*-acting upstream regulatory elements. Two distinct motifs have been identified within the alpha gene ICP4 (infected cell protein 4) enhancer that specifies response to VP16. Either motif can act independently to mediate *trans*-activation by VP16, but both combined allow maximal induction. Purified VP16 displays no substantial affinity for double-stranded DNA, implying that VP16-induced *trans*-activation occurs indirectly through host cell factors.

Recent work suggests that two host cell factors present in infected cells mediate VP16-dependent alpha gene induction and act by sequence-specific binding to the alpha gene *cis*-acting response elements. Triezenberg and co-workers analysed fractionated nuclear protein extracts from uninfected mammalian cells and established that certain cellular proteins bind directly to each VP16 motif. In studies of mRNA and protein expression using mutant forms of VP16 in transient co-transfections, Triezenberg and co-workers identified two domains of VP16 involved in *trans*-activation: a 78 aa region within the carboxy terminal that is required for VP16 stimulation of gene expression, and a separate area that confers a dominant interfering activity of VP16 mutants with this 78 aa region deleted. When the carboxy terminal *trans*-activating domain is not present, the mutant protein may compete with the wild-type VP16 for interaction with the *cis*-acting alpha gene response region, suggesting that the retained N-terminal VP16 sequences confer specificity for the interaction with that regulatory region.

HUMAN T-CELL LEUKEMIA VIRUS (HTLV) TYPES I AND II *tax* AND *rex*

HTLV-I and HTLV-II have been associated with human cancer and neurologic disease in a small proportion of seropositive individuals. HTLV-I causes adult T-cell leukemia/lymphoma (ATL), which is a rapidly fatal illness characterized by lymphadenopathy, lytic bone lesions, hypercalcemia and immunosuppression. HTLV-I has also been implicated in the pathogenesis of HTLV-I-associated myelopathy (HAM), which is an inflammatory demyelinating disease resembling multiple sclerosis (MS) that causes weakness and spasticity of the legs and urinary and bowel incontinence. HTLV-II has been found in several patients with rare T-cell malignancies, and has been identified in urban cohorts of intravenous drug abusers (IVDA), first serologically by ELISA assay, and more recently molecularly by polymerase chain reaction (PCR).

HTLV-I and -II are single-stranded RNA viruses, specifically type C retroviruses, with the same fundamental genomic structure of 5' and 3' long terminal repeats (LTRs) flanking open reading frames for *gag* (core proteins), *pol* (reverse transcriptase) and *env* (envelope proteins). The LTRs contain sequences mediating viral integration, replication and expression, and have three distinct domains, U3, R and U5 in 5' to 3' order. HTLV-I and -II also have two partially overlapping genes in the 3' end of the viral genome which encode two *trans*-acting regulatory proteins, Tax (for *trans*-activator) and Rex (for regulator of expression). HTLV-I and -II have an overall nucleic acid sequence homology of 65%, which is lowest in the LTR and highest in the *tax/rex* coding sequences. HTLV-I and -II produce three mRNA species: full-length 8.4 kb genomic RNA transcribed from the U3/R junction in the 5' LTR and terminating at the R/U5 junction in the 3' LTR, which encodes the *gag/pol* gene products and provides genomic RNA for packaging into virions; a singly spliced 4.3 kb mRNA species removing the 5' intron which encodes the *env* gene product; and a doubly spliced 2.1 kb mRNA which encodes both *tax* and *rex* from partially overlapping reading frames.

The HTLV-I and -II *tax* genes encode proteins of 40 and 37 kDa, respectively, which localize to the nucleus of HTLV-infected cells. As detailed below, work by several investigators has established that Tax *trans*-activates viral mRNA transcription through indirect interaction with promoter and enhancer elements in the U3 region of the 5' LTR. Initially, transcription from the HTLV-I LTR was found to be greatly stimulated in virus-infected cells when compared to non-infected cells. Deletion of sequences in the *tax/rex* genes was shown to render an infectious HTLV-II clone non-infectious, providing *in vivo* evidence that Tax and Rex are essential for viral replication. Co-transfections in mammalian cells of the HTLV-I and -II LTRs linked to an indicator gene, generally CAT, and a normal or mutated *tax* expression vector also confirm that functional Tax protein is required for *trans*-activation of LTR-linked genes. *In vitro*, Tax mutagenesis studies have shown that both N- and C-terminal sequences are required for full activity, and that certain N-terminal mutations (e.g. Pro 5 to Leu 5) produce a *trans*-dominant inhibitory phenotype in the mutant HTLV-I or -II Tax protein.

Tax-induced *trans*-activation in both viruses is mediated through *cis*-acting sequences in the U3 region of the 5' LTR; specifically, three imperfect 21 bp repeats upstream of the TATA box that are required for efficient transcriptional activation by Tax. The 21 bp repeat element of HTLV-I confers Tax-responsive *trans*-activation to otherwise unresponsive heterologous promoters independently of position and orientation, and the level of activation by Tax increases with increased numbers of 21 bp repeat elements. Co-transfection experiments have also identified a variety of heterologous promoters responsive to Tax, including adenovirus E1A, interleukin 2 (IL-2), a subunit of the the IL-2 receptor (IL-2Rα), and a variety of lymphokines including granulocyte-macrophage colony-stimulating factor (GM-CSF).

Tax does not appear to interact directly with the 21 bp response sequences in the HTLV LTR, since DNAase footprint patterns are similar with or without Tax; rather, it appears to act indirectly through host cell proteins. Several investigators, using DNA gel shift assays and oligonucleotide sepharose column separation of binding proteins, have identified multiple cellular proteins in HeLa nuclear extracts that bind to the HTLV-I 21 bp sequence. In addition, the 21 bp repeats of both viruses have some homology to AP-2 and NF-$_\kappa$B sites, which have been shown to mediate TPA activation, and contain the cAMP octanucleotide consensus element, which is required for cAMP activation. Site-directed mutagenesis in these regions abolishes both *trans*-activation by Tax and responsiveness to TPA or cAMP. Tax interaction with pre-existing cellular transcription factors may also help explain its ability to *trans*-activate many heterologous promoter enhancer elements that may require a similar complex of transcription factors for efficient transcription.

Rex in both viruses is a phosphorylated nuclear protein with predominantly nucleolar localization, which modulates *trans*-activation by Tax, primarily at a post-transcriptional level. The active form of Rex corresponds to the larger of the two protein species encoded by each virus, p27 and p21 in HTLV-I and p26 and p24 in HTLV-II. Since antisera to the carboxy termini will immunoprecipitate both species, and since deletion of an internal methionine codon in the HTLV-I *rex* open reading frame results in loss of HTLV-I p21, the smaller Rex presumably initiates from an internal methionine codon. No function has been found for the smaller Rex protein in either virus.

HTLV-I Rex appears to increase the relative amount of cytoplasmic non-spliced *gag/pol* and partially spliced *env* mRNA, and decreases the relative amount of doubly spliced *tax/rex* mRNA. Using co-transfection of mutant proviral HTLV-I constructs into a fibroblast cell line, Yoshida and co-workers observed a time-dependent change in cytoplasmic mRNA species, as assayed by Northern blot in the presence of Rex. Those kinetic studies showed that *tax/rex* mRNA appears first in the cytoplasm by 10 hours after transfection; by 16 hours, *gag*, *pol* and *env* mRNA increase significantly, with a subsequent dramatic decline in *tax/rex* mRNA, and then a lesser decline in *gag*, *pol* and *env* mRNA by 52 hours. RSV promoter-driven HTLV-I proviral constructs also showed an increase in cytoplasmic unspliced message without Tax in the presence of Rex, further demonstrating a post-transcriptional Tax-independent effect. Previous work by the same laboratory showed similar increases in unspliced cytoplasmic viral RNA even with the proviral constructs lacking a known HTLV-I splice acceptor, suggesting that the increase in cytoplasmic unspliced message was not due to direct inhibition of splicing. These observed effects of Rex in HTLV-I require a 300 bp region in the 3′ LTR which corresponds to a stable postulated stem loop and RNA structure. Other investigators observed a Rex-dependent increase in cytoplasmic *gag/pol* mRNA, and argue that Rex regulation in HTLV-I is due at least in part to facilitation of nuclear to cytoplasmic transport of unspliced message. The overall model proposed for Rex regulation in HTLV-I is that Rex increases expression of late structural *gag*, *pol* and *env* genes and decreases expression of early *tax/rex* genes. The decrease in Tax/Rex expression may also serve to diminish overall LTR-directed transcription, since less Tax would be produced, and may play a role in the induction of latency.

In HTLV-II, Shimotohno and co-workers have analysed total cellular RNA in co-transfection experiments in COS cells, and observed an increased in the ratio of unspliced to spliced mRNA from cytomegalovirus (CMV)-driven partial proviral constructs in the presence of Rex. This Rex effect required *cis*-acting sequences approximately 70 nucleotides (nt) downstream of the splice donor site in the HTLV-II LTR. As with HTLV-I, when viral mRNA transcription is driven by a non-HTLV enhancer, the increase in the ratio of unspliced to spliced viral mRNA still occurs with Rex, suggesting a post-transcriptional mechanism. In co-transfection experiments in lymphoid cells by our laboratory using the HTLV-II LTR linked to the CAT indicator gene, we have demonstrated: (i) marked potentiation of Tax-mediated *trans*-activation by low levels of Rex; and (ii) inhibition by high levels of Rex. In S_1 nuclease experiments using an oligonucleotide probe protecting mRNA initiating from the HTLV-II LTR cap site, the total cellular amount of viral HTLV-I remained stable despite marked changes in HTLV-II LTR-linked gene expression with or without Rex, suggesting a post-transcriptional mechanism of action. R/U5 deletion constructs linking the truncated HTLV-II LTR to the CAT gene also localized the *cis*-acting Rex-responsive sequences to the R/U5 region of the 5′ LTR. The precise mechanism of action of Rex in HTLV-II remains less well defined than in HTLV-I, although it is presumed to be similar.

Infection with HTLV-I and -II occasionally causes lymphoid malignancy. Although several cell types permit viral replication, only T-cells become transformed in cell culture, which corresponds to the clinical association of HTLV-I and -II with T-cell leukemia and lymphoma. Studies of ATL cells have established that malignant transformation by HTLV-I involves neither a recognized viral oncogene nor integration adjacent to a cellular oncogene in the host cell genome. Thus, attention has focused on the possible role of the HTLV *trans*-acting proteins, Tax and Rex, in this process. Tax *trans*-activates gene expression from the IL-2 and IL-2 receptor promoters, and the IL-2 receptor α chain is over-produced in most but not all ATL cell lines. Recent work using RNA PCR to detect low levels of viral mRNA have shown persistent *tax/rex* mRNA in fresh peripheral blood mononuclear cells of asymptomatic HTLV-I carriers and ATL patients, although the level of mRNA is too low to expect significant production of Tax and Rex. HTLV-I Tax, under control of the HTLV-I promoter, appears to induce tumors, albeit non-lymphoid (neurofibromas), in transgenic mice. Infection of fresh peripheral blood lymphocytes by a replication-competent transformation-defective herpesvirus *Saimiri* vector encoding Tax and Rex has resulted in immortalized but IL-2-dependent cells (HTLV-transformed T-cells are typically IL-2-independent) in tissue culture. Although these different observations indirectly link HTLV-I *tax* expression with malignant transformation, a precise mechanism for this process and the possible contribution by Rex remain unclear.

HUMAN IMMUNODEFICIENCY VIRUS TYPE 1 (HIV-1) *tat* AND *rev*

HIV-1 causes the acquired immunodeficiency syndrome (AIDS), a progressive fatal illness which is characterized by susceptibility to infection, by development of encephalopathy and by increased incidence of malignancy, particularly Kaposi's sarcoma and non-Hodgkin's lymphomas. AIDS has reached epidemic proportions among high-risk groups in the United States, including male homosexuals, intravenous drug abusers and hemophiliacs.

HIV-1 is an approximately 10 kb retrovirus, like HTLV-I and HTLV-II, but it has a more complex genomic organization, with at least six different non-structural viral proteins. The two most completely characterized *trans*-acting HIV-1 proteins are Tat and Rev, which, like Tax and Rex, are encoded on partially overlapping genes and act as essential regulatory proteins in the HIV-1 life cycle.

Tat is required for HIV LTR-linked gene expression, appears to increase steady-state levels of viral mRNA, and possibly increases viral mRNA translation as well. *In vitro* nuclear run-off studies suggest that the major effect of Tat is at the level of transcription initiation. Tat-mediated *trans*-activation requires *cis*-acting response regions of the HIV-1 5′ LTR between -17 and $+44$ of the cap site, the TAR region, which is capable of forming a stable stem loop RNA secondary structure, and −105 to −17, which contain an enhancer element, an SP1 site and the TATA box. Cellular transcription factors that bind to these elements are important in the regulation of basal and Tat-induced transcription in HeLa cells, suggesting that *trans*-activation involves interaction with these cellular proteins.

Rev is a 20 kDa phosphorylated protein located in the nucleus, in particular in the nucleolus of infected or transfected cells. Rev is required for expression of viral structural proteins and is essential for viral replication in culture. Several investigators have found an increase in the ratio of unspliced to spliced viral mRNA from total cell extracts in the presence of Rev, but since removal of known splice sites does not appear to change observed Rev effects on HIV-1 gene expression, direct inhibition of splicing by Rev appears unlikely. Other investigators evaluated nuclear and cytoplasmic RNA from transfected cells and observed an increase in unspliced viral mRNA in the cytoplasm relative to the nucleus in the presence of Rev, suggesting that Rev facilitates nuclear to cytoplasmic transport. This Rev effect requires a *cis*-acting region of approximately 230 nucleotides in the *env*-coding sequence downstream of the first splice acceptor site—the Rev-responsive element (RRE)—which is capable of forming a stable stem loop RNA secondary structure. Rev protein mutagenesis studies have identified an arginine-rich N-terminal region involved in nucleolar localization, and a C-terminal functional domain apparently mediating transport of unspliced viral message. Co-transfections of HIV Rev-deficient mutants with HTLV-I or HTLV-II *rex* vectors show rescue of p24 (HIV-1 *gag*) production, which is abrogated if the RRE is deleted, suggesting a similar mechanism of nuclear to cytoplasmic transport of unspliced viral message for Rex in HTLV-I and -II.

Beyond a critical role in HIV gene expression, HIV-1 Tat has been recently implicated as a possible transforming agent. Unlike HTLV-I and -II, HIV-1 has not been shown to directly cause cell transformation despite the significantly increased incidence of certain malignancies, particularly Kaposi's sarcoma in patients with AIDS. However, when a plasmid expressing HIV-1 Tat from the HIV-1 LTR was introduced into a transgenic mouse germ line, skin lesions resembling Kaposi's sarcoma were observed, suggesting that Tat expression may help induce Kaposi's sarcoma. Long-term cultures of Kaposi's sarcoma cells have been established using growth factors released by CD4-positive T-lymphocytes infected with HTLV-I, HTLV-II or HIV-1. Thus, retroviral *trans*-activating proteins may act either directly or indirectly through stimulation of growth factors to induce Kaposi's sarcoma.

CONCLUSIONS

Trans-acting viral proteins in many DNA and RNA viruses regulate the viral life cycle, and are capable of interacting with a variety of cellular genetic elements. The viruses discussed in this chapter all encode at least one viral protein localized to the nucleus that preferentially *trans*-activates viral promoter/enhancer elements, apparently through interaction with pre-existing cellular transcription factors that may directly bind to these *cis*-acting responsive sequences. Mutations in the functional domains of these regulatory proteins markedly decrease or abolish viral gene expression. In concert with stimulation of viral gene transcription, *trans*-acting viral proteins also trigger the switch from early viral life cycle, involving production of regulatory proteins and viral genome replication, to late viral life cycle, involving production of structural proteins and virion assembly. This switch may be mediated by the same transcriptional *trans*-activating proteins, as with SV40 T-antigen, or by other post-transcriptional *trans*-acting proteins, as with Rex in HTLV-I and -II and Rev in HIV-1.

The mechanisms underlying the switch from early to late viral life cycle are complex, and differ significantly between the viruses discussed. SV40 T-antigen appears to stimulate early gene transcription through a preferential interaction with specific *cis*-acting sequences, site I, at the initial lower levels of SV40 T-antigen expression, but diminishes transcription from the same SV40 promoter by interaction with other *cis*-acting sequences, sites II and III, when higher levels of SV40 T-antigen are attained. Rev in HIV-1 appears to act post-transcriptionally by sequence-specific nuclear to cytoplasmic transport of unspliced and partially spliced viral mRNAs (*gag*, *pol* and *env*) that are otherwise excluded from the cytoplasm. Although direct supporting evidence has not yet been published, most studies suggest a similar role for Rex in HTLV-I. In both cases, transport causes a cytoplasmic accumulation of *gag*, *pol* and *env* mRNA, thus, late cycle structural protein production. However, Rex in HTLV-I also causes a significant decline in overall doubly spliced mRNA, and thus Tax and Rex expression, which, due to decreased levels of the *trans*-activator, Tax, decreases levels of all viral mRNA species. In HTLV-II, the effects of Rex are less clear, but appear to involve both a post-transcriptional positive regulatory effect, with preferential accumulation of unspliced viral mRNA, and an overall negative regulatory effect at high levels of Rex that may be at the level of viral mRNA transcription or stability. Differences in Rev and Rex effects on total viral mRNA levels over time with persistent high-level *trans*-activation by Tat, as opposed to overall decreased viral mRNA in HTLV-I and -II with continued Rex action, may partially explain the tendency towards lysis in HIV-1 and non-lytic budding or latency in HTLV-I and -II.

Recent epidemiologic studies have demonstrated a significant rate of HTLV-II infection in a cohort of IVDA in New Orleans, a high HIV-1-risk population, which raises the possibility of co-infection with HTLVs and HIV-1. Co-transfection experiments using Rev-deficient HIV-1 mutants and HTLV-I and -II *rex* expression vectors have shown that HTLV-I and -II Rex can rescue HIV-1 p24 (*gag*) production, suggesting that crossover effects by *trans*-acting regulatory proteins might occur in co-infected cells. Peripheral blood T-cells infected with HIV-1 can also be induced to produce large quantities of HIV-1 after mitogenic stimulation with non-infectious HTLV-I virions. Thus, HIV-1 and HTLV-I or -II co-infection may change the clinical course of the dominant illness, like AIDS.

In addition to a crucial role in the viral life cycle, viral *trans*-acting proteins may contribute to cancer induction in some virally infected cells. Both E1a and SV40 T-antigen can bind the retinoblastoma gene product, which appears to act as an anti-oncogene by suppressing unregulated cell growth. A possible role for this interaction in the viral life cycle is that these DNA viruses replicate more efficiently if infected cells are stimulated to enter S phase, which might occur if the suppressive effect on cellular proliferation of the retinoblastoma gene product was abrogated.

Despite having neither a viral oncogene nor a specific proviral integration site near a cellular proto-oncogene, HTLV-I, HTLV-II and HIV-1 are also associated with human malignancy. Immunodeficient mouse models have been used to show tumor induction from transfected plasmids containing the appropriate viral LTR linked to *tat* or *tax*, and Kaposi's sarcoma cell lines have been developed using growth factors expressed by retrovirally infected cells. Both Tat in HIV-1 and Tax in HTLV-I and -II have been shown to *trans*-activate a variety of heterologous viral and cellular promoters, including promoters for several lymphokines and lymphokine receptors. Thus, results from different experimental systems suggest that autocrine stimulation by Tax- or Tat-induced growth factors may cause uncontrolled proliferation of certain infected cells, leading to malignancies such as ATL and possibly Kaposi's sarcoma.

Trans-activating viral proteins in general appear to have at least two distinct domains, one determining specificity of nucleic acid or protein interaction, and the second possessing an activation function, similar to the structure of many eukaryotic transcription factors. As has been shown with HSV-1 VP16 protein, mutations in the functional or activating domains of regulatory proteins may lead to a dominant inhibitory phenotype with *trans*-inhibition of activation by wild-type regulatory proteins. Baltimore has suggested that mutant regulatory proteins might eventually be used as 'intracellular immunogens' to inhibit wild-type regulatory proteins of pathogenic viruses, disrupting the viral life cycle and possibly altering the clinical course of the associated human disease, such as AIDS. Study of *trans*-acting viral genes can thus shed light on crucial aspects of viral pathogenesis and host cell transformation, and perhaps result in novel, effective therapies for serious virally induced human illnesses.

FURTHER READING

Baltimore, D. (1988) Intracellular immunization. *Nature*, **335**, 395–396.

Berk, A. J. (1986) Adenovirus promoters and E1a *trans*-activation. *Ann. Rev. Genet.*, **20**, 45–79.

Dynan, W. S. and Tjian, R. (1985) Control of eukaryotic messenger RNA synthesis by sequence-specific DNA-binding proteins. *Nature*, **316**, 774–778.

Everett, R. D. (1987) The regulation of transcription of viral and cellular genes by herpes virus immediate early gene products. *Anticancer Res.*, **4A**, 589–604.

Greene, W., Bohnlein, E. and Ballard, D. (1989) HIV-1, HTLV-I and normal T-cell growth: Transcriptional strategies and surprises. *Immunol. Today*, **10**, 272–278.

Ludlow, J., De Caprio, J., Huang, C. -M., *et al*. (1989) SV40 large T-antigen binds preferentially to an underphosphorylated member of the retinoblastoma susceptibility gene product family. *Cell*, **56**, 57–65.

Rosenblatt, J. D., Chen, I. S. Y. and Wachsman, W. (1988) Infection with HTLV-I and HTLV-II: Evolving concepts. *Semin. Hematol.*, **25**, 230–246.

Triezenberg, S., Kingsbury, R. and McKnight, S. (1988) Functional dissection of VP-16, the transactivator of herpes simplex virus immediate early gene expression. *Genes Dev.*, **2**, 718–729.

Varmus, H. (1988) Regulation of HIV and HTLV gene expression. *Genes Dev.*, **2**, 1055–1062.

Whyte, P., Williamson, N. and Harlow, E. (1989) Cellular targets for transformation by the adenovirus E1A proteins. *Cell*, **56**, 67–75.

Molecular Therapy: Antibodies

14 | Designer Antibodies

JOHN R. ADAIR
NIGEL R. WHITTLE
RAYMOND J. OWENS

ANTIBODIES AS CLINICAL REAGENTS

Antibodies have for a long time been viewed as potential agents for targeted drug delivery. The use of antibodies for the treatment of human tumours dates back to the work of Lindstrom who in 1927 used antiserum to treat chronic myelogenous leukaemia. Since the development of monoclonal antibody (MAb) technology in 1975 it has been possible in principle to produce a MAb to any antigen. A large number of rodent MAbs have been generated over the last 10 years which recognise a wide range of antigens. These include tumour-associated antigens, other cell-specific surface markers, viruses, bacteria and specific protein products, e.g. lymphokines and cytokines.

Monoclonal antibodies have made a significant contribution to cancer diagnosis, for example in immunoscintigraphy and immunohistochemistry. Considerable effort has also been invested in devising uses for antibodies in cancer therapy. In general, administration of antibody alone appears to have little effect on tumour regression *in vivo*. There are some notable exceptions. For example, the MAb 17-1A, a murine IgG2a which recognises a colon carcinoma associated antigen, has been shown to cause tumour cell lysis both *in vitro* and *in vivo*, probably via the host antibody-dependent cellular cytotoxicity (ADCC) system. In most cases, however, the antibody has been viewed as a highly specific targeting agent for the delivery of other effector or reporter moieties.

In this review we will briefly examine the key problems in the use of MAbs as therapeutic agents in cancer—immunogenicity, tissue penetration and the nature of the therapeutic effector—and for each area outline current approaches to improving the utility of these materials using recombinant DNA technology.

Genes and Cancer. Edited by D. Carney and K. Sikora
©1990 John Wiley & Sons Ltd

IMMUNOGENICITY

Antibodies as antigens

Most MAbs that have been used to date are derived from mouse or rat. While it should be possible to produce human MAbs against human antigens, technically this procedure has lagged behind the production of MAbs in rodents. A potential problem with the use of rodent MAbs as reagents for diagnosis and therapy—whether linked to an effector or reporter, or as the antibody alone or as an antibody fragment—is the xenogeneic source of the antibody. It has been noted in a number of studies that a consequence of administering repeat doses of xenogeneic immunoglobulin is that the recipient mounts an immune response against the antibody which may reduce the utility of the product. This response has been termed the HAMA (Human Anti-Mouse Antibody) response in the case where a mouse MAb is used in humans. Typically when serum is taken during the course of a study significant levels of HAMA can be detected; this consists of low affinity IgM, and also IgG. The antibody titre tends to increase with the kinetics expected for a secondary response, consistent with the presence of the pre-existing antibody. In some but not all cases the initial reactivity can be correlated with the presence of rheumatoid autoimmune factors which cross-react with murine antibodies. Antibody detected in the early phase of the response tends to be directed towards the Fc region of the MAb but during the course of the response reactivity against the $F(ab')_2$, and particularly the variable region, including the antigen binding site (anti-idiotype), can be detected. In some cases the anti-idiotype response can become a major component. For the antibody A5B7, which recognises the carcinoembryonic antigen (CEA), it was noted that serum HAMA levels above $30\mu g\ ml^{-1}$ led to accelerated clearance of antibody and absence of tumour localisation. However, it has also been observed that the response varies depending on the tumour type and patient. In cases where the disease condition leads to hypogammaglobulinaemia a reduced HAMA response has been noted.

It has also been clearly demonstrated that the HAMA response can have a significant effect when anti-T-cell antibody is used as an immunosuppressant in the treatment of acute allograft rejection. In the case of OKT3, a mouse MAb which recognises an antigen in the T-cell receptor-CD3 complex on most human T-cells, the data suggest that a significant HAMA response to both isotype and idiotype develops after 10 days of the start of a daily treatment regime. As the HAMA titre rises, CD3-positive T-cells reappear in the blood and rejection of the graft can occur. In some patients the anti-idiotype response was 50–60% of the total HAMA response.

An obvious way to reduce or remove the anti-antibody response is to replace as much as possible of the immunogenic non-human sequence with equivalent human sequence using the techniques of molecular biology.

Construction of chimaeric antibodies

Human and mouse antibodies (and by inference antibodies from other species, e.g. rat) have been shown to have conserved three-dimensional protein structures comprising discrete folding domains represented at the gene level as separate exons. This conservation of gene and protein organisation means that it is feasible for a particular MAb to be 'humanised' by replacing the DNA sequences from rodent heavy and light chain genes with suitable sequences from human antibody genes. If the constant regions only are replaced the resultant antibody is termed a chimaera, while if the constant regions and a significant part of the variable regions, not including those residues required for antigen binding, are replaced the resultant protein is termed a CDR (Complementarity Determining Region) grafted antibody. Careful choice of the constant region used in the construction of the chimaera may have a bearing on the efficacy of the resultant protein. Each antibody isotype differs in effector functions due to sequence variation in the Fc region of the antibody. For example IgG1 and IgG3 are more effective in ADCC and complement-mediated lysis than IgG2 or IgG4. Recently, sequences responsible for the binding of C1q, the first component of the complement cascade, have been identified. Similarly, sequences involved in the binding of antibody by cell receptors have begun to be identified. Using this information it should be possible to produce specifically tailored Fc regions containing all or some of the inherent Fc functions of antibody.

Early published data concentrated on the formation of chimaeric antibodies in model hapten systems, but the potential uses of the process in therapeutic situations has led to the publication of a number of papers describing chimaeric antibodies to various tumour-specific and other cell surface markers. Two strategies have emerged for the construction and expression of chimaeric genes. In one procedure genomic DNA from a hybridoma producing the MAb of choice is cloned and DNA fragments coding for the variable gene exon along with the signal sequence exon for each of the light and heavy chains are isolated using suitable restriction sites. The rodent genomic DNA is inserted in front of the required human constant region DNA and assembled in a suitable vector for expression. In this form of construct, expression of the antibody genes is usually achieved using the Ig promoter/enhancer in a myeloma line which has been selected for loss of expression of one or both of the resident antibody chains. The genes for light and heavy chain are usually introduced on separate plasmids and can be co-transfected or transfected separately in series. Yields of material ranging from 1 to 100 μg ml^{-1} have been quoted, bringing such transfectomas within the range seen for hybridoma cultures.

The second strategy that has been adopted involves construction of a cDNA library using mRNA derived from the hybridoma of choice (Figure 1). This library can be prepared using oligo-dT as primer for first strand synthesis to produce full-length cDNAs for the heavy and light chains, or specific primers can be used to clone the variable regions only. Following isolation by hybridisation screening the variable regions of the cDNAs are then fused to the constant region DNA of the human antibody of choice. The constant regions may be in the form of cDNA or genomic DNA and have been altered by silent site oligonucleotide-directed mutagenesis to provide usefully located acceptor restriction sites. In each case the variable region DNA becomes fused to the CH1 domain DNA of the human constant region. The chimaeric gene can then be inserted into an expression vector for expression in the cell type of choice. This procedure allows for the use of promoter/

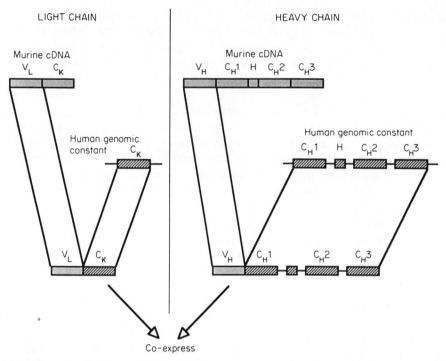

Figure 1. Diagramatic representation of the construction of chimaeric antibody. Genes for the light and heavy chain proteins are identified in a cDNA library prepared from mRNA from the hybridoma of choice. Useful restriction sites at or near the 3' end of the variable domain sequences are identified. In those cases where no useful sites are found a site can be introduced by oligonucleotide directed silent site mutagenesis. Oligonucleotide adapters are designed to link the variable region to the desired constant region. The constant region sequences have been modified to contain useful restriction sites for the construction of chimaeric or CDR grafted genes, and the heavy chain genes have been further modified so that construction of an Fd or Fd' fragment is a simple procedure. Once the genes have been reconstructed they are transferred to expression vectors and antibody is produced by co-expression of the antibody genes, initially in a COS cell transient expression system to demonstrate rapidly that the DNA manipulations have been successful, and then as a CHO stable cell line

enhancer systems other than the Ig promoter, and non-myeloid cells can be used for the expression of the genes. Expression in Chinese hamster ovary cells using the human cytomegalovirus major immediate early promoter/enhancer is currently favoured at Celltech.

More recently a refinement of the 'humanisation' procedure has been published, in which the DNA sequences for the hypervariable regions of the variable domains— the CDRs—are removed from the rodent antibody and substituted into the corresponding positions of the gene for a human myeloma. The CDRs code in the main for the surface loops which form the antigen-binding surface patch. The entire variable region DNA can be generated by gene synthesis or by using site-directed mutagenesis to replace existing hypervariable regions with new sequence. There may be circumstances in which the transfer of the hypervariable regions alone is not sufficient to restore antigen binding, and judicious alterations to the remainder of the variable domains may be needed to develop an active antibody. Once the variable gene DNA is constructed the antibody gene can be assembled and expressed using either of the strategies described above for the construction of chimaeric antibodies.

Clinical applications of humanised antibodies

At the time of writing reports are beginning to emerge relating to the clinical use of humanised rodent MAbs. Two recent conference papers describe results with chimaeric mouse-human versions of an anti-colorectal cancer antibody, 17-1A, and an anti-CD4 antibody which have been used in patient studies. The data suggest that anti-antibody was not detected under the circumstances of the studies. In the case of the chimaeric 17-1A the pharmacokinetics of the antibody were not affected, indicating that a significant immune response had not been generated.

The only other published example of the use of a humanised antibody describes a small study with the CDR grafted CAMPATH-1H antibody. This rat antibody recognises an antigen on virtually all lymphoid cells and monocytes but not on other cell types. The antibody has been used to treat lymphoid malignant disorders and to purge bone marrow of T-cells prior to transfusion so as to prevent a graft-versus-host reaction. Two patients with non-Hodgkin's lymphoma have been treated with CAMPATH-1H for up to 43 days with escalating doses ranging from 1 to 20 mg day^{-1} by intravenous infusion. In both cases a significant response was noted and no antibody response was detected during the course of treatment. However, the authors of the report stress that in this case the lack of response may be due to the fact that the antibody itself is immunosuppressive and the patients were already immunosuppressed as a result of their disease.

For the future, other avenues to circumventing the HAMA response are being explored. It has recently been shown that it is possible to rescue the genes for human monoclonal antibodies from early and potentially unstable human hybridomas and to introduce the genes into expression vectors as described above. This offers the advantage that the constant regions of the human MAb can be changed or modified, or defined fragments prepared as described below. Finally the development of mice which carry the cells of the human immune system offers the possibility of preparing effectively human hybridomas using 'classical' murine hybridoma technology.

TISSUE PENETRATION AND CLEARANCE

Antibody localisation

For an antibody or antibody-conjugate to be effective in cancer diagnosis or therapy, it must obviously reach and accumulate at the tumour site. This will be affected by a number of factors.

1. Firstly, the antibody must remain in the patient's circulatory sytem long enough to allow diffusion to the site of action to take place. In the case of targeting solid tumours, the antibody molecules must also freely penetrate throughout the tumour mass at a high concentration in order that a sufficient number of molecules can gain access to the surface of the neoplastic cells, where they can recognise and bind the specific tumour-associated antigen. Additionally, the binding must be stable and persist for sufficient time for the antibody or antibody-conjugate to be effective.

2. Secondly, the antibody must be cleared rapidly from the rest of the system in order to minimise the damage to non-binding cells and tissues.

These potentially conflicting requirements suggest that the most effective molecule would be a high-affinity antibody species with a high penetrative power, but possessing a brief biological half-life, being rapidly cleared by filtration through the kidneys, rather than via uptake and degradation by the reticuloendothelial system of the liver.

Penetration of the antibody into the tumour may be a key issue. In normal tissues the access of antibody molecules to cells is tightly controlled, and the barrier to the passage of antibodies varies on different tissues. For example in certain tissues, e.g. liver, spleen and bone marrow, there is little resistance to the passage of large macromolecules due to the presence of discontinuous endothelium containing a number of gaps and the absence of basement membrane beneath the cells. Administered immunoglobulin may then diffuse across the capillary wall, passing both across and between endothelial cells, and through the extracellular matrix to enter the extravascular space. The extravascular fluid here bathes the connective tissue, and in many tissues the cells are not usually tightly bound to each other by adhesions such as desmosomes and tight junctions. Antibody may therefore diffuse throughout the tissue and usually has free access to the surfaces of cells. Conversely in lung and skin there is poor permeability, and passage occurs via intracytoplasmic vesicles and trans-endothelial cell channels. The degree of antibody penetration may be profoundly affected by changes in the structure of tissues, such as the formation of tumours. In many instances tumours are poorly vascularised, minimising the flow of blood through them, and leading to the formation of a hypoxic necrotic core. In other tumours there is an efficient blood supply, but the density and connectivity of cells prevents diffusion of large solute molecules.

Use of antibody fragments

An IgG immunoglobulin is a 150 kDa tetrameric glycosylated protein molecule possessing a large Stokes radius, which may hinder its free diffusion across semi-permeable cellular barriers. A potential solution to the problem of penetration is the use of antibody fragments which retain the intact variable regions and therefore retain the antigen-specificity of the parent antibody molecule, but have had varying portions of the constant regions removed in order to reduce the molecular size; hence they lack the effector functions associated with whole immunoglobulin and which are factors in the clearance of whole antibody. For example, loss of the Fc receptor binding site may minimise uptake by the reticuloendothelial system, and hence reduce catabolism of the circulating antibody. Fc carbohydrate may also be involved in liver uptake of antibodies via the galactose receptor. In order to maintain the diagnostic or therapeutic utility of the molecule it may be necessary to replace one or more of these functions with an alternative effector agent (see below).

Antibody fragments can be made by proteolytic digestion using enzymes such as papain, which cleaves before the hinge domain to generate a monovalent Fab fragment, or pepsin, which cleaves after the hinge domain to generate a divalent F(ab′)$_2$ fragment, in each case with loss of the CH2 and CH3 domains. There are a number of instances in the literature of the generation and use of Fab fragments of tumour-specific antibodies in animal model systems or in clinical use to target tumour cells for diagnosis. It has been demonstrated that a better antibody localisation on tumours (i.e. an increased ratio of antibody binding to tumour over normal tissue) can be obtained using F(ab′)$_2$ and especially Fab fragments, as compared with whole antibody. This is presumably due to the increased penetrative ability of a small molecule. However, in all these studies the actual loading of antibody on the tumour was shown to decrease as the size decreased, presumably due to increased clearance and a diminished residence time in the systemic circulation. Thus Fab-based fragments appear to be the most promising reagents for human tumour immunoscintigraphy, if not for therapy. The advantage of the F(ab′)$_2$ species is that the divalent nature of the antibody is retained, enabling the fragment to bind to contiguous epitopes present at high density on the surfaces of target cells, and therefore the effective avidity of the antibody is high, resulting in more stable binding between the MAb and the cells. This may be particularly important where a low-affinity antibody is being used. The advantage of the Fab fragment is that the molecular weight and hence the size of the molecule is less than a third that of the whole antibody. However, clearance by the kidneys becomes correspondingly rapid, which may necessitate prohibitively large doses of antibody.

Proteolysis of antibodies in order to generate Fab fragments can be an unpredictable and difficult process, often producing problems such as clipping of the antibody, leading to loss of activity. There is also the need for reproducible batch production and processing of the antibody, which can cause regulatory problems and detract from clinical acceptability of the product.

Construction of antibody fragments

An improved system for the production of Fab fragments is by genetic engineering techniques, which then produce a defined product with little or no requirement for processing beyond the purification stage (Figure 2). At Celltech tumour-specific chimaeric antibody heavy chain genes have been constructed by site-directed mutagenesis and gene assembly in which the exons encoding the hinge, CH2 and CH3 domains have been removed from the chimaeric antibody and replaced with a translational stop codon in order to generate an Fd gene. Additionally, genes have been constructed in which DNA sequences encoding a particular IgG hinge sequence have been introduced adjacent to the Fd sequence in order to generate Fd′ genes containing any one of a number of possible hinges. When transfected together with the intact chimaeric light chain gene into mammalian cell expression systems as outlined earlier, the heavy and light chain genes are expressed, associate to form

CHIMAERIC ANTIBODY CONSTRUCTS

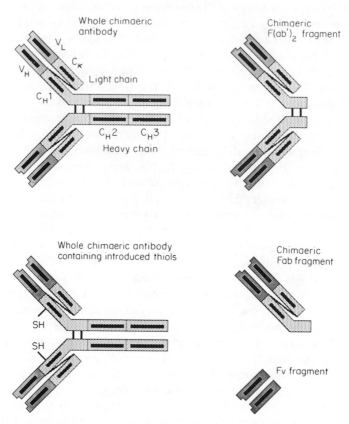

Figure 2. Diagrammatic representation of antibody or antibody fragments produced by recombinant DNA procedures. The antibody is represented as four hatched boxes which are subdivided internally into light and dark hatching. The dark hatching represents the variable domain from the rodent antibody and the light hatched region represents the domains obtained from a human antibody. Heavy black lines represent intra- or inter-chain disulphide bridges

either $F(ab')_2$ or Fab' fragments (Figure 2), and are secreted into the medium. Increasing the number of potential disulphide bridges capable of forming in the hinge by increasing the number of cysteines in the hinge sequence causes the formation of more $F(ab')_2$ than Fab'. The heavy and light chains then remain associated due to the presence of interchain disulphide bonds.

The smallest fragment of the antibody molecule that retains the antigen-binding activity is the Fv, composed of the variable regions of the heavy and light chains (Figure 2). Currently a number of groups are investigating the development of genetically engineered Fv fragments. The gene sequences for each domain have been constructed and expressed together in a number of systems, including *E. coli*, yeast and mammalian cell systems. In whole antibody, the two polypeptide chains of the variable region are not joined covalently; instead they associate through hydrophobic interactions. It has been shown in a number of cases that these hydrophobic interactions are sufficiently strong to stabilise the Fv molecule, at least in the presence of antigen. One possible route to the further stabilisation of these Fv molecules is the construction of a single gene containing a linking sequence arranged in such a way that translation *in vivo* leads to the production of a single polypeptide containing the two variable region protein domains correctly arranged and orientated. The major advantage of the use of Fv fragments is that due to their small size they should be highly penetrative and rapidly cleared from the rest of the system, hence giving a good signal/noise ratio. They also lend themselves readily to high-level production in microbiological systems.

THE THERAPEUTIC EFFECTOR

Antibody conjugates

Most applications of MAbs to cancer treatment require the attachment of effector (or reporter) molecules to the antibody. Three types of killing agent conjugated to antibodies are being evaluated:

1. Radionuclides, e.g. ^{90}Yttrium
2. Drugs, e.g. alkaloids
3. Toxins, e.g. ricin A chain

Currently, antibody labelling technology involves the non-selective modification of amino acid side-chains, e.g. tyrosine and lysine, in order to generate one or more randomly located attachment sites on the antibody. These are reacted with specific functional groups, for example thiols, on the effector molecule. The procedure can often lead to a decrease in the affinity of the antibody due to the modification of residues close to the antigen-binding site. This is particularly a problem for the preparation of antibody-drug conjugates. Cell killing requires the delivery of large amounts of the anti-cancer drug to the tumour target ($>10^6$ molecules/cell). Therefore each antibody has to be coupled to several drug molecules, increasing the chances of impairing the antigen-binding activity. Antibodies will obviously vary in their resistance to chemical substitution, depending upon the sequences at the antigen-binding site, thus the production of conjugates is a largely empirical and unpredictable business.

Site-specific attachment of effector to antibody

In view of the limitations of current technology, a simple reproducible method for attaching effector molecules to a wide range of MAbs is highly desirable. The value of labelling antibodies site-specifically has recently been demonstrated using Fc carbohydrate side-chains as the points of attachment. Antibody conjugated in this way retains the antigen-binding activity of the unmodified control, whereas randomly labelled antibody shows reduced activity. However, this method involves periodate oxidation of sugar residues to reactive aldehydes, a procedure that may also modify a number of amino acids, particularly methionine. In addition since the method depends upon labelling Fc carbohydrate, it cannot be used to label Fab' or F(ab')$_2$ fragments.

At Celltech, an alternative approach to labelling antibodies has been taken using the thiol groups of cysteines as the points of attachment. To avoid the problems of random/multiple coupling, the possibility of engineering cysteine residues into an antibody at predetermined positions has been explored. It has been shown that cysteine residues can be substituted into the CH1 domain of the heavy chain by site-directed mutagenesis without adversely affecting the binding properties of the antibody (Figure 2). However, it has been found that the availability of the thiol groups of the cysteines for labelling depends upon the topographical position of the introduced residues. Thus cysteines located in surface 'pockets' can be used for site-specific attachment to the antibody, whereas those at more accessible sites appear to be blocked. This procedure has been used to link a tumour-specific MAb to a radionuclide-chelator complex. The resulting complex has been shown to localise specifically to human tumour cells in a mouse xenograft model.

The above study illustrates the possibility of building attachment sites into antibodies using recombinant DNA techniques. This technology can be combined with suitable chemistry to construct antibody conjugates with drugs, toxins or radioisotopes using a variety of different antibodies or antibody fragments.

Genetic fusion of antibody to effector

For antibody conjugates involving protein effector molecules, it is attractive to consider linking the two elements at the genetic level. This is particularly relevant to immunotoxins, which are highly potent and require the antibody to deliver as little as one molecule to the target cell to cause cell killing. Pioneering work by Neuberger and co-workers in 1984 demonstrated the principle that a bi-functional molecule could be produced from fusion of an antibody gene to that of a novel effector, in this case either a bacterial nuclease or DNA polymerase. The genetic hybrids were constructed using the DNA sequence encoding the Fd fragment of the heavy chain. Similar antibody-enzyme chimaeras have been made between the serine protease domain of tissue plasminogen activator and a fibrin-specific MAb. Using a similar approach it seems possible that a genetic hybrid could be made between a tumour-specific MAb and a toxin. It would obviously be necessary to ensure that the conjugate did not prove toxic to the cells in which it was to be produced. In this context recent work at the NIH by Pastan and co-workers has involved construction of a 'cytotoxin' by replacing the cell-binding domain of *Pseudomonas* exotoxin with the cytokines, IL-1 or IL-2. The toxin conjugate was produced in *E. coli* and shown to specifically target the toxin to T-lymphocytes expressing either the IL-1 or IL-2 receptor.

Bi-specific antibody

An alternative to covalently or genetically linking the antibody to the effector would be to make use of the bivalent nature of the antibody. In this sytem a bi-specific antibody is used in which one Fab arm of the antibody recognises the target cell whilst the other binds to an effector, e.g. a drug or toxin. The bi-specific antibody can be prepared by fusing two hybridomas expressing the two required specificities and selecting the desired hybrid from the randomly segregated heavy and light chains.

Alternatively, chemical cross-linking can be used to join the dissociated heavy chains or the Fab fragments of the two antibodies. The yield of bi-specific antibody from both these methods can be limited. To date no recombinant DNA approach to producing bi-specific antibodies has been reported.

A limitation of this system is the reliance on non-covalent interactions to link antibody and effector, which may not be sufficiently stable *in vivo*. In addition, binding of the bi-specific antibody to the tumour cell will be monovalent and hence possess reduced avidity. If tumour cell uptake depends upon cross-linking the antigen at the cell surface the bi-specific antibody may not easily penetrate the target cell.

CONCLUDING REMARKS

The exquisite specificity of antibodies means that they have potential as therapeutic reagents. The problems inherent in the clinical use of a large, multi-subunit, glycosylated protein complex are being addressed using recombinant DNA procedures. In this chapter we have identified some of the key problems and outlined current strategies for overcoming them. An effective therapeutic molecule will undoubtedly possess some or all of the engineered modifications described here.

FURTHER READING

Burton, D. R. (1985) *Mol. Immunol.*, **22**, 161.
Byers, V. S. and Baldwin, R. W. (1988) *Immunology*, **65**, 329.
Colcher, D., Milenic, D., Roselli, M., *et al.* (1989) *Cancer Res.*, **49**, 1738.
Hale, G., Dyer, M. S., Clark, M. R., *et al.* (1988) *Lancet*, **ii**, 1391.
Kabat, E. A., Wu, T. T., Reid-Miller, M., *et al.* (1987) In: *Sequences of Proteins of Immunological Interest*. U S Department of Health and Human Services, N I H, USA.
Neuberger, M. S., Williams, G. T. and Fox, R. O. (1984) *Nature*, **313**, 604.
Neuberger, M. S., Williams, G. T., Mitchell, E. B., *et al.* (1985) *Nature*, **314**, 268.
Roitt, I. M., Bostoff, J. and Male, D. K. (1985) In: *Immunology*. Gower Medical, London.
Skerra, A. and Pluckthun, A. (1988) *Science*, **240**, 426.
Whittle, N., Adair, J., Lloyd, J. C., *et al.* (1987) *Protein Engineering*, **1**, 499.

15 Antibodies to Synthetic Peptides

PAUL W. SHEPPARD

The investigation of cellular proteins of extremely low abundance and/or short biological life, such as most oncoproteins (see Part A: Oncogenes), often proves extremely difficult due largely to the absence of appropriate probes possessing the desired specificity. Whilst antibodies could serve as specific probes, the route to their production using conventional techniques has been difficult, if not impossible.

ANTIBODIES TO UNDEFINED PROTEINS

Recombinant DNA technology has made the isolation, characterisation and sequencing of genes a relatively straightforward matter, as witnessed by the volume of sequence data now appearing in the literature and on commercially available sequence databases. Based upon this abundance of sequence data, there are two approaches that might be considered for raising antibodies to undefined proteins with well characterised genes, namely the xenoprotein and synthetic peptide approaches.

The *xenoprotein approach* involves the isolation or synthesis of all or part of a gene of interest, which is inserted into an appropriate expression vector, cloned and subsequently used to transform bacteria. Once transformed, the bacteria are induced to express the xenoprotein, which is isolated and purified. Having obtained sufficient protein, it is used to raise antibodies in the usual manner. This method has proven itself useful in antibody production. However, it is both labour intensive and time consuming, and unfortunately the probes obtained often lack the desired degree of specificity.

Genes and Cancer. Edited by D. Carney and K. Sikora
©1990 John Wiley & Sons Ltd

The second strategy, known as the *synthetic peptide approach* to antibody production, involves the synthesis of peptides selected from the amino acid sequence of the protein, which has been inferred from the nucleotide sequence of the gene of interest. The essential feature of the approach is the predetermined and site-directed nature of the antibodies obtained. However, in order to achieve the desired degree of success many points need to be considered and addressed.

The ease, economy and reproducibility of peptide immunisation has shown it to be a most practical approach to obtaining a desired antibody, and in many cases it has produced antibodies that might otherwise have proven unobtainable. Synthetic peptides have some major advantages over proteins as antigens, not least of which is their routine availability in large quantities. In contrast, the isolation of a natural antigen may not prove practical for a number of reasons, e.g. a protein's existence may only be predicted from gene expression studies; it may be synthesised in only a few copies per cell; or it may be derived from a pathogenic organism. Moreover, with peptide immunogens, the reproducibility and assurance of the immune response is normally guaranteed. Another great advantage of synthetic peptides is that not only is it possible to purify and characterise fully before use, but that it is possible to design the antigen for the purpose intended. A linker amino acid residue may be incorporated into the peptide for conjugation purposes, or a radiolabelled amino acid may be included to permit quantitation during peptide-carrier protein conjugation. Finally, the use of peptides as immunogens enables an investigator to select precisely the part or domain of the protein to which antibodies might subsequently react.

METHODOLOGY

If antibodies of a desired specificity are to be produced using the synthetic peptide approach it is imperative that certain points be considered and appropriately addressed during the production process. A summary of the synthetic peptide approach to antibody production is presented in Figure 1. Points requiring particular consideration are the selection, synthesis and conjugation of synthetic peptides, immunisation procedures, and the purification and characterisation of resulting antibodies. Each of these points will be considered briefly.

Peptide selection

Without doubt, one of the most important and difficult steps in the entire approach is the selection of regions from the protein sequence that are likely to give rise to antibodies capable of reacting with the native protein. There is no single set of rules that will *guarantee* success; however, if certain guidelines are followed the likelihood of a successful outcome is greatly enhanced. First and foremost, it is important that the region selected be immunologically accessible, i.e. on the exterior of the protein. Many so-called predictive methods of protein sequence analysis have been proposed to aid in achieving this end; none are of particular use in isolation, but when combined they do provide a starting-point.

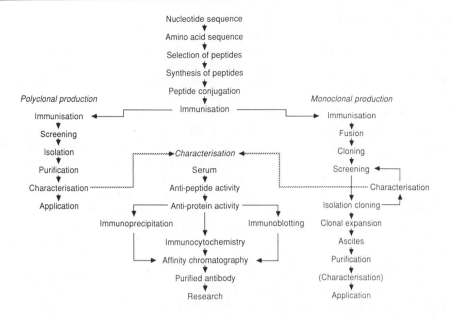

Figure 1. Synthetic peptide approach to protein antibody production

Hydrophilicity and hydropathicity analysis, in which values are assigned to each of the 20 amino acids depending upon the nature of their side-chains and used to progressively evaluate the protein sequence, defines polar and non-polar regions of the molecule. Polar regions are more likely to be surface located than non-polar and are therefore more likely to be immunologically accessible. The major problem is that such predictive analysis frequently reveals far too many potentially interesting regions than can be considered for synthesis.

Considerations of secondary structure as predicted from primary sequence were thought to be useful, as turns were often found to exist as protrusions from the main body of a protein. The value of such an interpretation was severely questioned when it was found that identical peptide sequences could possess completely different structures within different proteins. In fact, the structure of a particular sequence is just as likely to be determined by its interactions and environment than by its own constituent amino acid sequence.

It has been reported that mobile segments of a protein might prove to be suitable candidates, as such regions stand a greater chance of being recognised in the form of peptides due to the increased number of degrees of conformational freedom permitted. Two approaches applied in this area are those of segmental mobility and flexibility analysis. From crystallographic data, temperature coefficients are calculated from which the location of potentially mobile regions may be determined. The lack of detailed crystallographic data for the vast majority of proteins is a serious limitation. A predictive analytical method has been developed to define flexible segments from primary sequence data. Flexibility coefficients are derived from known protein structures and assigned to each amino acid. These values are used to progressively evaluate the protein sequence in a similar fashion to that used for hydropathicity analysis. The method has yet to be fully evaluated.

The termini of a protein may be conformationally less restricted in a native protein than other parts of the same molecule and therefore should be recognised by a larger fraction of a complementary peptide-derived antibody population. Studies have demonstrated the superiority of terminally derived antibodies over those derived from internal regions. However, this just as likely demonstrates the problems associated with peptide selection in general rather than any absolute point. It should also be noted that antibodies may be raised against almost any part of a protein using the peptide approach, although protein reactivity success rates have been found to vary enormously.

Given that no single method appears satisfactory and even when used in combination the results obtained seem inadequate, how then are suitable sequences selected? A region of the protein sequence with hydrophilic character but carrying a reasonably balanced overall charge is to be preferred. If a hydrophilic region is identified containing some hydrophobic amino acids then it would be preferred to one without such characteristics. The presence of a proline residue within a sequence places that sequence under a conformational constraint that is more likely to be represented within a homologous peptide and is to be encouraged. Additionally, proline is useful from a practical point of view as its incorporation into peptides during synthesis has been shown to prevent aggregation problems known to limit synthetic success. Cysteine-rich regions of a protein should be avoided as such residues are likely to be involved in disulphide bonding with similar residues elsewhere in the protein, thereby forcing an unpredictable conformation upon any proximal regions. Sites of known or potential (i.e. predicted) protein modification, for example glycosylation, phosphorylation and myristylation, should also be avoided. The C-terminus of a protein is often a good choice and may be preferred over the N-terminus and any internal regions, although this is highly dependent upon the individual characteristics of the amino acid sequences under consideration. A peptide length of between 12 and 20 amino acids is recommended with the norm being around 15. For a protein of the order of 500 amino acids in length, three to four peptides would routinely be selected for synthesis, giving a good coverage of the various protein domains. A further constraint applied by chemists is that the selected sequence(s) should be synthetically achievable; there is little value to be gained in selecting a peptide that is going to prove problematic during synthesis and purification. Finally, in selecting peptides for synthesis it is important to consider the route by which conjugation to a carrier protein will be effected and to 'design in' an appropriate linker residue.

In conclusion, therefore, peptide selection is very much a case of inspired guesswork which, if subsequently proven correct, might be regarded as 'directed serendipity'!

Synthesis of peptides

There are three methods of peptide synthesis in current usage to a greater or lesser extent, namely solution-phase, solid-phase and enzymatic peptide synthesis. For the present purpose, namely the preparation of small quantities of several medium-sized peptides, the solid-phase approach to peptide synthesis proves to be the fastest, most efficient and most cost-effective method available.

In solid-phase peptide synthesis the peptide chains are assembled from the carboxy terminus, one amino acid at a time, working towards the amino terminus. The C-terminal amino acid is covalently attached to an insoluble supporting resin via a cleavable linker. Remaining amino acids are added one at a time until peptide assembly is complete. Subsequent cleavage of the peptide-resin bond allows isolation of the product.

There are two modes of solid-phase peptide synthesis in current usage: the Merrifield approach using Boc/benzyl protected amino acids and a polystyrene resin, and the Sheppard approach using Fmoc/t-butyl protected amino acids and a polyamide resin. The Fmoc-polyamide mode now offers the best chance of obtaining a desired product at the first attempt. Recent developments such as continuous flow technology, real-time monitoring of reaction progress and full automation, make this approach the method of choice for specialist and non-specialist peptide producer and user alike. The essential features of the Fmoc-polyamide mode of solid-phase peptide synthesis are summarised in Figure 2. In brief, the method utilises a polar support, an orthogonal protecting group strategy, efficient activation and much increased flexibility over other methods.

The importance of peptide purification and analysis should not be understated. Antibody production is a time-consuming and costly matter; it is unwise to proceed further with the approach unless one is assured of the integrity of the peptides being used. The old computer axiom applies well here—'Garbage in, garbage out!' If necessary, peptides may be purified by one method, or a combination of methods, including size exclusion, ion-exchange and high performance liquid chromatography (hplc), with the onus these days being on reverse-phase hplc due to its very high resolving capability. Analysis of synthetic peptides should routinely include thin-layer chromatography, reverse-phase hplc, amino acid analysis after acid hydrolysis and, wherever possible, fast atom bombardment mass spectrometric analysis. Detailed descriptions of all the above mentioned purification and analytical techniques and their application are widely described in the technical literature.

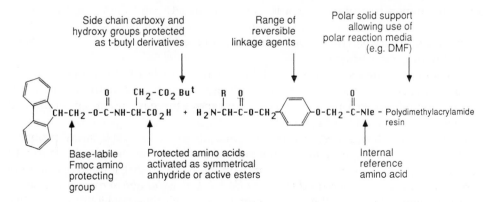

Figure 2. Fmoc-polyamide solid-phase peptide synthesis

Conjugation of peptides

Although invariably antigenic, peptides are seldom immunogenic in their own right. Immunogenicity is usually conferred by conjugating a peptide to a large protein molecule that is itself immunogenic. In order to optimise the conjugation process it is necessary to consider the coupling method, the carrier protein and the likely properties of the resultant conjugate. Ideally, attention should be made to the intended mode of conjugation at the time of peptide selection and synthesis in order that various points be correctly addressed. A specific, stable and covalent linkage is preferred between the peptide and the carrier protein, ideally through a single point of attachment thereby minimising any modification to the peptide. An optimal approach involves the incorporation of a linker residue into the peptide during synthesis, at either the carboxy or amino terminus. In this way a 'designer antigen' may be built specific for the purpose intended, and presenting the peptide in such a way that it is most likely to represent that region of the protein from which it was selected.

There are a great many conjugation procedures to be found in the scientific literature but only three are currently widely favoured and recommended. Glutaraldehyde is a homobifunctional coupling reagent capable of linking compounds containing primary amino groups. It is useful in conjugating peptides N-terminally through the free alpha amino group. Its use should be avoided when there are lysine residues present within the body of the peptide sequence as coupling will additionally, if not preferentially, occur through the epsilon amino group of lysine side-chains. This may lead to substantial modification of the peptide sequence. bis-diazotised tolidine is used to cross-link peptides to carrier proteins primarily through tyrosine side-chains via a diazo linkage. The method is not as specific as one would like, having side-reactions with cysteine, histidine and lysine residues. Under appropriate conditions these side-reactions may be minimised and a good conjugate produced. One should be wary of adding tyrosine residues to peptide termini for conjugation purposes simply because tyrosine is reported to be a highly immunodominant amino acid and that its incorporation may substantially alter the way in which the peptide induces antibodies. The preferred method of conjugation involves the incorporation of a cysteine residue into the peptide during synthesis, at either carboxy or amino terminus, depending upon which is most appropriate, and then using a hetero-bifunctional reagent, *m*-maleimidobenzoic acid N-hydroxysuccinimide ester, as coupling agent between the sulphydryl moiety of the cysteine side-chain and amino groups within the carrier protein.

In general, the limited choice of suitable reactive groups on the peptide and the nature of the carrier under consideration dictates the coupling method to be used. It is rare to find a situation in which one of the above three methods cannot be used to give a well-defined conjugate.

So long as a potential carrier protein is immunogenic its exact nature probably matters very little. Keyhole limpet haemocyanin (KLH) has been much favoured in recent years; however, bovine serum albumin (BSA) thyroglobulin, ovalbumin and many others have been used to good effect. If the use of one of the more unusual carrier proteins is proposed then it is important to consider the availability of potential attachment sites. For example, tuberculin PPD, which is finding increasing use as a carrier protein in monoclonal antibody production, has a molecular weight of ~10 000 and does not have as many potential attachment sites as KLH with a molecular weight of ~900 000. Consequently, it is likely that peptide:carrier ratios will be much lower for PPD conjugates than for those of KLH.

Some reports have drawn attention to the solubility of conjugates. Certainly, BSA conjugates are more likely to be soluble than those of KLH, but this seems to make little, if any, difference to their efficacy as immunogens.

If a long immunisation schedule is being considered it is unwise to assume that any conjugate will be stable for extended periods of time. Various methods have been suggested for analysing conjugates including weighing (!), spectrophotometric analysis and amino acid analysis. The most accurate results, however, are obtained using a radiolabelled peptide, thereby facilitating accurate quantification of incorporation of peptide into a conjugate. However, this approach is quite costly, requiring an intrinsically labelled peptide. It is unwise to rely on the radio-iodination of peptides containing tyrosine or histidine as a source of radiolabelled peptide. Iodination grossly affects the physical and chemical properties of a peptide and may result in misleading results being obtained. Use of tritiated or carbon-14-labelled peptides is greatly preferred.

Immunisation

The procedures used in immunisation will obviously vary depending upon whether the goal is a polyclonal or monoclonal antibody. It is worth pointing out that, if the literature is to be believed, the chances of success in raising good protein-reactive monoclonal antibodies using synthetic peptides are small. That is not to say that success is impossible to achieve, indeed recent work has produced some excellent monoclonal antibodies to a variety of oncoproteins, but there are certain problems that may not be easy to overcome. The number of known effective immunisation schedules is enormous and they are to be found well documented in the scientific literature. Peptide immunisation does, however, have some peculiarities which must be appreciated as high-quality antibodies with well-defined characteristics are seldom arrived at by chance. Detailed and precise protocols have to be developed and optimised in order to guarantee success. The major points may be addressed under the four 'S headings'—species, site, schedule and stopping.

Species. For polyclonal antibody production, rabbits are a very convenient choice. However, much commercially oriented work is carried out in sheep because of the larger quantity of serum obtainable. Immunisation of mice, and increasingly rats, is used in monoclonal antibody production programmes. With outbred animals, such as sheep and goats, and even with certain inbred animals such as rabbits, the question of strain selection is not a major issue. However, with highly inbred species, such as mice and rats, strain choice becomes a most important consideration. It is recommended that mice from a minimum of two, and preferably three, strains are immunised in any study due to the varying responses obtained. The number of animals to be immunised always represents a compromise between financial constraint and experimental desire. However, experience would suggest that each immunogen should be placed into ten mice of each strain, five rabbits or three to five sheep, depending upon the nature of the programme under way, in order to maximise the chance of achieving the desired goal.

Site. Route and site of injection will vary depending upon the species being immunised, the volume being administered and the required release time for the immunogen. The welfare of the animal is of paramount importance: a healthy and happy animal is much more likely to respond well to immunisation than a sick or distressed one. Intramuscular or subcutaneous administration of immunogens at multiple sites in the flanks and hindquarters of sheep and rabbits is recommended, with subcutaneous or intraperitoneal administration being favoured for mice.

Schedule. A schedule is composed of several parts, including amount of immunogen, use of adjuvants and time scale. The optimum dose of an immunogen proves extremely difficult to elucidate in that the effective dose is unlikely to bear little relationship to the actual dose introduced at immunisation due to variable rates of clearance from the site of administration. Doses of 50–200 μg of peptide-carrier protein conjugate per initial immunisation and subsequent boost have produced good effects in sheep, rabbit and mouse despite the great differences in body mass. The use of adjuvants has been shown to be essential in inducing a strong immunological response to soluble antigens. For peptide-derived immunogens, Freund's adjuvants find almost universal application, although alum precipitates are also used to good effect for intraperitoneal administration in mice. The preparation of the immunogen, i.e. the emulsifying of the peptide conjugate solution in adjuvant, is probably the single most important step in the entire synthetic peptide approach. If the emulsion is not prepared correctly it places the entire project in jeopardy. The final point to be considered is timing. It appears that the initial antibody response to peptide immunisation is directed predominantly to peptide reactivity. After three to five boosts, the anti-peptide response appears to plateau whilst the protein-reactive antibody response appears to increase. It is important that the planned schedule takes this observation into account. A two-weekly immunisation programme with test bleeding during the intervening week appears to be a reasonable compromise between effort and return.

Stopping. Determining when to stop the study is a critical matter, seemingly requiring a considerable degree of both foresight and hindsight!

Characterisation

Throughout the immunisation period test bleeds are screened for peptide reactivity using a simple enzyme-linked immunosorbent assay (ELISA) in order to follow the effect of continued immunisation. Peptide reactivity is, of course, not the goal of the process and it is therefore essential to screen for protein reactivity by a variety of relevant methods. In particular, it is important to screen antibodies for reactivity in the system for which they are ultimately intended. Protein reactivity is routinely

Discovery and characterisation of gene products
Demonstration of protein similarity
Distinction between similar proteins
Subcellular localisation of proteins
Study of proteolytic processing
Study of protein function
Protein purification
Assay of proteins
Monoclonal antibodies as therapeutics

Figure 3. Application of antipeptide antibodies

determined using immunoblotting, immunoprecipitation and immunocytochemical procedures.

Purification

A variety of techniques may be applied as appropriate to provide antibody in varying degrees of purity. Simple salt precipitation affords total globulin, removing the bulk of contaminating proteins. Immunoglobulin classes may be fractionated using ion-exchange or staphylococcal protein A chromatography, whilst affinity chromatography using immobilised peptide as the ligand results in isolation of all peptide-reactive antibody populations. Such purification techniques should be undertaken with care, as and when deemed necessary, as they may result in substantial modification of the antibody population. Indeed, affinity purification may result in antibodies that have affinity for the peptide and little, if any, for the protein of interest. Furthermore, a required protein-reactive population may have little affinity for the immobilised peptide and will not therefore bind to the affinity matrix. For this reason it is essential to screen both bound and unbound fractions during affinity purification. Nevertheless, a combination of the above approaches usually results in a highly purified antibody possessing the desired specificity.

APPLICATION

Many examples of the application of protein-reactive antibodies raised via the synthetic peptide route exist in the literature. It is well beyond the constraints of this chapter to consider specific applications in any detail. A summary of the major applications is presented in Figure 3.

CONCLUSION

Over recent years tremendous effort has been directed at the development of reagents for use in developmental and cancer research in the expectation that such products might lead to the development of clinically useful diagnostics, prognostics and therapeutics. Recent developments utilising the synthetic peptide approach to antibody production may help to bring these goals a little nearer.

FURTHER READING

Doolittle, R. F. (1986) *Of URFs and ORFs*. University Science Books.
Harlow, E. and Lane, D. (1988) *Antibodies: A Laboratory Manual*. Cold Spring Harbor Laboratory.
Reddy, E. P., Skalka, A. M. and Curran, T. (eds.) (1988) *The Oncogene Handbook*. Elsevier.
Sheppard, R. C. (1983) Continuous flow methods in organic synthesis. *Chemistry in Britain*, **402**.

16 Targeted Mono-clonal Antibodies for Cancer Therapy

R. H. J. BEGENT

Many agents can kill cancer cells but are too toxic to normal tissues for effective treatment of common cancers. Targeted treatment, in which the therapeutic agent concentrates in the tumour relative to normal tissues, is an attractive means of overcoming this problem.

Cell surface antigens, which are abundant in tumours relative to normal tissues, provide targets against which many monoclonal antibodies have been raised. This chapter will deal with targeting to these cell surface antigens, the parameters determining the efficiency of such systems, the therapeutic agent to be delivered and therapeutic effects in animals and man.

HISTORY

Soon after the properties of antibodies were described by Behring and Kitasato in 1890 it was appreciated that they might be used to discriminate between cancerous and normal tissues. Treatment of cancer with antibodies raised against human tumours was reported by Hericourt and Richet in 1895. They immunised dogs and donkeys with extracts of human carcinomas and sarcomas and gave repeated injections of the resulting antisera to the patients against whose tumours the antisera were raised. Responses were reported but the treatment did not become established.

In the 1950s Pressman and Korngold, and Bale and colleagues, established the specificity of antibody targeting by showing that radiolabelled antibodies directed against transplantable animal tumours localised in the appropriate tumour to a greater

Genes and Cancer. Edited by D. Carney and K. Sikora
©1990 John Wiley & Sons Ltd

extent than non-specific antibody. Monoclonal antibodies have now produced a host of antigen-antibody systems for tumour targeting and give the prospect of large-scale production of reproducible reagents. These have been extensively investigated in the congenitally T-cell-deficient nude mice bearing xenografts of human tumours, as first employed for this purpose by Mach.

In the early 1970s, attempts at gamma camera imaging of human tumours with intravenous radiolabelled antibodies were unsuccessful, probably because the persistence of radiolabelled antibody in the blood and normal tissues obscured any specific localisation in tumours. The subtraction technique used by Goldenberg overcame this problem for antibodies to carcinoembryonic antigen (CEA) and was equally successful with anti-HCG.

The specificity of antibody localisation in man has also been established by comparison with non-specific antibodies, and superior localisation in tumour shown in a variety of tumour types and antibody-antigen systems.

BIODISTRIBUTION

When an antibody is given intravenously, highest concentrations are generally found in the blood for the first few hours or days; however, some diffuses into normal and neoplastic tissues whether or not a specific antigen is present. If a specific reaction occurs between the antibody and a tumour-associated antigen, antibody is retained and may continue to accumulate over the next 8 h to 7 days. Concentrations of non-specific antibody are often as high as those of specific antibody for the first day or two but decline more rapidly. By contrast, specific and non-specific antibody are cleared relatively rapidly from normal tissues. Thus the tumour to normal tissue ratio increases with time for specific antibodies and not for the non-specific. Antibody targeted therapy of cancer requires that a favourable distribution of antibody is sustained in tumour relative to normal tissues.

The principal factors determining efficiency of tumour targeting are shown in Table 1.

REGULATORY CONSIDERATIONS

The safety, quality and efficacy of monoclonal antibodies must be assured before they can be considered for use in man. Guidelines covering the whole of this area have been published by the Commission of the European Communities and the Food and Drugs Administration of the USA. When monoclonal antibodies are produced by academic research units in small quantities, ie. compared to industrial

Table 1. The principal factors determining efficiency of tumour targeting

1. The concentration of antibody in tumour interstitial fluid (a measure of antibody available to bind to tumour-associated antigen)
2. The extent of binding
3. Loss of antibody from the specific binding site
4. The difference between the above factors in tumour and vulnerable normal tissues

facilities, less stringent guidelines have been accepted in order to allow clinical trials under the UK Department of Health doctors and dentists exemption scheme.

STRATEGIES FOR THERAPY

Natural effector mechanisms

It has been proposed that an anti-tumour effect can be produced by complement activation or antibody-dependent cell-mediated cytotoxicity. The concept of using the antibody–antigen reaction to initiate a cytotoxic cascade of the body's own natural effector mechanisms is attractive for its potential power, if it can be manipulated precisely. Knowledge of the appropriate components of the immune system is growing rapidly but the subject is beyond the scope of this chapter. There is, however, optimism that specific activation of cytotoxic effector mechanisms at the site of antibody–antigen reaction in tumour may give effective anti-tumour therapy.

Various targets and therapeutic strategies are being investigated. Anti-idiotype antibodies directed against the idiotype of the monoclonal immunoglobulin secreted by B-cell lymphomas has been used to treat B-cell lymphomas. This has the attraction that the target is theoretically truly tumour specific. Although sustained responses are reported they seem to be exceptional and the mechanisms producing them are not understood.

The idea that human immunoglobulins may be more effective at activating natural effector mechanisms in man has been investigated. Chimeric antibody with a rat immunoglobulin-derived hypervariable region directed against the human lymphoid cell antigen CAMPATH-1, and with human immunoglobulin constant regions, has been produced by recombinant DNA technology. This produces anti-tumour effects in non-Hodgkin's lymphoma.

In an alternative approach, it is proposed that an anti-tumour effect observed against colon carcinoma in some patients given 17-1A antibody is mediated through the idiotypic network. This is based on the network hypothesis of Jerne and uses idiotypic determinants on antibodies as substitutes for conventional tumour antigens. Anti-idiotype antibodies (Ab2) directed against the binding region of the anti-tumour antibody (Ab1) are produced by the host. Some types of Ab2 are an internal image of the antigen, and if it is used for immunisation an antibody is produced which is directed against the antigen. Thus, monoclonal beta Ab2 antibodies can be used to immunise against tumours or infections. Herlyn and colleagues have treated patients with colorectal cancer with polyclonal anti-idiotype antibodies against 17-1A mouse monoclonal antibody to colorectal carcinoma. The patients developed a humoral anti-tumour response and some improvements in tumour measurements were reported. The nature of the antibody responses requires more precise characterisation but the results are encouraging.

Radioimmunotherapy

This technique, in which an alpha- or beta-emitting radionuclide is linked to the antibody, has been investigated since the 1970s. The targeting efficiency can be

Table 2. Factors in radioimmunotherapy

Tumour
   Intrinsic radiosensitivity
   Potential doubling time
   Capacity to repair non-lethal radiation damage

Radionuclide
   Emission spectrum
   Physical half-life
   Ability to link to targeting agent

Biodistribution
   Macroscopic
   Microscopic

monitored by following the distribution of radioactivity and anti-tumour effect, and normal tissue toxicity can be estimated by measurements of cumulative radiation dose. The resulting information is valuable for understanding other forms of antibody-targeted therapy. Table 2 lists the parameters on which radioimmunotherapy depends. The isotope does not have to be delivered to every cell. This may be a crucial advantage over other forms of antibody-targeted therapy because of differences in antigen expression and variation in antibody penetration to different parts of the tumour.

Figure 1 summarises the parameters of antibody and radionuclide distribution. The falling levels in the blood are associated with rising values in tumour and normal tissue interstitial fluid until equilibrium is reached. Interstitial fluid levels will then fall roughly in parallel with blood values. Specific binding to tumour and normal tissue will continue while there is antibody in the interstitial fluid and antigen is not saturated. Release of antibody through dynamic equilibrium and catabolism will eventually reduce tumour radionuclide levels. A favourable therapeutic ratio depends

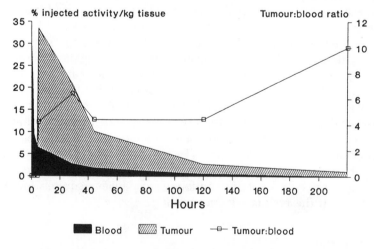

Figure 1. Graph showing the relationship of tumour and blood levels of antibody in a patient with particularly good tumour localisation of ^{131}I-antibody to CEA. Tumour activity was taken from gamma camera imaging, blood from venous blood samples

on exploiting the time when specific binding dominates over interstitial fluid levels of antibody. The distribution of antibody shown in Figure 1 produced a partial response in the liver metastasis and is probably the least that is needed for effective therapy.

The sensitivity of cells in different tumours may vary according to innate radiosensitivity, rate of cell division and rate of repair of radiation-induced damage. Sensitivity of tumour relative to normal tissues also varies, and these factors have to be integrated into any formula for effective radioimmunotherapy.

Animal studies. Delay in growth of xenografts of human carcinomas has been shown in experimental animals with intravenously administered antibodies labelled with the beta-emitting radionuclides, iodine-131 and yttrium-90. The alpha emitter, astatine-211 has also been effective in an animal lymphoma model.

Clinical studies. A series of over 100 patients with hepatoma have been treated with ^{131}I-antibody to ferritin at Johns Hopkins Hospital. The response rate was 48%, with 7% complete remissions, but the effect of the ^{131}I-antibody therapy cannot be assessed because external beam radiation and cytotoxic drugs were also used in the protocol. The same group also reported 40% response in Hodgkin's disease treated only with ^{131}I-antibody to ferritin. Clinically useful activity has also been shown in non-Hodgkin's lymphoma in patients who are unresponsive to conventional therapy. ^{131}I-antibody therapy has also been used to treat melanoma, colon carcinoma and neuroblastoma. Although responses are reported it appears exceptional for these to be sustained. ^{90}Y-labelled antibody has been used for treatment of hepatoma, and radiation dose to the tumour appears to be at a level capable of producing responses.

Levels of radioactivity in tumour and normal tissues can be quantified accurately by three-dimensional single photon emission tomography with correction for Compton scatter. In this way serial imaging can be used to give a graph of levels of radioactivity in tumour and normal tissues. Cumulative radiation dose is then estimated by integration of the curves. A study of 16 patients treated for colorectal carcinoma at Charing Cross Hospital with ^{131}I-labelled antibody to CEA showed that maximum concentrations of radioactivity were found in tumour 8 hours after administration. Activity in tumour varied up to nine-fold in different patients. Gamma camera images of a patient receiving ^{131}I-antibody to CEA are shown in Figure 2.

Measurements of cumulative radiation dose to tumour and normal tissues were made to assess the possibilities for effective therapy. The patient with the highest tumour activity had a beta-radiation dose to tumour of 5.1 cGy per mCi injected, with a whole body dose of 0.25 cGy per mCi injected, a ratio of 20.4:1. Dykes has predicted that a ratio of 30:1 is needed for effective therapy, assuming that a whole body dose of 200 cGy is tolerable. By these criteria effective therapy may be in range for some patients.

Bone marrow radiation is the dose-limiting toxicity factor with ^{131}I-and ^{90}Y-labelled antibody. A higher bone marrow dose might be acceptable with appropriate facilities to support a myelosuppressed patient. It is likely that recovery would be usual with 400 cGy to bone marrow, and that even higher doses would be tolerable with autologous bone marrow transplantation.

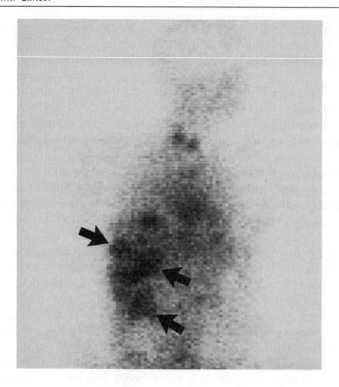

Figure 2. Anterior gamma camera image of a patient with colon carcinoma showing the concentration of ^{131}I in liver metastases (arrowed) after the administration of 50 mCi ^{131}I-antibody to CEA 3 days previously. There is little activity in other parts of the body except the thyroid gland, which can be seen as a bilobed structure towards the top of the image

In the best patient in the Charing Cross study, a tumour dose of 1020 cGy would be given for a blood dose of 200 cGy. Responses of cutaneous T-cell lymphoma and B-cell lymphoma have been reported with ^{131}I-labelled antibody therapy delivering a tumour dose estimated between 100 and 500 cGy. These responses are perhaps better than might be expected with external beam radiotherapy and may be the result of an underestimate of dose delivered to cancer cell nuclei.

Autoradiographic study of microscopic distribution of antibody within the tumour shows localisation on and around tumour cells relative to stromal and necrotic areas of tumour as discussed previously. The extent of the advantage produced by this factor is unknown.

Cytotoxic drugs

The extensive knowledge of the metabolism and toxicity of cytotoxics makes their investigation attractive to clinicians. Mathé began the study of cytotoxic drugs linked to antibodies by treating L1210 leukaemia cells with methotrexate coupled to antibody binding to the cells. Conjugates with many different drugs, including methotrexate, chlorambucil, adriamycin, daunorubicin, vindesine, alpha amanitin, mitomycin C and neocarzinostatin, have been shown to have activity *in vitro* or in animal tumour models.

The potency of cytotoxic drugs is low by comparison with toxins, and attempts to deliver a large amount of drug on each antibody molecule can lead to loss of immunoreactivity of the antibody. Carrier molecules (such as albumin and dextran) linked to the antibody, to which many drug molecules are coupled, have been investigated. Internalisation of the cytotoxic drug is necessary and tumour cells may have the ability to develop resistance to cytotoxic drugs. Nevertheless, any increase of therapeutic ratio of a cytotoxic drug by antibody targeting is likely to be useful in clinical practice. This is supported by a clinical trial with antibody to colorectal carcinoma linked to neocarzinostatin given via the hepatic artery to patients with liver metastases. Three of eight patients had a reduction of tumour volume on CT scan.

Immunotoxins

Various toxins of plant and bacterial origin can be linked to antibodies to form immunotoxins (for review see Vitetta *et al.*, 1987, under Further Reading). In general they act enzymatically once internalised into the tumour cell and are extremely potent. The lectin B chain of ricin causes the molecule to bind non-specifically to many cell types, the molecule then being internalised for the A chain to have its cytotoxic effect. For antibody therapy the isolated A chain can be linked to antibody or the linkage arranged so that the B chain is not active. The conjugate will then localise specifically to tumours. The A chain catalytically inactivates the 60S ribosomal subunit of eukaryotic cells by modifying nucleoside residues of the 28S ribosomal RNA. *In vitro* ricin A-antitumour antibody conjugates can be of the order of 10^3–10^4 times as toxic to tumour cells as ricin A chain alone. This activity depends on internalisation of ricin A chain and on its reaching the ribosomes once inside the cell.

In vivo, ricin A immunoconjugates initially suffered from rapid clearance from the circulation with poor tumour uptake. This has been shown to be caused by uptake of the immunoconjugate by Kupffer cells in the liver, which bind mannose-terminating oligosaccharides of ricin A chain. Deglycosylation of ricin A chain and production of unglycosylated recombinant ricin A chain go some way to overcoming this problem.

One clinical study with ricin A chain linked to an anti-melanoma antibody reported responses, but it is not yet established that these are mediated through the ricin A chain rather than natural effector mechanisms. A further study in colorectal cancer is also in progress. Treatment of graft versus host disease with an immunotoxin directed against the CD5 antigen of T-cells has had a beneficial effect in one reported patient, suggesting that targeting of immunoconjugates in another context is effective.

IMPROVING THE THERAPEUTIC RATIO

Antibody-targeted therapy is presently limited in man by three major factors: the therapeutic ratio is not high enough; a therapeutic dose is not delivered to the target;

or repeated therapy cannot be given. Much work is in progress to overcome these problems.

Local therapy

Systemic toxicity of antibody-directed therapy can in theory be diminished, and anti-tumour effect enhanced, by giving the immunoconjugate into a body cavity to which the tumour is confined. Alternatively it is given into the artery supplying a localised tumour. The tumour is thus exposed to higher concentrations of immunoconjugate than it would with intravenous administration. Systemic exposure should be similar or less and the therapeutic ratio therefore improved. Success depends on retention of immunoconjugate within the cavity targeted or area perfused. This is probably achieved when radiolabelled antibody is given into the cerebrospinal fluid. Responses have been reported when patients with meningeal involvement by primary neural tumours and common epithelial malignancy were treated with intrathecal ^{131}I-labelled antibodies. Intraperitoneal and intrapleural therapy of ovarian carcinoma with ^{131}I-labelled antibody has been reported to produce remissions in patients with lesions of less than 2 cm diameter.

Intra-arterial therapy with radiolabelled antibody has been investigated for hepatic metastases of colorectal carcinoma via the hepatic artery, and for brain glioma by the carotid artery. This strategy has not been shown to be significantly superior to intravenous therapy, possibly because the slow clearance of antibody from the circulation means that most of the exposure of the tumour is to antibody which has recirculated rather than antibody on its first pass direct from the arterial catheter.

Second antibody

A second antibody directed against the first (anti-tumour) antibody will accelerate its clearance from the circulation without causing a corresponding reduction in antibody in the tumour, and this has been shown to be effective in radioimmuno-therapy. Studies of cumulative radiation dose delivered by ^{131}I-labelled antibody in animal systems show, however, that the effective reduction of radiation dose to bone marrow, the most vulnerable tissue, is no more than 50%. Findings are similar in studies in man.

Two-phase systems

Natural effector mechanisms. When antibodies bind to their specific antigen they may change their conformation so as to activate systems such as the complement cascade or antibody-dependent cell-mediated cytotoxicity, which destroy the antigen-bearing cell or organism. This confines the toxic action to the target site.

Prodrug activation. An anti-tumour antibody linked to carboxypeptidase has been used to localise to tumour. After waiting for clearance of this conjugate from the blood a prodrug is given which is activated by carboxypeptidase to form a benzoic acid mustard. This is released at the tumour site and can eradicate xenografts of human choriocarcinoma in some nude mice. There is potential for production of other pairs of enzyme and prodrug. Systemic toxicity is thus minimised by generating a cytotoxic agent with a short half-life at the tumour site.

Neutron capture therapy. In neutron capture therapy anti-tumour antibodies are labelled with boron. A tumour thus containing targeted boron will emit alpha particles when irradiated with thermal neutrons. This technique is limited to tumours which are localised, by the limited availability of suitable neutron beam machines and by doubt about whether it would be possible to target enough boron.

Bispecific antibodies. Glennie and colleagues have constructed an $F(ab')_2$ in which one arm is directed against the tumour and the other against saporin, a ribosome-inactivating toxin. This was investigated in an animal tumour model system and it was found that although administration of antibody and saporin at separate sites had an anti-tumour effect, mixing saporin and the antibody before administration gave better results.

REPEATED THERAPY

It is highly likely that repeated antibody-targeted therapy will be needed to produce major tumour responses. This is prevented by the formation of human anti-mouse antibody (HAMA) after one or more injections of mouse monoclonal anti-tumour antibody. This causes hypersensitivity reactions and prevents anti-tumour antibody from localising in the tumour. Suppression of the response to immunoglobulin can be achieved with cyclosporin A making repeated therapy possible in man. Antibodies with low immunogenicity, such as human-mouse hybrid antibodies or IgG with a mouse variable region and human constant region, have been made. These are likely to be less immunogenic than whole murine antibodies but it is unclear whether they will lead to the generation of an anti-idiotypic response.

CONCLUSIONS

There is now abundant evidence that antibodies can be targeted specifically to tumour cells. One of the greatest obstacles to using this for tumour eradication is the difficulty of targeting to sufficient tumour cells to eradicate the disease. The fact that most success has been in lymphoma may be related to the target antigens being present on a high proportion of tumour cells. When fewer tumour cells bear the target antigen, strategies such as the use of beta-emitting radionuclides which will kill 'bystander' cells may be effective, but improvement of the radiolabelled antibody therapy reported to date is needed. The toxicity to normal tissues through which radiolabelled antibody inevitably circulates is difficult to avoid altogether. However, much information about the macroscopic and microscopic distribution of antibodies is being obtained by monitoring radioactivity. The potential of targeted toxins and cytotoxic drugs has been only partly explored to date, and study of natural effector mechanisms and prodrug systems is at an even earlier stage.

A degree of patience is needed with the preclinical and clinical investigations of antibody-targeted therapy. All techniques require a number of different conditions to be fulfilled for tumour killing to occur. However, the progress being made in the field does justify optimism for the future.

ACKNOWLEDGEMENTS

The author is supported by the Cancer Research Campaign and is grateful to his colleagues in the Cancer Research Campaign Laboratories, Department of Medical Oncology, Charing Cross and Westminster Medical School.

FURTHER READING

Bagshawe, K. D., Springer, C. J., Searle, F., *et al*. (1988) A cytotoxic agent can be generated selectively at cancer sites. *Br. J. Cancer*, **58**, 700–703.

Begent, R. H. J. (1985) Recent advances in tumour imaging; Use of radiolabelled antibodies. *Biochim. et Biophys. Acta.*, **780**, 151–166.

Begent, R. H. J., Ledermann, J. A., Green, A. J., *et al*. (1989) Antibody distribution and dosimetry in patients receiving radiolabelled antibody therapy for colorectal cancer. *Br. J. Cancer* (in press).

Embleton, M. J. (1987) Drug-targeting by monoclonal antibodies. *Br. J. Cancer*, **55**, 227–231.

Epenetos, A. A., Monro, A. J., Stewart, S., *et al*. (1987) Antibody-guided irradiation of advanced ovarian cancer with intraperitoneally administered radiolabeled monoclonal antibodies. *J. Clin. Oncol.*, **5**, 1890–1899.

Hale, G., Dyer, M. J. S., Clark, M. R., *et al*. (1988) Remission induction in non-Hodgkin lymphoma with reshaped human monoclonal antibody CAMPATH-1H. *Lancet*, **ii**, 1394–1399.

Lashford, L. S., Davies, A. G., Richardson, R. B., *et al*. (1988) A pilot study of 131I monoclonal antibodies in the therapy of leptomeningeal tumors. *Cancer*, **61**, 857–868.

Ledermann, J. A., Begent, R. H. J., Bagshawe, K. D., *et al*. (1988) Repeated antitumour antibody therapy in man with suppression of the host response by cyclosporin A. *Br. J. Cancer*, **58**, 654–657.

Order, S. E., Stillwagon, G. B., Klein, J. L., *et al*. (1985) Iodine-131 antiferritin, a new treatment modality in hepatoma: A Radiation Oncology Group study. *J. Clin. Oncol.*, **3**, 1573–1582.

Riechmann, L., Clark, M., Waldmann, H. and Winter, G. (1988) Reshaping human antibodies for therapy. *Nature*, **332**, 323–327.

Rosen, S. T., Zimmer, M., Goldman-Leikin, R., *et al*. (1987) Radioimmunodetection and radioimmunotherapy of cutaneous T-cell lymphomas using an 131I-labeled monoclonal antibody: An Illinois cancer council study. *J. Clin. Oncol.*, **5**, 562–573.

Spitler, L. E., Rio, M., Khentigan, A., *et al*. (1987) Therapy of patients with malignant melanoma using a monoclonal antimelanoma antibody-ricin A chain immunotoxin. *Cancer Research*, **47**, 1717–1723.

Stevenson, G. T. (1980) Preliminary experience in treating lymphocytic leukaemia with antibody to immunoglobulin idiotypes on the cell surface. *Br. J. Cancer*, **42**, 495.

Takahashi, T., Yamaguchi, T., Kitamura, K., *et al*. (1988) Clinical application of monoclonal antibody-drug conjugates for immunotargeting chemotherapy of colorectal carcinoma. *Cancer*, **61**, 881–888.

Vitetta, E. S., Fulton, R. J., May, R. D., *et al*. (1987) Redesigning nature's poisons to create anti-tumor reagents. *Science*, **238**, 1098–1104.

17 Immunotherapy with Monoclonal Antibodies

V. HIRD

A. A. EPENETOS

Since Kohler and Milstein described the development of monoclonal antibodies (MAbs) in 1975, the concept of their use to target therapy to malignant lesions while sparing normal tissues has been an attractive and elegant one.

Although advances have been made in the therapeutic use of MAbs, many problems have also arisen. Their solutions have led to a greater understanding of the art of using monoclonal antibodies as a treatment entity, but as yet cancer treatment using MAbs is not the 'magic bullet' optimistically envisaged by the early workers in the field.

Antibodies are sequences of amino acids linked to form two heavy, and two light chains. Each light chain is connected to a heavy chain by a disulphide bridge, and the two heavy chains are connected by disulphide bridges. Separation at these sites yields portions called Fab (monomeric), F(ab')$_2$ (dimeric) and Fc (crystallizable) fragments (Figure 1).

Monoclonal antibodies (MAbs) are produced using hybridoma technology to produce antibodies from a single clone of cells. A mouse is immunized with human tumour cells to which it makes antibodies. These are produced by B-lymphocytes, large numbers of which are found in the spleen. Spleen cells are removed, and fused with myeloma cells, so that cell proliferation derived from a single hybridoma will result in a single clone of cells producing antibodies.

To treat a particular tumour using MAbs, the tumour must express an identifiable tumour-associated or tumour-specific antigen to which a MAb can be raised. The distribution of the tumour within the body, access to it, its vascularity, its sensitivity to drugs and radiation, and the quantitative expression of antigens on the tumour surface are all factors which will influence the way in which treatment will be

Genes and Cancer. Edited by D. Carney and K. Sikora
©1990 John Wiley & Sons Ltd

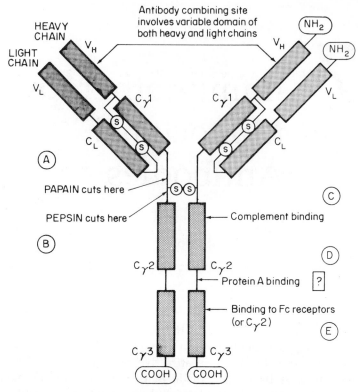

A   Papain cuts here to give two univalent Fab fragments which bind antigen but do not crosslink it on the cell surface

B   Pepsin cuts here to give one divalent $F(ab')_2$ fragment which retains the antigen binding properties of the original IgG

C   Complement binding (classical pathway) is initiated by binding C1q to $C_\gamma 2$ domain: later C4 binds to $C_\gamma 1$ or V_H

D   Protein A binding probably occurs here

E   Binding to Fc receptors on cell surface is usually via the $C_\gamma 3$ domain; $C_\gamma 2$ domain is sometimes also involved

Figure 1. A schematic representation of an antibody molecule

approached. Individual patient evaluation may be necessary for the optimal use of therapeutic MAbs.

Tumour-specific antigens have not been defined in most malignancies. The MAbs commonly used for radioimmunoscintigraphy and treatment are directed against epitopes on tumour-associated antigens. These antigens are also present on some normal tissues, but their differential expression on tumour tissue is greater, so that targeting can be achieved. Most MAbs in clinical use are of mouse origin, although human antibodies have been developed, and recombinant DNA techniques are being used to manufacture chimaeric antibodies where the Fc portion is of human origin and the Fab arms are derived from mouse cells. Murine MAbs administered to patients have been well tolerated at doses ranging from less than 1 mg to over 1 g.

Unconjugated antibody, as well as immunoconjugates, have been administered, although clinical responses to unconjugated antibody have not so far been very encouraging. Radioisotopes, toxins or drugs may be attached, to provide a theoretical means of specific, tumour-directed treatment.

Although many *in vitro* and animal studies have been performed in order to evaluate proposed treatments, clinical data have been slow to accumulate. Nude mice containing human tumour xenografts are the most widely used animal model. The data obtained from mouse studies are useful, but cannot be directly translated to apply to the human situation. A 1 cm (1 g) tumour makes up roughly 5% of the total mass of the mouse, while in man it would constitute only 0.0014%. The rapid metabolic rate and short circulation time of these small animals exaggerate the pharmacokinetics of the antibodies. Whereas over 10% of the intravenously administered Ab may be found per gram of tumour in the mouse, the same has not been seen in human biodistribution studies, where the percentage of injected dose per gram of tumour is of the order of 0.005–0.01%. Trends seen in small animal studies may be useful when planning clinical trials, but it must be borne in mind that the differences in tumour bulk, vascularity and other factors in humans may be very different.

UNCONJUGATED MAbs

Many studies have been performed in animal models using unconjugated MAbs, and inhibition of tumour cell growth has been demonstrated in some cases. Complement fixation does not seem to be necessary for the anti-tumour effects, which vary depending on the Ig subclass and isotype. Therapeutic effects on large well-established tumours are unimpressive. Clinical trials have also taken place, mostly in the form of phase 1 studies which do not claim to be assessing responses. However, encouraging responses have been seen—in some cases of leukaemia, B-cell lymphoma and melanoma.

Unconjugated MAbs may be administered in an attempt to generate an anti-idiotypic response, and in effect make antibodies whose variable regions are directed against an antigen on the tumour cell surface. A human anti-mouse antibody response (HAMA) is seen in almost all patients who have received mouse antibodies. The antibody response is often directed against the Fc portion of the molecule, which is antigenic, but bears no relation to the epitope which is being targeted. When antibodies are made to the antigen-binding site of the administered MAb, they are called anti-Id-1 antibodies. Should these act as antigens, then the subsequent antibodies formed (anti-Id-2 Abs) may be directed against the tumour cell surface antigen which was originally targeted (Figure 2).

This attractive idea has yet to be fully implemented. An obvious stumbling block is the fact that most tumours express a variety of tumour-associated antigens. Administering an antibody to some, but not all, may result in selecting out groups of cells which cannot be targeted.

Repeated administrations of antibody are necessary to generate an anti-idiotypic antibody, but this may also lead to immune complex formation. As the HAMA generated by the administration of whole antibody is commonly directed against

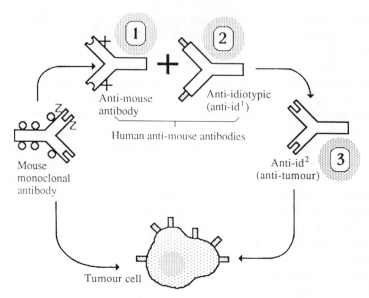

Figure 2. A diagrammatic representation of the anti-idiotypic network

the Fc portion, and not against the variable regions, administering antibody may be more advantageous, and studies are currently under way to investigate this.

IMMUNOCONJUGATES

Monoclonal antibodies may be conjugated to drugs, toxins or radioisotopes. Very few clinical studies have been performed using antibody-targeted chemotherapy; the drugs most often used are methotrexate, adriamycin and the vinca alkaloids.

Preliminary data from one group using monoclonal antibodies conjugated to adriamycin showed markedly different toxicities for the conjugated drug compared to the free drug. Doses of up to 750 mg adriamycin were administered over a 3-week period without alopecia or severe bone marrow depression being seen.

Recently a two-step approach has been used, where a prodrug is activated at the tumour site by a non-mammalian enzyme conjugated to an antibody. Initially the antibody-enzyme conjugate is injected, and allowed to localise to the tumour. After a certain length of time, when the conjugated antibody has cleared from non-specific binding sites, a prodrug is administered, which is relatively stable and is only activated by the enzyme at the tumour sites. The prodrug is converted to a highly toxic agent which can enter tumour cells, but which has a short half-life, so that its toxicity to normal tissue is minimised. MAbs may also be conjugated to toxins such as ricin, abrin, diphtheria toxin and *Pseudomonas* exotoxin.

The aim in conjugating MAbs to radioisotopes is to administer radiation to the tumour, while sparing the surrounding tissues. Radiolabelling of antibodies is used constantly in radioimmunoscintigraphy, where tumour localisation by antibodies can be demonstrated. Isotopes which are alpha- or beta-emitters can be considered for use to deliver radiation in a therapeutic setting. The more commonly used beta-emitters for therapy are iodine-131 and yttrium-90.

Iodination of antibodies is a well-established technique. ^{131}I is a beta-emitter, with a particle range of 1–2 mm and a half-life of 8 days. It is used in the management of carcinoma of the thyroid, therefore medical, physics and nursing staff are all used to handling it. Dehalogenation of the antibody takes place *in vivo*, and free iodine is excreted. For non-thyroid malignancies uptake of the isotope must be prevented by thyroid blocking. Patients need to be nursed in a radiation-controlled environment for a variable period of time, depending on the dose of ^{131}I administered.

^{90}Y is a pure beta-emitter, with a half-life of 64 hours. The high-energy particles have a penetration of up to 11 mm, which seems attractive for the treatment of small volume disease. It can be linked to the antibody using DTPA. However, the chemical bond is not stable *in vitro* or *in vivo*. This leads to some of the resulting free ^{90}Y becoming deposited in bone after *in vivo* administration, and can contribute to myelosuppression.

Clinical studies have been reported using both these isotopes, with some tumour regression seen. The dose-limiting organ is bone marrow, with severe myelosuppression occurring with doses of radiation below an estimated tumoricidal level.

If alpha-emitters, e.g. astidine and bismuth, are to be used for radioimmunotherapy it is essential that there should be a uniform distribution in the tumour because of their short range (50–90 μm). This renders the isotope relatively safe to non-targeted tissues, with a high linear energy transfer at the target. Astidine is a halogen, and therefore could potentially have the same dehalogenation problems *in vivo* as iodine. Bismuth has a short half-life (60.6 minutes), and until recently it was thought that this might be a disadvantage. However, recent studies with Tc-labelled fragments (technetium also has a short half-life) indicate that it might be possible to achieve good tumour:normal tissue ratios in a short space of time.

ROUTES OF ADMINISTRATION

Labelled MAbs may be administered systemically by intravenous injection, or injected into a body cavity, e.g. intraperitoneally, intrapleurally or intrathecally. Local administration aims to increase the availability of the antibody to the tumour before it enters the circulation. The kinetics of the administered antibody depend on the route of administration, and the degree of myelotoxicity depends on the kinetics (the area under the curve on the graph of % dose in blood vs. time) (Figures 3 and 4).

Another approach which may theoretically increase the amount of antibody initially available to tumour is to inject it into a vessel (artery) which directly supplies a tumour, as in intra-carotid injection in gliomas or when hepatic vessels are cannulated in an attempt to control liver metastases. Intralymphatic administration may be considered in an attempt to treat lymph node metastases.

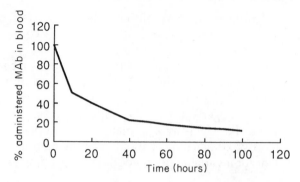

Figure 3. The pharmacokinetics in blood following intravenous administration of whole antibody radiolabelled with indium-111

PROBLEMS

Animals studies, mostly carried out in nude mice bearing human tumour xenografts have shown that effective localisation of tumour by an appropriate MAb is possible, with amounts of the order of 10% of the administered antibody localising per gram of tumour, and tumour:normal tissue ratios of 10+. Tumour regression has been demonstrated in tumour-bearing mice treated with yttrium-labelled antibody (though bone marrow suppression was a problem). In man, however, the situation is somewhat different, with much smaller amounts of antibody localising to the tumour target (approximately 0.005% of the injected dose per gram of tumour, irrespective of the route of administration). If conjugated antibodies are to be an effective means of treatment, then ways of localising larger amounts of antibody to the tumour must be found.

One way of achieving this might be to give larger doses of antibody, as long as that does not result in increased toxicity to the host. labelled antibodies have been given repeatedly, using cyclosporin and corticosteroids to suppress the immune response to the mouse antibody.

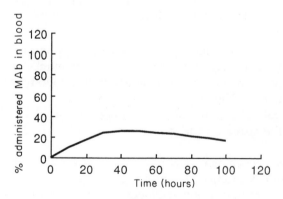

Figure 4. The pharmacokinetics in blood following intraperitoneal administration of whole antibody radiolabelled with iodine-131

Biotin and streptavidin have an extremely high affinity for one another, and biotin is a very small molecule that can diffuse rapidly through most tissues. Using streptavidin antibodies followed after an appropriate period by radiolabelled biotin should result in an increased amount of radiolabel on the tumour. This has been shown to improve the tumour:non-tumour ratio considerably.

It would appear that tumour penetration by the administered antibody is limited to superficial cells. Bulky tumours appear to have less uptake in terms of percentage of the injected dose per gram. This could potentially limit the use of immunoconjugates to small volume disease only. Tumoricidal levels of radiation have been reported in intraperitoneal treatment of malignant ascites by radiolabelled antibodies. The model of malignant cells in suspension is an ideal one for radioimmunotherapy with a low-power beta-emitter like iodine-131.

As stated previously, the majority of administered MAbs are murine in origin, and will excite a HAMA response. It is not known whether any clinically useful responses with immunoconjugates are mediated partly by the immune system, and so its intervention may not always be disadvantageous. Should repeated administration of MAbs appear appropriate, immunization will mean faster clearance of the antibody, which may result in reduced myelotoxicity but with the risk of immune complex formation and deposition. The development of human MAbs may allow repeated treatments. Also, bone marrow rescue or the use of GMCSF may be useful if treatment proves effective in causing tumour regression.

There are still many hurdles to be overcome before the use of MAbs becomes a practicable means of treating patients on a large scale, and many clinical studies are at present under way. These should identify the problems, and increase our understanding so that solutions may be found.

FURTHER READING

Bagshawe, K. D., Springer, C. J., Searle, F., *et al.* (1988) A cytotoxic agent can be generated selectively at cancer sites. *Br. J. Cancer*, **58**, 700–705.

Courtenay-Luck, N. S., Epenetos, A. A., Larche, M., *et al.* (1988) Development of primary and secondary immune responses to mouse monoclonal antibodies used in the diagnosis and therapy of malignant neoplasms. *Cancer Res.*, **46**, 6489–6493.

Dillman, R. O. (1987) Antibody therapy. In: Oldham, R. K. (ed.) *Principles of Cancer Biotherapy*. Raven Press, New York.

Epenetos, A. A., *et al.* (1984) Antibody guided irradiation of malignant lesions. *Lancet*, **30**, 1441–1443.

Epenetos, A. A., *et al.* (1986) Limitations of radiolabelled monoclonal antibodies for localization of human neoplasms. *Cancer Res.*, **46**, 3183–3191.

Sivolapenko, G. B., *et al.* (1989) Radiolabelled monoclonal antibodies in the management of cancer. In: Waxman, J. and Sikora, K. (eds.) *The Molecular Biology of Cancer*. Blackwell Scientific Publications, Oxford.

18 Endothelial Cell Attack as a Novel Approach to Cancer Therapy

JULIE DENEKAMP

Most cancer therapists have as their ultimate goal the eradication of every cancer cell in the body. This they hope to achieve by making use of some difference between the chemosensitivity or radiosensitivity of malignant and normal cells, or by identifying an antigenic characteristic of the tumour cell which is not expressed to the same extent by any normal cells in the body. Since general biochemical or immunological differences between normal and malignant cells have not emerged it has been necessary to try to develop strategies for each individual histological type of tumour. Many tumours proliferate more rapidly than the normal cell of origin, but this property is difficult to use, in practice, with systemic therapy because of the rapid cell turnover that is also seen in intestine, bone marrow and hair follicles. However, all solid tumours do have one common feature, which distinguishes them from normal adult tissues. For any solid tumour to grow, it must either infiltrate surrounding normal tissue to parasitize its blood supply, or it must induce the vascular network to expand locally in order to supply its additional nutritional requirements. All solid tumours show some degree of neovascularization, although lymphomas may obtain more of their vasculature by infiltration than most carcinomas and sarcomas.

ANGIOGENESIS

The new vascular network that is produced in response to the tumour's demands is inadequate in many respects. The new vessels have poorly formed, thin walls,

Genes and Cancer. Edited by D. Carney and K. Sikora.
Published 1990 by John Wiley & Sons Ltd.

with perhaps just a basement membrane and endothelial cells. They have a wider lumen than normal capillaries and do not develop normal innervation. The new vessels lengthen as the tumour grows and, therefore, the quality of the blood carried in them is often poor, being depleted of oxygen and nutrients, particularly towards the centre of large tumour masses. As a result, many tumour cells die and large necrotic areas can often be found, in which cords of viable tumour cells are visible as a thin rim around individual blood vessels (Figure 1). This inadequacy of the vasculature has been recognized for many years. It has been identified as the reason why 10–20% of tumour cells may be radioresistant (because of their hypoxia) and many are resistant to cycle-specific chemotherapy (because of their inability to proliferate, and the difficulty of drug access) (Figure 2). Much effort has been focused on trying to overcome these disadvantages. Hyperbaric oxygen, high LET radiations such as neutron beams, or chemical sensitizers have been used to control hypoxic radio-resistance in radiotherapy and systemic vasoconstrictors have been administered, along with chemotherapy, in the hope of increasing passive blood flow to the unresponsive tumour vessels.

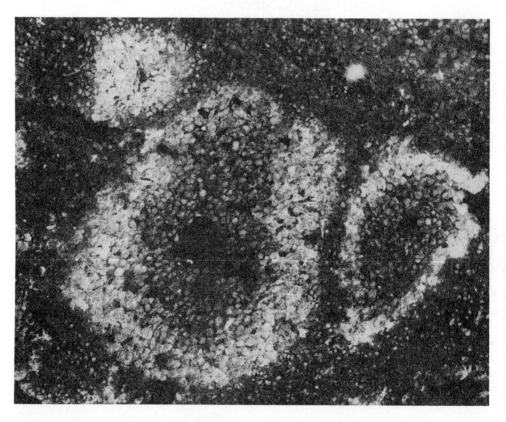

Figure 1. Photomicrograph of cords in a mouse mammary tumour. Three cords are visible in a sea of necrosis. The central vessel in each cord is displaced too far from adjacent vessels to fulfil the nutritional requirements. The light staining areas represent hypoxic cells identified immunofluorescently because they have bioreduced and bound a nitroimidazole (photomicrograph courtesy of R. J. Hodgkiss)

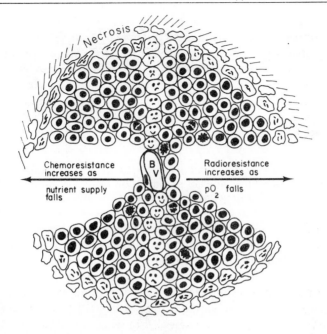

Figure 2. Schematic representation of a tumour cord illustrating the relationship between the architecture and the sensitivity to cytotoxic drugs and to radiation

However, it has recently been suggested that a poor blood supply should be seen as an advantage, for if it can be made a little worse the results for the dependent tumour cells will be quite catastrophic.

VASCULAR INSUFFICIENCY IN TUMOURS

Normal tissues have a more than adequate vascular network, so that all cells have a sufficient supply of nutrients, and there is a reserve capacity for times of stress. This reserve operates if the blood flow is varied (vasodilation or vasoconstriction) or additional vessels which are always present, but do not always have blood flowing through them, open up. By these means the blood flow to normal skin and muscle, in response to a stimulus such as moderate heat or exercise, can increase by a factor of ten. Tumours do not have this capability. Their lack of innervation to the blood vessels prevents them, in general, responding to vasoactive stimuli. Furthermore, since the blood vessels are barely coping with the nutritional demands of the tumour, there are no reserve vessels that can be called into service when needed. Thus, when a mouse tumour is heated the blood flow can only increase by a factor of 1.1 to 1.5, in contrast to the very large increases seen in some normal tissues.

THE IMPACT OF VASCULAR OCCLUSION

If a localized occlusion of a small blood vessel occurs in a normal tissue, the effect will not be very significant, since adjacent collateral vessels may supply the cells

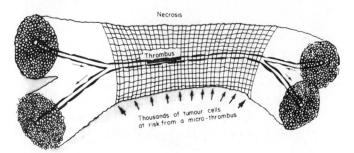

Figure 3. Illustration of the large number of cells at risk in a tumour cord, whose sole source of nutrients will disappear if the capillary becomes occluded by a thrombus. If branches are less frequent, more cells will be at risk

around the infarcted vessel. However, a similar occlusion in a tumour vessel will lead to ischaemic death of all the tumour cells downstream from the infarct to the next vessel branch and upstream of the infarct to the previous vessel branch (Figure 3). This is because many of the dependent tumour cells already exist at the diffusion limits for nutrients from each vessel, and are extremely unlikely to be able to obtain an alternative supply if that vessel fails. From the occlusion of a single capillary the death toll could be 10^3 or even 10^4 tumour cells. Hence, it appears that the vasculature is the vulnerable point or 'achilles heel' of solid tumours.

TUMOUR ANGIOGENESIS FACTORS

Since new blood vessels are being formed and existing vessels are elongating in tumours, it seems obvious that the component cells must proliferate to provide additional vessel walls. Early workers identified low oxygen tension, lactic acid from glycolysis and the resultant low pH, as factors which stimulate vessels to proliferate. However, in the last decade, work pioneered by Folkman and his colleagues, has resulted in the extraction, from tumours, of specific growth factors that stimulate the migration and proliferation of vascular endothelial cells. These have been termed tumour angiogenesis factors (TAFs) and methods of inhibiting their production or activity, as a means of preventing further angiogenesis in tumours, have been sought. The initial approach was to block TAF activity immunologically, but then heparin was found to play an inhibitory role in the growth of vessels. Curiously, both a heparin antagonist (protamine) and a fragment of heparin itself (combined with high-dose cortisone) have been shown to inhibit angiogenesis in model systems and have caused the regression of certain rodent tumours. This is an area of active research, but unfortunately not all research groups have obtained such dramatic results with the cortisone–heparin combination. The reasons why experimental results differ between laboratories and tumour lines are not yet understood.

ENDOTHELIAL CELL PROLIFERATION

Although it has been generally accepted that tumour blood vessels are proliferating, there have been remarkably few quantitative studies of the proliferation rates of

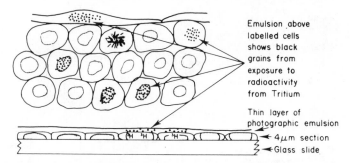

Figure 4. Principle of autoradiography to detect cells which have incorporated tritiated thymidine, a precursor of DNA, in preparation for the next mitosis

stromal cells in tumours, in marked contrast to the many cell-kinetic studies of malignant cells and their normal parenchymal counterparts. Tannock first showed that mouse mammary carcinomas contain blood vessels in which 11% of the endothelial cells are in active DNA synthesis at any time. This was demonstrated using a radioactive precursor of DNA (tritiated thymidine) which is only taken up by cells preparing for the next mitosis. The labelled cells are identified from the grains in a photographic emulsion laid over the section (autoradiography—Figure 4). Tannock demonstrated that the rate of generation of new endothelial cells closely matched the rate at which the tumour volume was increasing. Thus, it appeared that vascular expansion might be a major factor determining the tumour growth rate. Subsequent studies showed that high endothelial labelling indices were found in all tumours (Table 1), and that there was no obvious correlation between the vascular growth rate and the rate of doubling of tumour volume.

Table 1. Uptake of tritiated thymidine into endothelial cells in rodent tumour blood vessels

Tumour	L.1%	Author
Mammary carcinoma C3H	11.4	Tannock, 1970
Mammary carcinoma C3H	14.0	Gunduz, 1981
Mammary carcinoma RH	4.5	Hirst *et al.*, 1982
Mammary carcinoma KHH	17.7	Hirst *et al.*, 1982
Mammary carcinoma KHU	17.9	Hirst *et al.*, 1982
Anaplastic sarcoma RIB5	32.3	Denekamp & Hobson, 1982
Fibrosarcoma KHJ	18.0	Denekamp & Hobson, 1982
Lymphoma KHAA	3.6	Denekamp & Hobson, 1982
Rhabdomyosarcoma KHKK	16.5	Denekamp & Hobson, 1982
Fibrosarcoma KHTD	16.7	Denekamp & Hobson, 1982
Mammary adenocarcinoma TB	10.2	Denekamp & Hobson, 1982
Mammary adenocarcinoma AD	14.1	Denekamp & Hobson, 1982
Mammary carcinoma KHLL	9.5	Denekamp & Hobson, 1982
Mammary adenocarcinoma BAC	9.0	Denekamp & Hobson, 1982
Squamous carcinoma SQ D	7.1	Denekamp & Hobson, 1982
Mammary adenocarcinoma KHLI	7.7	Denekamp & Hobson, 1982
Mammary adenocarcinoma KHHH	8.0	Denekamp & Hobson, 1982
Hepatoma KHI	10.5	Denekamp & Hobson, 1982
Mammary adenocarcinoma RHf	6.6	Denekamp & Hobson, 1982
Fibrosarcoma SA Sf	3.9	Denekamp & Hobson, 1982

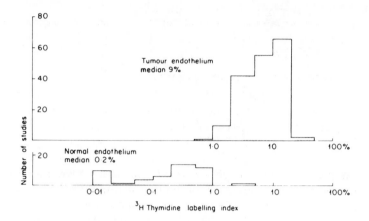

Figure 5. Histogram to show the labelling index in endothelial cells of tumour blood vessels (top) or normal blood vessels (bottom). The median values are grossly different and there is almost no overlap of the histograms. (Note: the horizontal scale is logarithmic.)

COMPARISON OF NORMAL AND TUMOUR BLOOD VESSELS

The cell proliferation studies were extended to compare a wide variety of different rodent tumours with normal tissues; the results are summarized in Figure 5. Most of the rodent tumours showed endothelial labelling indices (percent of cells labelled after a short exposure to ^{3}HTdR) of between 10 and 20%. All but one of 200 tumours showed values above 1%, and the median value was 9%. In marked contrast, very few endothelial cells in normal blood vessels took up tritiated thymidine at all. Most tissues had only one labelled endothelial cell in 500; others one in 10 000. Indeed, only one published study has referred to a normal value in excess of 1%. This finding was obtained for rat mesenteric vessels and was not confirmed in a detailed study of the mouse mesentery.

Figure 5 shows, on a logarithmic scale, the very large difference between the labelling indices of endothelial cells in all tumour vessels and those in all normal tissues. There is virtually no overlap of the histograms and the median values differ by a factor of almost 50; extreme values differ by a factor of about 3000. Thymidine uptake in normal vessels is always very low, regardless of the rate of parenchymal-cell turnover. Thus, it is similar in intestine, skin, brain and kidney. The only normal tissues in which high values have been observed are the placenta and wound tissue after surgical insult.

HUMAN TUMOUR ENDOTHELIUM

A number of human tumours have also been labelled with tritiated thymidine, either by incubating biopsy material *in vitro* or, more rarely, by administering the tracer to the patient. The endothelial labelling indices in human tumours are remarkably similar to those of rodent tumours. They range from 2 to 20%. This similarity is even more remarkable when it is realized that the human tumours were growing in many different sites, were sometimes much larger, and had a much slower growth rate than the experimental mouse tumours.

CONTINUOUS LABELLING STUDIES

A more sophisticated method of measuring the cell proliferation rate is to supply the tracer repeatedly over a period of time, so that every cell that enters DNA synthesis during that time will be labelled. In this way a more accurate picture can be built up of the proliferation characteristics, including the potential doubling time of the population and the fraction of cells which are actively cycling. This technique has been used to study five different types of mouse tumour and ten different normal tissues. The way in which the labelling index increases with repeated 8-hourly injections of tritiated thymidine is shown in Figure 6.

Within four days, 50% of the endothelium is labelled in the five different types of mouse tumour studied by us (upper panel) and tumours studied by Gunduz.

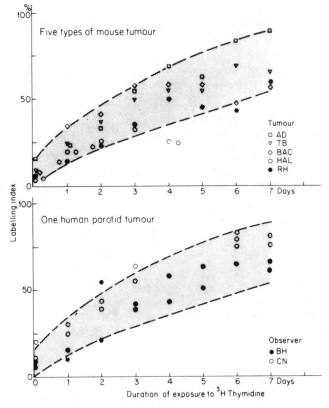

Figure 6. Uptake of tritiated thymidine into tumour endothelium when administered repeatedly for 7 days. *Upper panel*: Five types of mouse mammary carcinoma. Shading includes 95% values. *Lower panel*: Biopsies from two different regions of a human salivary gland tumour, assessed by two different observers. Shaded area reproduced from upper panel

The lower panel shows the data obtained from a human salivary gland carcinoma in a patient who received a local infusion of tritiated thymidine, via the carotid artery, continuously over a 7-day period. The tumour was biopsied every day and the ³HTdR uptake into two different regions assessed by two observers. There is an extraordinary similarity between the pattern of uptake in this human tumour and in the mouse tumours. Data from ten different normal tissues show that almost all the normal adult endothelium remains unlabelled, even after a week of exposure to ³HTdR. However, the uptake in placenta and in granulation tissue of wounds is even higher than in any of the tumours. It is possible that the uterine capillaries during the oestrous cycle may also show rapid proliferation at certain stages, but there are no data on these.

APPROACHES TO ATTACKING TUMOUR BLOOD VESSELS

The rapid proliferation of tumour endothelial cells, vulnerability of tumour cells (because of their dependence on a single blood vessel with no collateral reserve), and intimate contact between endothelial cells and the bloodstream, make the vasculature a feasible target for therapy. It has been shown, with interventional radiology, that deliberate occlusion of the major vessels supplying tumours can lead to massive tumour regression, resulting in debulking for surgery or in prolonged palliation.

Hyperthermia, at temperatures above 42°C, is known to cause collapse of tumour vasculature, leading to ischaemic cell death. The same temperature causes hyperaemia in normal tissues. In the last five years, many agents have been shown to cause reductions in tumour blood flow, as indicated in Figure 7. The width of the arrows is a rough indicator of the strength of the evidence that the observed

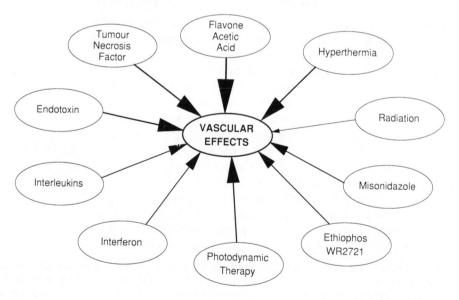

Figure 7.

effects (on endothelial cells, on blood-borne cells or on tumour blood flow) are directly and causally related to tumour cell death. Haemorrhagic or ischaemic necrosis are notable features of the response to heat, to photodynamic therapy (laser light exciting haematoporphyrin to produce toxic singlet oxygen) and to several of the cytokines, particularly tumour necrosis factor. Vascular shutdown occurs after radiation, but seems minor compared with direct cell kill. However, the radiation sensitizer misonidazole, which is also a bioreductive cytotoxin, causes massive vascular collapse after high doses. The assumption that its chemotherapeutic effect on tumours might result from hypoxic metabolism to a cytotoxin may therefore be a misinterpretation of ischaemic cell death following cessation of blood flow. The radioprotector WR2721, shown to have preferential uptake in normal tissues, may have its differential effect because it is dephosphorylated from the prodrug form by endothelial alkaline phosphatases in normal vessels which are reduced or absent in tumour endothelium.

Evidence exists for vascular changes after some conventional cytotoxic drugs, e.g. the vinca alkaloids, but the most striking antivascular agent so far is the novel compound from Lipha, flavone acetic acid (FAA). FAA causes massive tumour regression (and even cures) after single doses in many rodent tumours. Histology within the first 6–24 hours shows haemorrhagic necrosis, with occasional tumour cords surviving, whilst adjacent cords have totally necrosed. Vascular shut down is seen within 1–4 hours and this is associated with changes in the coagulation parameters of the systemic blood. An initial decrease in clotting time is followed by an increase, associated with evidence of platelet depletion, perhaps indicating a consumptive coagulopathy. In a panel of tumours showing a range of sensitivities to FAA the sensitivity is correlated with the blood flow reduction, and with platelet depletion. The whole body toxicity is also correlated with the tumour sensitivity. It seems likely that FAA influences the endothelial control of the procoagulant status in blood. This may also be influenced by tissue factor produced or induced by the adjacent tumour cells. These mechanisms may also be involved in the action of FAA, endotoxin and other cytokines, since the histological pattern is very similar.

Initially the studies of endothelial proliferation led to the concept that the endothelial cells in tumour vessels could be used as a target in monoclonal antibody targeting. They would have the advantage over current anti-tumour strategies of having no barrier between them and the blood-borne antibodies. However, many other aspects of the differences between tumour and normal blood vessels may be manipulable to give a therapeutic benefit. Existing agents need to be re-evaluated to see whether they exert anti-angiogenic activity. If they do their scheduling may need to be totally different from that predicted for a strategy of direct cell kill. This may have been the case with FAA which was disappointing in its early clinical trials. In the screening of new agents, screens using cells *in vitro*, disseminated lymphomas or leukaemias, or solid tumours treated *in vivo* immediately after transplantation (i.e. prevascularisation) are all inappropriate for the detection of vascular mediated injury.

However, if a conscious effort is made to direct therapy at the tumour endothelium, a step forward may be achieved which would be relevant to all solid tumours, since the endothelial cells in each tumour are simply normal cells responding to a common angiogenic stimulus. Very large tumours have the most vulnerable vascular networks, but all tumour masses in excess of a few hundred cells are already inducing endothelial proliferation. It may be possible to attack them by modifying the pharmacokinetics of known cancer chemotherapy agents. The bioavailability of a drug could be reduced so that it did not diffuse freely through all soft tissues, but was retained within the bloodstream. Thus, the cell layer which would receive the highest exposure dose, and which had the largest surface area/volume ratio for exposure, would then be the endothelial layer. If the drugs were ineffective on quiescent cells the desired objective of specificity for tumour endothelial cells might be achieved. But other drugs, with activities that are totally unrelated to proliferative activity, may also become important because of differential redistribution of blood flow, altered viscosity, coagulation or changes in systemic or interstitial pressures.

INTERDISCIPLINARY COLLABORATION

For an endothelial approach to work there must be change in the focus of attention and an increased interaction between specialists of different disciplines. The fundamental first step is to consider that the inadequacy of tumour vasculature is a potential advantage. From that it follows that manoeuvres designed to maximize the killing of tumour cells by vessel occlusion must concentrate on endothelial cell biology, rather than on differences between normal and malignant cells. The participation of the endothelial cell in producing and modulating the complex factors in the clotting cascade, the movement of all bloodborne molecules across the semiselective endothelial cell barrier, and the endothelial cell's avidity for certain chemicals (e.g. low-density lipoproteins) are all factors that may assist us in achieving our goal. By concentrating on the endothelial cell we may find the means for systemic eradication or persistent control of all solid tumours, including both macro- and micro-metastases, without toxicity to normal tissues.

FURTHER READING

Crum, R., Szabo, S. and Folkman, J. (1985) *Science*, **230**, 1375–1378.
Denekamp, J. (1982) *Br. J. Cancer*, **45**, 136–139.
Denekamp, J. and Hill, S. A. (1990) *Radiother Oncol.*, in press.
Denekamp, J. and Hobson, B. (1982) *Br. J. Cancer*, **46**, 711–720.
Fajardo, L. F. (1989) *Am. J. Clin. Pathol.*, **92**, 241–250.
Folkman, J. (1974) Tumour angiogenesis factor. *Cancer Res.*, **34**, 2109–2113.
Folkman, J. *et al.* (1983) *Science*, **221**, 719–725.
Folkman, J., Taylor, S. and Spillberg, C. (1983) Development of the vascular system. *Ciba Found. Symp.*, **100**, 132–149.
Gunduz, N. (1981) *Cell Tissue Kinet.*, **14**, 343–363.
Hill, S. A., Williams, K. B. and Denekamp, J. (1989) *Eur. J. Cancer Clin. Oncol.*, **251**, 1419–1424.
Hirst, D. G., Denekamp, J. and Hobson, B. (1982) *Cell Tissue Kinet.*, **15**, 251–261.
Hobson, B. and Denekamp, J. (1984) *Br. J. Cancer*, **49**, 405–413.
Jain, R. K. (1989) *J. Natl Cancer Inst.*, **81**, 570–576.
Kalinowski, F., Schaefer, C., Tyler, G. and Vaupel, P. (1989) *Br. J. Cancer*, **60**, 555–560.
Song, C. W. *et al.* (1984) *Trans. Biomed. Engin.*, **31**, 9–16.
Stern, D., Nawroth, P., Handley, D. and Kisiel, W. (1985) *Proc. Natl Acad. Sci. USA*, **82**, 2523–2427.
Tannock, I. F. (1970) *Cancer Res.*, **30**, 2470–2476.
Thomlinson, R. H. and Gray, L. H. (1955) *Br. J. Cancer*, **9**, 539–549.
Wallace, S., Chuang, V. and Swanson, D. (1981) *Radiology*, **138**, 563–570.
Zwi, L. J., Baguley, B. C., Gavin, J. B. and Wilson, W. R. (1990) *Br. J. Cancer*, in press.

Molecular Therapy: Drug Resistance

19 Drug Resistance

J. F. SMYTH

The term 'drug resistance' encompasses a variety of different situations which, if strictly defined, would comprehensively include almost every situation in which cytotoxic drugs were non-curative. However, in common terminology there are two categories of drug resistance, referred to as 'intrinsic' and 'acquired'. Intrinsic resistance describes the situation where a tumour is totally insensitive to a given cytotoxic drug; acquired resistance describes the situation of a previously chemosensitive tumour progressing or recurring and proving resistant to further exposure of the same cytotoxic drug. For example, colon cancer and melanoma are intrinsically resistant to virtually all cytotoxic drugs, whilst small cell lung cancer exemplifies the phenomenon of acquired resistance, being initially sensitive to a variety of drugs but universally recurring and then proving resistant on further exposure to the same agents.

Relatively little is known about the reasons for intrinsic resistance at the molecular level; much more is known about different types of acquired resistance. Much of this work has stemmed from the development of techniques for growing human tumours under laboratory conditions, facilitating the repeated exposure of tumour cells to the same stimulus and studying the physical, biochemical and genetic consequences of this on cell survival. Research over the past decade has demonstrated some fundamental principles concerning the difference between intrinsic and acquired drug resistance.

With acquired resistance, a variety of highly sophisticated changes in a tumour cell can result from repeated exposure to the same cytotoxic drug. These changes include: alterations in membrane permeability; alterations in the transport, both in and out of the cell, of the cytotoxic drug; changes in patterns of intracellular metabolism, including alterations in the kinetics of target enzymes and genetic amplification of the quantity of target enzymes and substrates; and intranuclear alterations in genetic susceptibility to the damage invoked.

Concerning intrinsic resistance, whilst knowledge is still sparse as to the mechanisms for metabolic protection of such cells, the development of monoclonal antibodies has greatly enhanced understanding of the heterogeneity of tumour

Genes and Cancer. Edited by D. Carney and K. Sikora
©1990 John Wiley & Sons Ltd

tissues. It is therefore becoming clear that in the clinical situation, where many tumours were previously thought to be essentially sensitive to a cytotoxic drug and developed acquired resistance by the mechanisms identified above, it is now becoming apparent that tumours may contain clones of both sensitive and intrinsically resistant cells. Initial chemotherapy may eliminate the sensitive clones, leaving the subpopulation of intrinsically resistant cells to propagate and emerge as the recurrent or progressive tumour which has 'apparently' become resistant to further chemotherapy.

In describing the phenomenon of drug resistance, emphasis is usually placed on events at the cellular or molecular level. However, it is important to remember the multiple factors which influence the efficacy of a cytotoxic drug, including those that determine whether or not an adminstered drug successfully reaches the tumour tissue in a biologically active form and at the required concentration. The pharmacokinetic parameters of route of administration, variation in absorption, distribution, metabolism and excretion may all contribute to the efficacy or inefficacy of the prescribed drug and falsely imply drug resistance at the tumour level.

ROUTE OF ADMINISTRATION

Primary failure of response to a drug (intrinsic resistance) may be partly influenced by the route of its administration. For orally prescribed drugs patient compliance is an obvious but sometimes forgotten reason for treatment failure, and should always be considered. Similarly, the emetogenic properties of many anti-neoplastic drugs may result in inadequate time for absorption in the upper gastrointestinal tract. This is particularly relevant to the use of combinations of oral and parenterally administered drugs where, for example, the co-administration of cisplatinum, a highly emetogenic drug, with oral VP-16 may result in inadequate plasma levels of the epipodophyllotoxin. The use of antiemetics themselves may influence absorption and drug distribution as recently shown for the effect of metoclopramide enhancing the rate of absorption of the nitrosourea TCNU as a result of more rapid gastric emptying. Other factors which will influence the absorption of orally prescribed cytotoxic drugs include previous surgery to the gastrointestinal tract and subacute or chronic malabsorption syndromes. It should be recognised that alterations in the physiology of the upper gastrointestinal tract may influence the metabolic activity of a drug either positively or negatively in terms of end result. Malabsorption may influence primary response or develop as a result of previous chemotherapy and thus present as a form of acquired resistance. For example, it has been shown that both primary and acquired malabsorption of oral methotrexate can develop in patients receiving maintenance treatment for acute lymphoblastic leukaemia. Wide inter-patient variations in the absorption of drugs such as melphalan, cyclophosphamide, methotrexate and hexamethylmelamine have been described. These differences may be due to variability in membrane transport across the gut wall or to the other factors previously mentioned, such as antiemetic drugs or the effect of narcotic drugs which may similarly influence gastric and jejunal motility.

Most cytotoxic drugs are prescribed parenterally, but apparent drug resistance may result from the inappropriate administration into body cavities of drugs that require hepatic metabolism for activation—the most obvious example being the use of intraperitoneal or intravesical cyclophosphamide, an illogical but still not uncommon practice. The converse situation allows the administration of some cytotoxic drugs into body cavities in order to enhance the local concentration of drug, at least until absorption takes place. Thus, for example, the intraperitoneal administration of cisplatinum may influence the intrinsic sensitivity (resistance) of human ovarian carcinoma by allowing a high local concentration in direct contact with tumour prior to its systemic absorption.

SCHEDULE AND DOSE

By analogy with the use of anti-microbial drugs, and as confirmed by *in vitro* selective-pressure experiments, the repeated administration of the same cytotoxic drug or drugs, can produce acquired resistance. Some of the likely explanations of this are considered later when discussing events at the molecular level. However, the phenomenon of cytotoxic drugs inducing their own metabolism may be relevant to the development of acquired drug resistance. For example, it has been shown that the repeated administration of cyclophosphamide to children is associated with a decrease in plasma half-life $(T_{1/2}\beta)$ and urinary excretion, indicating that cyclophosphamide may reversibly induce its own metabolism. In patients receiving repeated doses of cyclophosphamide at 30–60 day intervals the $T_{1/2}\beta$ and apparent volume of distribution did not vary appreciably from infusion to infusion, but the fraction of administered dose excreted in the urine increased with each successive treatment. Daily administration of cyclophosphamide resulted in decreased $T_{1/2}\beta$ and urinary elimination indicating that the former was not a consequence of the latter.

The effect of dose on drug resistance is controversial. It seems probable that the repeated administration of low doses of cytotoxic drugs enhances the development of acquired drug resistance, and this is one of the reasons for recommending the administration of cytotoxic drugs intermittently and at high concentration. There is experimental evidence to suggest that increasing the dose of the given drug can overcome drug resistance, but this has proved difficult to confirm in clinical practice due to our relative inability to escalate drug dosage safely without inducing unacceptable host toxicity. Experimentally it is possible to demonstrate a dose-response relationship for alkylating agents and for some anti-metabolites. One obvious reason for wishing to increase the plasma concentration of any cytotoxic drug at any given time is to increase the permeation into large tumour masses, where relative avascularity may result in subtherapeutic doses of drug reaching the centre of large tumours in comparison to small ones. However, the clincial use of very high doses of methotrexate following the development of folinic acid rescue has not made a clear-cut impact on the problem of methotrexate resistance. Similarly, neither the introduction of mesna to facilitate the use of higher concentrations of iphosphamide, nor the development of autologous bone marrow harvesting to allow the use of very high doses of alkylating agents such as melphalan or cyclophosphamide, has significantly overcome the resistance patterns encountered with more conventional doses of these agents. Studies of this type are limited by host toxicity, and current research is focused on the use of haematopoietic growth factors such as G-CSF and GM-CSF to spare bone marrow toxicity thus allowing clinical trials of higher doses of a number of agents previously limited by bone marow toxicity. Whether or not such dose escalation will overcome the apparent resistance to drugs such as the anthracyclines has yet to be determined.

RESISTANCE IN DIFFERENTIAL SITES

The phenomenon of 'sanctuary sites' is now well appreciated where, for example, tumour cells in the central nervous system or the gonads may appear to be resistant to chemotherapy by virtue of the fact that they are biologically protected from the drug in the plasma circulation. It is less clear why differential responses in different organs of the body are seen in sites not thought to be protected by known factors, such as the blood–brain barrier. For example, it is not infrequently found that metastatic carcinoma of the breast will respond differently to the same cytotoxic drugs in the same patient depending on the site—e.g. skin, lymph nodes or bone. Similarly, in malignant melanoma, although the condition is usually intrinsically resistant in sites such as the liver, metastates in lymph nodes or in the lung may respond. Tumour mass does not explain these differential responses since, for example, in testicular teratoma metastatic to the lung, even large metastases may completely resolve whilst in the same patient smaller tumour deposits in liver or abdominal lymph nodes may persist.

Tumour bulk alone may contribute to drug resistance in different sites on the basis of differentially impaired vascular supply; this is thought to be a major contributing factor to the refractoriness of many tumours that have been previously irradiated in sites such as the head and neck and uterine cervix. Nevertheless, fibrosis alone cannot be the reason for this apparent drug resistance since there are studies showing that previously unirradiated carcinoma of the cervix may be sensitive in metastatic sites but not at the site of the primary. For example, complete remissions in carcinoma of the cervix, metastatic to lung, soft tissue or liver, have been achieved with cisplatinum, vincristine, mitomycin C and bleomycin without affecting the primary tumours at all.

The role of the blood–brain barrier remains controversial. It is still thought that many cytotoxic drugs that do not readily penetrate the blood–brain barrier will be intrinsically inactive against primary cerebral tumours. Recent results, however, have shown that metastatic tumours, particularly from small-cell lung cancer and carcinoma of the breast, appear to have disturbed the blood–brain barrier sufficiently to allow effective penetration of cytotoxic drugs to effect useful tumour response. The central nervous system should no longer be considered a generalised sanctuary site, particularly for metastatic carcinoma.

A further explanation for variable drug resistance/sensitivity in different sites may result from altered disposition and metabolism of cytotoxic drugs in different target organs. For example, 30 minutes after a standard administration of adriamycin, human tumour biopsies of breast carcinoma tissues showed concentrations almost five times as high as biopsies of colorectal carcinoma tissue. It is well established that breast carcinomas are sensitive and colorectal carcinomas resistant to adriamycin, and part of the explanation for this apparent intrinsic resistance may relate to the fact that adriamycin does not penetrate colorectal tissues as effectively as malignant breast tissue. One explanation may relate to the presence of P-glycoprotein in colorectal tissue, which effectively excludes cytotoxic drugs such as adriamycin. Apart from variable tissue distribution of adriamycin in human cancer tissues it has been shown that there are major inter-patient variations in the pharmacokinetics and biodistribution of drugs such as adriamycin, which clearly will also influence whether or not a tumour is sensitive or resistant in an individual patient.

DRUG RESISTANCE AT THE CELLULAR LEVEL

A great deal of work has been carried out to investigate the phenomenon of drug resistance using experimental tumours *in vitro* or in animals. Whilst this has contributed significantly to our understanding of the possible mechanisms by which tumours may circumvent the effects of chemotherapy, there remain major uncertainties as to the application of such knowledge to clinical practice. The development of techniques for growing human tumours in the laboratory assists with this, but as yet it has proved extremely difficult to grow normal host tissue counterparts under laboratory conditions in order to investigate changes in the therapeutic ratio of drug response. The importance of this lies in the fact that while emergence of resistance in tumours is common, the equivalent effect in host tissues such as bone marrow (i.e. the development of tolerance), is virtually never seen. In fact in clinical practice the reverse effect is more common, with tolerance decreasing over time; thus the development of a relatively small degree of drug resistance in the tumour may restrict further chemotherapy since the dose of drug can neither be escalated nor, in some cases, held steady due to persistent and possibly increased sensitivity of host tissues to toxicity.

It was, of course, such considerations that underpinned the search for techniques to protect host tissues, such as the use of folinic acid in association with methotrexate, and mesna for iphosphamide and other alkylating agents. Methotrexate is probably the cytotoxic drug which has received greatest study and about which there is most information regarding different potential mechanisms of resistance.

Methotrexate resistance

Methotrexate enters the cells by an energy-dependent carrier-mediated process which is common to the influx of other reduced folates but separate from that of folic acid. It has been shown in mouse lymphoma cells that one mechanism of resistance to methotrexate is by reduced transport of the drug into cells (whilst the level of the target enzyme dihydrofolate reductase and its affinity for methotrexate remain unchanged). This transport deficit is due to a decreased affinity (increased K_m) of the drug for the carrier. It has been shown that in this situation transport of folic acid is not impaired, suggesting that one way to overcome methotrexate transport resistance would be to develop antifolates which enter the cell via the folate pathway. Another mechanism of methotrexate resistance has been shown to result from the increased activity of dihydrofolate reductase (DHFR). In enzyme-resistant cell lines increases in DHFR arise both as a result of accelerated synthesis and delayed turnover of the enzyme. DHFR occurs in two forms: as the free enzyme (form 1) or containing an equimolar amount of non-covalently bound NADPH (form 2). In resistant cells the delayed turnover of DHFR has been attributed to stabilisation of form 2 by NADPH and to stabilisation of DHFR by bound methotrexate. The increased rate of synthesis of DHFR has been shown to derive from elevated levels of the appropriate mRNA, which arise directly as a result of an increase in the genes coding for DHFR—the phenomenon of gene amplification. Work on Chinese hamster and human lung carcinoma cells has shown that elevated DHFR levels are seen in cells with homogeneously staining regions (HSRs) of metaphase chromosomes; the selectively amplified DHFR genes are clustered in these regions. Using highly resistant cells selected with actinomycin D, daunorubicin or vincristine, it has been shown that vincristine-resistant cells likewise contain an HSR, indicating gene amplification. As described in subsequent chapters the phenomenon of gene amplification is now known to be applicable to the development of resistance against several classes of cytotoxic drugs. In the experiments with Chinese hamster sub-lines with acquired resistance to actinomycin D, daunorubicin and vincristine, it was shown that there was decreased permeability to the drugs associated with mutual cross-resistance. The demonstration of cross-resistance to structurally very different compounds has now been explained on the basis of the amplification of genetic material giving rise to abnormal expression of a P-glycoprotein on the tumour cell surface. This P-glycoprotein is a minor constituent of the normal cell surface, but multiple drug resistance (a frequently observed clinical situation) may result from the genetic amplification of this material, which influences the retention of cytotoxic drugs within the cell.

CONCLUSIONS

The term 'drug resistance' encompasses the major problem facing the clinical development of cytotoxic drugs for the treatment of human cancers. Mechanisms for the extreme sensitivity of some human cancer cells, such as those found in leukaemia and teratoma, are no better understood than the reasons for the apparent resistance of cells such as those found in malignant melanoma or colon carcinoma. It is likely that progress to develop effective therapies for the intrinsically resistant carcinomas must await novel strategies; it is unlikely to be influenced by minor refinements of the use of existing cytotoxic drugs. Despite this, however, it is essential to remember the pre-cellular factors associated with route of administration, absorption, metabolism and excretion, referred to in this chapter, which may influence whether or not a tumour tissue receives a potentially therapeutic dose of any given administered drug. These factors are particularly important in the treatment of chemosensitive tumours where the difference between cure and palliation is largely the result of the development of apparent acquired resistance. If the latter is due solely to the emergence of a sub-clone of intrinsically resistant cells in the original tumour then current strategies will only influence results in a very modest way. On the other hand, the data explaining the multiple mechanisms of acquired drug resistance at the cellular level do support the development of therapeutic strategies to delay or overcome such acquired resistance. Thus the development of analogues with different transport mechanisms, the avoidance of repeated administration of subtherapeutic doses of drug sufficient to induce resistance, and the development of strategies such as the haematopoietic growth factors to allow higher doses of drug to be administered, hold genuine promise for improving the therapeutic ratio of cytotoxic chemotherapy.

FURTHER READING

Allegra, C. J., Grem, J. L., Yeh, G. C. and Chabner, B. A. (1988) Antimetabolites. In: Pinedo, H. M., Longo, D. L. and Chabner, B. A. (eds.) *Cancer Chemotherapy and Biological Response Modifiers*. Elsevier Science Publishers, Amsterdam.

Chabner, B. A. (1982) *Pharmacologic Principles of Cancer Treatment*. W. B. Saunders, Philadelphia.

Clark, P. I. and Slevein, M. L. (1987) The clinical pharmacology of etoposide and teniposide. *Clinical Pharmacokinetics*, **12**, 223.

Cummings, J., Milstead, R., Cunningham, D. and Kaye, S. (1986) Marked inter-patient variation in adriamycin biotransformation to 7-deoxyaglycones: Evidence from metabolites identified in serum. *European Journal of Cancer and Clinical Oncology*, **22**, 991–1001.

Cummings, J. and Smyth, J. F. (1988) Pharmacology of adriamycin: the message to the clinician. *European Journal of Cancer and Clinical Oncology*, **24**, 579–582.

Fine, R. L. (1988) Multidrug resistance. In: Pinedo, H. M., Longo, D. L. and Chabner, B A. (eds.) *Cancer Chemotherapy and Biological Response Modifiers*. Elsevier Science Publishers, Amsterdam.

20 The Cell Membrane and Drug Resistance

JANE A. PLUMB
STAN B. KAYE

Although the phenomenon of drug resistance is well documented we know very little about the mechanisms behind such resistance. From studies with cell lines grown *in vitro* it is apparent that repeated exposure to one drug will result in resistance not only to that drug, but also to certain others—a phenomenon known as pleiotropic drug resistance. These drugs are often unrelated and have diverse structures and mechanisms of action. However, most are lipid soluble and, in general, have to cross the cell membrane in order to be cytotoxic. The degree of resistance induced *in vitro* depends on the selecting agent and the selection procedure. Resistant cells are known to show collateral sensitivity to several local anaesthetics, steroid hormones and some non-ionic detergents. The cytotoxic mechanisms of these compounds are unknown but all are thought to affect plasma membrane function. In many instances resistant cells have been shown to accumulate less drug than the parental cell line from which they were derived. Based on these observations, Takashi Tsuruo of the Japanese Foundation for Cancer Research looked for membrane-active agents that might interfere with drug uptake into or drug efflux from resistant cells. Verapamil, a calcium antagonist known to inhibit the secretion of a number of hormones, was shown to inhibit drug efflux and to increase the sensitivity of drug-resistant cells. Subsequently, several other calcium antagonists and a number of unrelated compounds were also shown to possess this property (Table 1).

It was noted that in order for cells to maintain their drug-resistant phenotype they required a source of energy. When exposed to drug in the absence of glucose and in the presence of a metabolic inhibitor, such as sodium azide, drug-resistant cells

Genes and Cancer. Edited by D. Carney and K. Sikora
©1990 John Wiley & Sons Ltd

Table 1. Non-cytotoxic agents capable of circumventing pleiotropic drug resistance in experimental models

Bepridil	Quinidine
Cyclosporin A	Reserpine
Dilazep	Tamoxifen
Dipyridamole	Tiapamil analogues
Nifedipine	Trifluoperazine
Perhexiline	Verapamil

were unable to maintain a reduced intracellular drug concentration. In order to explain this observation it was proposed that drug-resistant cell membranes contained either an energy-dependent drug efflux pump or an energy-dependent permeability barrier. All of the above observations point to the cell membrane as a potential site for the development of a drug resistance mechanism and much attention has focused on differences in the membrane of drug-resistant cells.

IDENTIFICATION OF P-GLYCOPROTEIN

The first studies on the role of the cell membrane were carried out on Chinese hamster cells, either ovary or lung, where drug resistance was induced by repeated exposure to a specific drug. June Biedler's group at the Sloan Kettering Institute for Cancer Research demonstrated the presence of a family of membrane glycoproteins of M_r 150 000 in Chinese hamster lung cells resistant to daunomycin and vincristine. Independently, Victor Ling's group at the Ontario Cancer Institute in Toronto also identified a novel glycoprotein species of M_r 170 000 (P170) in Chinese hamster ovary cells resistant to colchicine. A number of other laboratories identified similar high molecular weight glycoproteins in multi-drug-resistant cell lines, both animal and human, and it became apparent that this was a common feature. Following development of a monoclonal antibody to P170, Victor Ling was able to show that these groups had all identified a highly conserved gene product. Further evidence to support the involvement of this gene product in the multi-drug-resistant phenotype was also provided by Ling's group. They isolated part of the chromosome from the Chinese hamster genome containing the P170 gene and transferred it into drug-sensitive cells. These cells became drug resistant and expressed P-glycoprotein in the cell membrane. This could not be taken as proof that P-glycoprotein is involved in drug resistance since the transferred DNA contained more than one gene. However, in 1986 Ira Pastan and Michael Gottesman of the National Cancer Institute, together with Igor Roninson of the University of Illinois, isolated the human gene encoding for P170 (the MDR1 gene). They were then able to demonstrate conclusively that a cloned MDR1 gene on a retrovirus can transfer the complete drug-resistant phenotype to drug-sensitive cells.

STRUCTURE OF P-GLYCOPROTEIN

The MDR1 gene encodes a 1280 amino acid protein. A model of the molecule has been proposed based on the known amino acid sequence. Much of the molecule appears to be intracellular, with 12 membrane-spanning domains and only short sequences exposed on the cell surface. There is a 43% sequence homology between the two halves of the molecule, suggesting that the entire MDR1 gene arose from a gene duplication. Furthermore, the mouse and human sequences are 80% identical, implying a high degree of conservation between species. Although P170 is a glycoprotein the site of glycosylation is not conserved between species and the carbohydrate moiety is not necessary for the function of the molecule. When human leukaemic lymphoblasts are grown in the presence of tunicamycin, which inhibits glycosylation of membrane proteins, the cells retain their resistance to anthracyclines and vinblastine.

There are two proposed intracytoplasmic nucleotide-binding sites that bear a close sequence homology to ATP-binding subunits of multicomponent bacterial transport proteins. Indeed, there is a marked sequence homology between P-glycoprotein and an _E. coli_ membrane protein HlyB (M_r 107 000) required for export of haemolysin. Tsuruo has purified the P-glycoprotein molecule by antibody affinity chromatography and demonstrated that it has ATPase activity. This clearly lends support to the suggested function of the molecule as an energy-dependent drug efflux pump.

DRUG BINDING TO P170

As yet the drug binding site has not been identified. It is known that P-glycoprotein can bind cytotoxic drugs. Marilyn Cornwell and colleagues at the National Cancer Institute have shown that P170 can be labelled with a photoaffinity analogue of vinblastine, N-(p-azido-3 ^{125}I-salicyl)-N'-(B-amino ethyl) vindesine. This label can be displaced by daunomycin, vinblastine, verapamil and quinidine, but not by colchicine or actinomycin D. Since not all of the MDR drugs inhibit binding of the label it appears that there may be more than one drug binding site. Furthermore, resistance modifiers can also displace the label, suggesting that these agents may act by preventing binding of the cytotoxic drug to the efflux pump present in drug-resistant cells. However, more recent evidence indicates that the activity of resistance modifiers is more complex. Skovsgaard's group at Harlev University Hospital in Denmark have studied the binding of cytotoxic drugs to membrane vesicles prepared from drug-resistant cells. They showed that the ability of a resistance modifier to displace vincristine from the vesicles did not necessarily relate to the ability of the modifier to increase the drug sensitivity of the cell line from which the vesicles were prepared. Both verapamil and trifluoperazine increase the phosphorylation state of P-glycoprotein in a human multi-drug-resistant leukaemia cell line (K562/ADM). It is possible that this phosphorylation occurs by activation of protein kinase C, but other kinases may well be involved.

When cells are made resistant to one of the MDR group of drugs they also develop resistance to other members of the group, but the degree of resistance differs between the drugs. It appears that these differences in sensitivity can be explained by single amino acid changes. In multi-drug-resistant KB cells a valine at position 185 of the P-glycoprotein sequence favours resistance to colchicine. However, both the parental cell line and vinblastine-resistant KB cells have a glycine at position 185. This selectivity for colchicine could be reproduced by transfection of sensitive cells with an MDR1 cDNA expression vector with a valine at position 185.

Membrane vesicles prepared from drug-resistant but not drug-sensitive cells will transport vinblastine. Drug transport is ATP-dependent and can take place against a concentration gradient. There is, thus, ample evidence to indicate a role for P-glycoprotein as an energy-dependent drug efflux pump that is present in drug-resistant but not drug-sensitive cells.

THE ROLE OF P-GLYCOPROTEIN IN CLINICAL DRUG RESISTANCE

The presence of P170 in multi-drug-resistant cell lines *in vitro* is now well documented. What is not clear is the relevance of this mechanism to drug resistance in the clinic. Fine and co-workers at the National Institute of Health in Bethesda have determined the drug sensitivity of a number of cell lines derived from tumours removed from patients who had received chemotherapy and from untreated patients. They reported the presence of pleiotropic drug resistance in both human breast and small-cell lung cancer lines, but were unable to show the presence of a high molecular weight glycoprotein in these cells. It is now possible to address the problem more specifically following the production of monoclonal antibodies raised against the P-glyocprotein molecule and the generation of cDNA probes to the MDR1 gene. Both approaches have been used to detect the presence of P-glycoprotein in clinical specimens of both normal and tumour tissue. A surprising finding was that the molecule appears to be present in a variety of normal tissues (Table 2). The initial studies by Tito Fojo and colleagues at the National Cancer Institute used a cDNA probe to detect MDR1 mRNA. Although most tissues had low or undetectable levels, significant amounts were found in others. The problem with this approach is that no information is obtained as to the cellular location and distribution of the molecule within a tissue. A more detailed study of these tissues, lead by Ira Pastan, with a monoclonal antibody provided evidence to suggest that P-glycoprotein may function as a transport mechanism in normal tissues. The P170 molecule was shown, to be

Table 2. MDR1 expression in normal and tumour tissue

Tissue	MDR1 expression		
	High	Intermediate	Low
Normal	Adrenal gland Kidney medulla	Liver Lung Small intestine Colon	Brain Prostate Skin Bone marrow Ovary Stomach
Tumour	Phaeochromocytoma Adrenal Colon Kidney Liver Pancreas Carcinoids		Leukaemia Breast Ovary Thyroid Neuroblastoma Sarcoma Non-Hodgkin's lymphoma

situated on the bile canalicular surface of hepatocytes, the brush border of proximal tubules, the mucosal surface of small and large intestine and on the luminal surface of pancreatic ductules. Organs such as liver, kidney and intestine are the sites from which cytotoxic natural products present in the diet or introduced into the body are removed from the body. Thus it is proposed that P-glycoprotein is part of a natural defence mechanism.

Significant levels of MDR1 mRNA expression have been detected in adeno-carcinomas derived from liver, kidney, adrenal gland and intestine. These tumours are known to be intrinsically resistant to a wide range of chemotherapeutic agents, including those relating to the multi-drug-resistant phenotype. Thus there appears to be a link between the normal level of P-glycoprotein within a tissue and the drug sensitivity of tumours derived from the tissue. Of those tumours derived from tissues not normally expressing P170, detectable levels of the protein have been obtained in some cases of ovarian cancer, breast cancer, sarcoma and acute leukaemia.

What we do not know is the level of expression that is significant in terms of clinical drug resistance. Estimation of MDR1 mRNA in a tumour biopsy reflects the average level of all cell types, both normal and tumour, within the tissue. More detailed studies with *in situ* hybridization techniques and antibody staining will hopefully reveal more about the distribution of expression between the normal and tumour cells and between tumour cells within the same biopsy. So far, very few laboratories have reported significant levels of P-glycoprotein in lung tumours, suggesting that this may not be a major mechanism of drug resistance in this tumour type.

THE ROLE OF MEMBRANE LIPIDS

In addition to studies of membrane glycoproteins the membrane lipids have also received attention. It has been suggested that the novel glycoproteins act by stabilizing the membranes of drug-resistant cells. Clearly, membrane fluidity is an important determinant of the ability of a molecule to diffuse through the lipid domain of the cell membrane. This is particularly relevant to lipophilic drugs, such as adriamycin, which are thought to enter the cell by non-ionic passive diffusion through the membrane lipids. Studies of membrane fluidity have been carried out either by fluorescence polarization or by electron spin resonance spectroscopy. Both increased and decreased membrane fluidity have been observed in association with anthracycline resistance. Local anaesthetics which are known to increase membrane fluidity have been shown to increase the rate of entry of adriamycin into cells and to increase the sensitivity of some cells to adriamycin.

Plasma membranes of murine leukaemia cells (P388) resistant to adriamycin demonstrate a higher structural order than those of drug-sensitive cells. The cholesterol to phospholipid ratio, an important determinant of membrane fluidity, is similar but there are differences in the amounts of specific phospholipids present which could account for differences in membrane fluidity. Thus, unsaturated fatty acids are known to increase membrane fluidity whereas saturated fatty acids produce a rigid crystalline membrane structure. Drug-resistant P388 cells can be made drug-sensitive by treatment with Tween 80, a detergent known to increase membrane fluidity and to increase the intracellular drug concentration. Other non-cytotoxic agents known to affect membrane lipids, such as perhexiline, have a similar sensitizing effect.

Factors which determine membrane fluidity are complex and any hypotheses relating to drug resistance are difficult to test. As a result, whilst this is an area of potential interest it has received little attention.

MEMBRANE TRAFFICKING

Direct transport or diffusion through the plasma membrane is not the only route by which substances are taken up and removed from cells. Following the observation that in some drug-resistant cell lines membrane fluidity is increased, attention was focused on membrane endocytosis—a process known to be affected by changes in membrane fluidity. Adriamycin, a weak base, is thought to enter cells by passive diffusion. However, Skovsgaard's group have proposed that once in the cell, adriamycin could become trapped by protonation within acidic compartments such as lysosomes. The contents of lysosomes can be exported from the cell by energy-dependent exocytosis, and in this manner the drug would be removed from its site of action. The group have shown enhanced endocytotic activity in both Ehrlich ascites tumour cells and P388 leukaemia cells in association with resistance to anthracyclines. Furthermore, the resistance modifier, verapamil, can alter lysosomal activity. Verapamil increases the cytotoxicity of epidermal growth factor-linked *Pseudomonas* exotoxin by inhibiting the breakdown of the complex which accumulates in the lysosomes. Both verapamil and some calmodulin inhibitors delay the degradation of cellular proteins and low-density lipoproteins by the lysosomal enzymes. It is far from clear how all these observations fit together, but they do indicate that alternative explanations exist to account for drug resistance in cell lines that do not express P170 but are sensitised by verapamil.

THERAPEUTIC IMPLICATIONS

From our knowledge of the involvement of the cell membrane in drug resistance, expression of P-glycoprotein in drug-resistant tumours is an obvious target for therapeutic intervention. Of the agents which have been shown to inhibit the drug efflux pump *in vitro*, verapamil has received most attention in the clinic. The major trials are still at an early stage and initial reports of improved response to chemotherapy have yet to be confirmed. However, what is apparent is that the dose-limiting cardiotoxicity of verapamil may prevent achievement of the required plasma concentrations for resistance modification. Agents such as quinidine and nifedipine may be more effective since they are active at concentrations which can be achieved clinically.

SUMMARY

Of the many proposed and identified mechanisms of drug resistance, activity of the drug efflux pump is the best understood. It is clear from studies *in vitro* that multiple mechanisms of resistance can be induced in any given cell, and the relative activity of each mechanism differs between drug-resistant cell lines. The importance of P-glycoprotein to clinical drug resistance is not known. However, there is sufficient evidence already to encourage clinical studies with agents that can interfere with the efflux mechanism of drug resistance.

FURTHER READING

Ames, G. F-L. and Higgins, C. F. (1983) The organisation, mechanism of action, and evolution of periplasmic transport systems. *Trends in Biochemical Sciences*, **8**(3), 97–100.

Beck, W. T. (1987) The cell biology of multiple drug resistance. *Biochemical Pharmacology*, **36**, 2879–2887.

Bradley, G., Juranka, P. F. and Ling, V. (1988) Mechanisms of multidrug resistance. *Biochimica et Biophysica Acta*, **948**, 87–128.

Cornwell, M. M., Pastan, I. and Gottesman, M. M. (1987) Certain calcium channel blockers bind specifically to multidrug-resistant human KB carcinoma membrane vesicles and inhibit drug binding to P-glycoprotein. The Journal of Biological Chemistry, **262**, 2166–2170.

Gerlach, J. H., Endicott, J. A., Juranka, P. F., *et al.* (1986) Homology between P-glycoprotein and a bacterial haemolysin transport protein suggests a model for multidrug resistance. *Nature*, **324**, 485–489.

Goldstein, L. J., Galski, H., Fojo, A., *et al.* (1989) Expression of a multidrug resistant gene in human cancers. *Journal of the National Cancer Institute*, **81**, 116–124.

Gottesman, M. M. and Pastan, I. (1988) Resistance to multiple chemotherapeutic agents in human cancer cells. *Trends in Pharmacological Sciences*, **9**, 54–58.

Moscow, J. A. and Cowan, K. H. (1988) Multidrug resistance. *Journal of the National Cancer Institute*, **80**, 14–20.

Sehested, M., Skovsgaard, T., van Deurs, B. and Winther-Nielsen, H. (1987) Increase in nonspecific adsorptive endocytosis in anthracycline- and vinca alkaloid-resistant Ehrlich ascites tumour cell lines. *Journal of the National Cancer Institute*, **78**, 171–177.

Thiebaut, F., Tsuruo, T., Hamada, H., *et al.* (1987) Cellular localisation of the multidrug resistance gene product P glycoprotein in normal human tissue. *Proceedings of the National Academy of Sciences*, **84**, 7735–7738.

21 | DNA Repair and Drug Resistance

ADRIAN L. HARRIS

GENETIC APPROACHES TO ANALYSIS OF DNA REPAIR

The majority of chemotherapeutic agents interact directly with DNA (e.g. alkylating agents, cisplatin, intercalating agents, bleomycin), with DNA binding proteins (VP16, intercalators), or inhibit key steps in DNA synthesis (antimetabolites). It is therefore reasonable to investigate if differences between normal tissues and tumour tissues, in their ability to modify the DNA damage, could account for differential toxicity and also drug resistance. However, it is presumably the 'resistance' of normal tissues that allows the use of chemotherapy and radiotherapy.

In order to investigate the heterogeneity within and between tumours in their response to chemotherapy and the relationship of repair to the normal tissue distribution of toxicities for each agent, it is necessary to have an understanding of normal tissue DNA repair mechanisms.

Most of our knowledge of DNA repair derives from the analysis of *Escherichia coli* mutants defective in DNA repair pathways. This knowledge has allowed cloning of the relevant genes, purification of repair enzymes and reconstitution *in vitro* with defined substrates. However, to show conclusively the role of specific repair enzymes in drug resistance, it will be necessary to have mutants defective in one or other pathway and to show that they are more sensitive to cytotoxic drugs. Genes responsible for basal resistance mechanisms can then be isolated by transfecting human DNA into the cells and selecting resistant clones. Transfection of cloned genes into wild-type or normal cells may make them more resistant. Once such probes are available, the role of repair enzymes can be investigated in normal tissues and tumours, and intratumour heterogeneity can be analysed by *in situ* hybridization, or antibodies to synthetic peptides based on DNA sequences.

Genes and Cancer. Edited by D. Carney and K. Sikora.
Published 1990 by John Wiley & Sons Ltd.

MUTANT CELL LINES HYPERSENSITIVE TO DNA-DAMAGING AGENTS

Several human genetic diseases are associated with hypersensitivity to DNA-damaging agents. Cell lines from patients with ataxia telangiectasia (AT) are hypersensitive to X-irradiation, bleomycin, neocarzinostatin, streptonigrin, and VP16. The dose of radiation required to reduce survival to 37% differs only two-fold from normal cells, yet fatal adverse reactions to radiation occur in these patients.

In xeroderma pigmentosum (XP) there is a wider range of sensitivity, two- to ten-fold, and nine different genetic types. They are defective in excision repair. There is a high incidence of skin and visceral cancers.

In cell lines from patients with Fanconi's anaemia, there is hypersensitivity to mitomycin C and cisplatin, and there is a defect in cross-link repair.

There are over 20 human diseases or variants of the above associated with hypersensitivity to DNA-damaging agents. Since these must be compatible with life, this suggests that an even greater number of gene products are essential for the repair of or recovery from DNA damage. Only one defect has so far been defined and that is in Bloom's syndrome, where there is a defective DNA ligase I. It is clear that differences of only two- to three-fold in DNA damage and repair are relevant to toxicity and carcinogenicity in humans. This contrasts with the many-fold resistance induced *in vitro*, in cell lines used to study resistance mechanisms.

OTHER MAMMALIAN CELL LINES

Much more rapid progress has been made by isolating Chinese hamster cell lines hypersensitive to various DNA-damaging agents. At least six different complementation groups for UV light sensitivity have been described, and several for mitomycin C, bleomycin, doxorubicin and methylating agents.

The first human repair gene has now been cloned and sequenced (ERCC1), based on the ability of human DNA to correct the defect in a mutant Chinese hamster ovary cell line hypersensitive to UV light. The gene has a striking homology to a previously cloned yeast repair gene and to an *E. coli* repair gene. Its mechanism of action remains to be elucidated, but several other human genes are now in the process of being isolated by this method.

The number of mutants is over 40 and none of them seems to be the counterpart of the human genetic syndromes, again emphasizing the complexity of the process. The patterns of cross-sensitivity differ for the various cell lines, some being quite similar to those seen in human tumours (e.g. BLM-2 is cross-sensitive to cisplatin, VP16 and bleomycin).

REPAIR MECHANISMS AND ENZYMES INVOLVED IN DNA REPAIR AND DRUG RESISTANCE

Inducible responses to DNA damage

In *E. coli*, there are three major inducible DNA repair pathways. One is induced by alkylating agents (the adaptive response), the others are induced by a wide range of drugs, including anti-metabolites, in what is known as the 'SOS' response. The mechanisms induced are excision repair of DNA adducts (Figure 1) and recombination repair. Defects in these pathways make the cells hypersensitive to DNA damage. There is evidence for inducible repair of DNA damage in mammalian cells. Virus survival after plating on mammalian cells is reduced if the viruses have been pretreated with cytotoxic drugs, UV light or X-rays. Pretreatment of the host cells with X-rays, UV light or mitomycin C can enhance recovery. Heat shock can also enhance virus recovery in some cases, suggesting an overlap in stress response (as in *E. coli*). Differences are potentially important in normal and malignant tissue responses to DNA damage, but cannot yet be analysed without further characterization of the biochemical processes involved.

Repair of potentially lethal damage

If cells are exposed to suboptimal growth conditions after DNA damage, survival may increase. It is postulated that repair processes take place, enhancing survival. Thus, potentially lethal damage is repaired. This phenomenon is well described for radiation resistance and may relate to the degree of radiosensitivity of different human tumour types. A similar phenomenon occurs with bleomycin, doxorubicin, AZQ and actinomycin D. The increase in survival is several-fold and could be important in tumours, compared with normal tissues, because the effect is obtained under suboptimal growth conditions.

Recombination

The various DNA rearrangements (recombinations) known to occur in mammalian cells include homologous events which depend on extensive sequence homology and non-homologous events which require no sequence homology or only one or two base pairs of homology. Examples of the former include genetic recombination

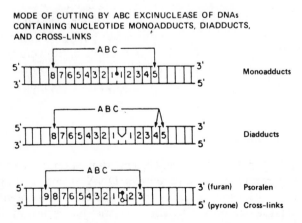

Figure 1. Sites of incision of damaged DNA by inducible excision repair enzymes. Sites vary depending on the adduct

in meiosis (the basis of genetic mapping) and sister chromatid exchange. Examples of the latter include chromosome translocations and certain gene amplification events.

Recombination is critical for the repair of DNA double-strand breaks and is involved in repair of DNA inter-strand crosslinks. It is also involved in the mechanism of gene amplification. Since the latter is one mechanism involved in the activation of oncogenes and in resistance to most antimetabolites or specific enzyme inhibitors, an understanding of recombination will be helpful to many areas of cancer biology. Many genes are involved in *E. coli* and the mechanism is fairly well understood. In mammalian systems, no genes have yet been isolated, although several *in vitro* assays have been described.

Since gene amplification does not seem to occur in normal tissues, interfering with recombination may be more toxic to tumour cells or may prevent the emergence of further heterogeneity and drug resistance by amplification.

O^6-Alkylguanine-DNA alkyltransferase (O^6AT)

The best characterized DNA repair protein is O^6AT. This enzyme removes covalently bound alkyl lesions from the O^6 position of guanine in DNA, leaving an intact DNA molecule. The alkyl lesion, which can be a methyl, ethyl, hydroxyethyl or chloroethyl group, is covalently bound to a specific sulphydryl group on the protein, which is then inactivated. Therefore, one O^6AT molecule is required to remove one alkyl group from DNA—a very high energy cost. Human cell lines defective in O^6AT are much more sensitive to a range of methylating agents (e.g. DTIC, streptozotocin) and chlorethylnitrosoureas, including some new compounds in phase I/II trials (clomesone, cyclodisone, mitozolamide). Cell lines are classified as mer$^+$ if they possess O^6AT and mer$^-$ in its absence. O^6AT is inducible by DNA damage in *E. coli* (part of the adaptive response) but not to any similar extent in mammalian cells. It is inducible in the livers of animals exposed to bleomycin and γ-rays.

A clear indication that the enzyme is a component of resistance to alkylating agents is the transfection of the functional gene into cell lines defective in O^6AT, which greatly enhances their resistance to methylating agents. Assay of O^6AT in human tumours shows a wide variation, which can be greater or lesser than normal adjacent tissue. It will be of interest to correlate this activity with response to the appropriate cytotoxic drug. The work with O^6AT is an example of how elucidation of the mode of DNA repair, at a molecular level, derived from work on *E. coli*, can be applied in the clinical and therapeutic situation. This approach will be needed for the many other DNA repair mechanisms.

Topoisomerase II (topoII)

Topoisomerase II is an ATP requiring enzyme that can produce single- and double-stranded DNA strand breaks and allows DNA strand passage, knotting and unknotting of DNA. The strand breaks are associated with covalently bound enzyme via tyrosine residues (Figure 2). The enzyme has roles in DNA replication, transcription, release of mRNA and sister chromatid exchange, and possibly excision repair of UV-induced DNA damage. TopoII is the target for most intercalators and

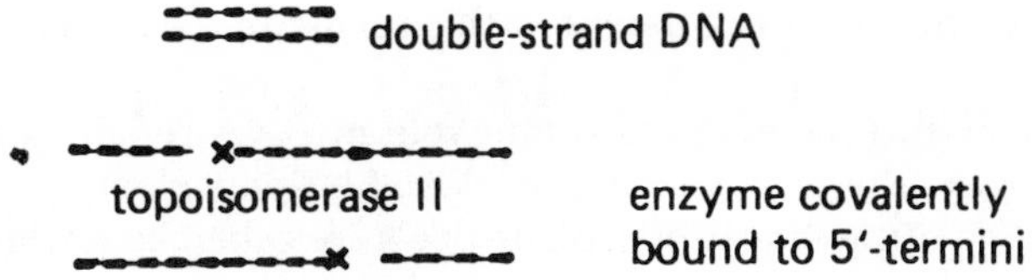

double-strand DNA

topoisomerase II   enzyme covalently
                                bound to 5'-termini

Figure 2. Topoisomerase II induced DNA strand breaks have covalently bound enzyme at 5', overhanging by four base pairs

VP16, which 'poison' the covalent DNA-protein complex so that completion of the reaction with DNA cannot occur. The enzyme remains trapped as a covalent DNA-protein complex masking a DNA single- or double-strand break. There is a good correlation between these protein-associated breaks and cytotoxicity for individual drugs.

Since the toxicity of the drugs depends on the amount of topoII, which is regulated during the cell cycle, there is a possibility of modulating topoII concentrations and hence drug efficacy.

DNA topoisomerases may be inhibited by novobiocin. This has been used as a way to assess whether topoisomerases are involved in DNA repair. Unfortunately, novobiocin inhibits other targets apart from topoisomerase II. Although there is increasing evidence that there are mutant mammalian cell lines which are hypersensitive to topoisomerase II inhibitors and to X-rays, the direct relationships remain unproven. Bacterial mutants in the equivalent enzyme gyrase are hypersensitive to UV radiation.

More recently topoisomerase I has been investigated. This enzyme produces only single-stranded breaks in DNA. Bacterial mutants in this enzyme are hypersensitive to ultraviolet light and it seems much clearer that in these cells there is a role in DNA repair. With the use of specific inhibitors of topoisomerase I, such as camptothecin, it will be possible to detect the role of topoisomerase I in mammalian DNA repair.

In Raji cell lines made resistant to nitrogen mustard, topoisomerase expression was increased, and this was associated with collateral sensitivity to topoisomerase II inhibitors. Similarly, novobiocin was able to enhance cross-links due to alkylating agents in murine cell lines. However, because of the multiple sites of action of novobiocin it is difficult to be clear that this is due to inhibition of topoisomerase II alone.

Glutathione transferases

Free radicals are produced by X-irradiation and a wide range of cytotoxic drugs (e.g. doxorubicin, bleomycin, streptonigrin, mitomycin C). Free radicals produce DNA damage via a variety of mechanisms that include the production of modified bases. These bases can produce covalent links with proteins.

Although glutathione transferases are usually considered as enzymes that conjugate carcinogenic and cytotoxic drugs to inactivate them, they have many other substrates. One type can convert the free radical damaged base, 5-hydroperoxymethyl-uracil to 5-hydroxymethyluracil. The latter is a substrate for a further repair system that excises base damage (glycosylases). Expression of transferases may thus be important for the repair of DNA as well as for its detoxification.

Glutathione may also have an important role in DNA repair. It is a necessary substrate in the biosynthesis of deoxyribonucleotide triphosphates by ribonucleotide reductase. Although nucleotide triphosphate pools are generally not limiting in repair this will be dependent on the rate of DNA biosynthesis in an individual cell. Furthermore, glutathione may protect various enzymes involved in DNA biosynthesis from free radical and other types of damage. In cisplatinum-resistant ovarian cancer cell lines depletion of glutathione levels decreased the rate of repair of platinum-induced DNA damage. This could be overcome by the addition of glutathione. In addition, the use of an antimetabolite, aphidicolin, to inhibit DNA polymerase α and reduce repair was further enhanced by lowering glutathione levels. This is a modulation that could, potentially, be investigated clinically in cisplatinum resistance.

Poly ADP-ribose polymerase (ADPRP)

ADPRP is a nuclear enzyme that is activated by DNA strand breaks. It converts nicotinamide adenine dinucleotide (NAD) to a polymer, poly ADP-ribose, releasing nicotinamide (Figure 3). The poly ADP-ribose is attached covalently to various acceptor proteins, including histones H_1, H_2, and the polymerase itself. There are several nicotinamide analogues (e.g. 3-aminobenzamide [3AB], 3-acetamidobenzamide) that are specific inhibitors of the enzyme at concentrations below 5 mM. They can potentiate cell killing produced by methylating agents, including the active metabolite of DTIC. More DNA strand breaks appear in the presence of 3AB, but the mechanism is controversial. It has been postulated that one type of DNA ligase (II) is activated by poly ADP-ribosylation. Prevention of this modification would prevent ligase activity increasing and hence potentiate damage. Other workers have suggested that inhibiting ADPRP activates an endonuclease.

Human ADPRP has recently been cloned and transfer of the gene into normal cells increased their rate of repair of X-ray induced DNA strand breaks. It will now be possible to analyse the above mechanisms more definitively.

Use of the inhibitors therapeutically may be expected to have some differential effects in tumours, since nutritionally deprived cells have lower NAD concentrations and cells with less substrate should be more susceptible to a competitive inhibitor.

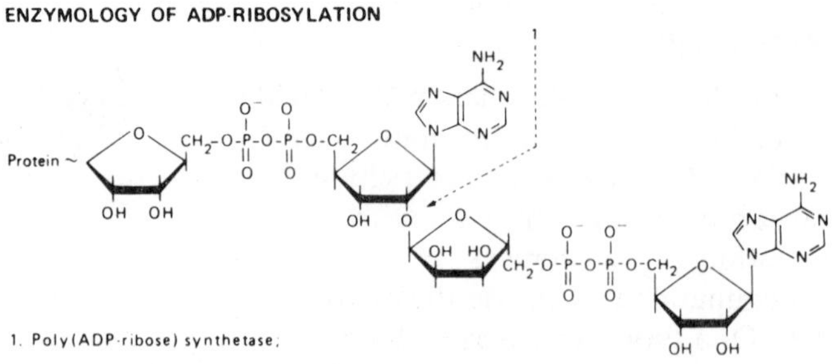

Figure 3. The structure of poly ADP-ribose

Use of antimetabolites to inhibit DNA repair

Excision repair is important in the removal of covalent DNA damage, which is produced by most cross-linking agents and alkylating agents, and the types of damage produced by X-irradiation, other than double-strand breaks. As shown in Figure 1, after excision of several bases on either side of the damage, it is necessary to resynthesise DNA using DNA polymerase α, β or δ, followed by ligation of the new patch into the DNA. The different DNA polymerases seem to have different roles, depending on the size of the lesion and the nature of the lesion. DNA polymerase α is considered to be one of the most important, with DNA polymerase δ being recently assigned an important role in UV excision repair in mammalian cells.

Inhibition of these enzymes would obviously potentiate DNA damage by inhibiting repair DNA synthesis. Alternatively, depleting nucleotide pools such that there were insufficient to fill in the patches would also potentiate the damage. These approaches have been successful *in vitro* in inhibiting excision repair using either hydroxyurea to deplete nucleotide pools or araC to inhibit DNA polymerase α. Aphidicolin also inhibits the latter enzyme, and it is in a phase I trial. In general *in vitro*, it is necessary to use both hydroxyurea and araC to obtain maximum inhibition of repair DNA synthesis. However, levels required *in vitro* can be achieved clinically and an application where this would be most relevant is in cisplatinum repair. High levels of antimetabolites would be required. With hydroxyurea levels of at least 1 mM can be achieved with high dose infusions.

Analysis of DNA repair *in vivo*

DNA repair can be measured directly by using antibodies to determine the number of specific adducts and monitoring their rate of disappearance, although it does not elucidate the mechanisms involved. *In vivo*, platinum adducts in leucocyte DNA correlated with disease response in ovarian cancer patients receiving platinum-based chemotherapy. Further application of these techniques, particularly to haematological neoplasms and malignant ascites, will be necessary to evaluate the role of adduct repair in drug resistance. The differences so far reported may be due to pharmacokinetic variation in drug handling, or to changes in the half-life of the granulocytes. However, it may be that DNA repair processes in leucocytes reflect those in other tissues and in tumours. This would imply that the degree of expression of DNA repair is under the genetic control that is retained within tumours.

If so, then heterozygosity for some of the many DNA repair deficiencies may be important in drug toxicity, tumour response, and cancer susceptibility. It has recently been reported that AT heterozygotes have an increased risk of breast cancer.

CONCLUSIONS

DNA repair is certainly vital in basic resistance of normal tissues to endogenous and exogenous DNA damage. The relevance of DNA repair to drug resistance can only be determined with the use of specific assays of mechanisms relevant to specific drugs applied to clinical material.

Modulation of cell growth may be able to enhance toxicity by increasing a proliferation-related target, topoII. DNA repair inhibitors may be selectively toxic via ADPRP but current inhibitors are poorly water soluble and have a short plasma half-life.

Analysis of the mechanisms of repair by recombination and the role of recombination in gene amplification may produce new therapeutic targets. The pace of development of mammalian repair is such that probes for the above investigations will be available in the near future.

FURTHER READING

Barranco, S. C. and Townsend, C. M., Jr. (1986) *Cancer Res.*, **46**, 623–628.

Cantwell, *et al.* (1989) *Cancer Chemoth. Pharmacol.*, **23**, 252–254.

Collins, A. and Johnson, R. T. (1987) *J. Cell Sci.*, **Suppl. 6**, 61–82.

Creissan, D. and Shall, S. (1982) *Nature*, **296**, 271–272.

Day, R. S., III, Babich, M. A., Yarosch, D. B. and Scudiero, D. A. (1987) *J. Cell Sci.*, **Suppl. 6**, 333–352.

Debenham, P. G., Webb, M. B. T., Jones, N. J. and Cox, R. (1987) *J. Cell Sci.*, **Suppl. 6**, 177–190.

Downes, C. S. and Johnson, R. T. (1988) *BioEssays*, **8**, 179–184.

Dresler, S. L. and Robinson-Hill, R. M. (1987) *Carcinogenesis*, **8**, 813–817.

Fichtinger-Schepman, A. M. *et al.* (1987) *Cancer Res.*, **47**, 3000–3004.

Hoeijmakers, J. H. J. (1987) *J. Cell Sci.*, **Suppl. 6**, 111–126.

Kraemer, K. H. *et al.* (1987) *Arch. Dermatol.*, **12**, 241–250.

Lopez, B., Rousset, S. and Coppey, J. (1987) *Nucl. Acids Res.*, **15**, 5643–5654.

Lunn, J. M. and Harris, A. L. (1988) *Br. J. Cancer*, **57**, 54–58.

Margison, G. P. and Brennand, J. (1987) *J. Cell Sci.*, **Suppl. 6**, 83–96.

Plooy, A. C. M. *et al.* (1986) *Cancer Res.*, **46**, 4178–4814.

Reed, E. *et al.* (1987) *Proc. Natl. Acad. Sci. USA*, **84**, 5024–5028.

Robson, C. N., Harris, A. L. and Hickson, I. D. (1985) *Cancer Res.*, **45**, 5305–5309.

Robson, C. N. *et al.* (1987) *Cancer Res.*, **47**, 1560–1565.

Sarasin, A. (1985) *Cancer Invest.*, **3**, 163–174.

Sedgwick, B. (1987) *J. Cell Sci.*, **Suppl. 6**, 215–224.

Stark, G. R. and Wahl, G. M. (1984) *Ann. Rev. Biochem.*, **54**, 1151–1193.

Swift, M. *et al.* (1987) *New Engl. J. Med.*, **316**, 1289–1294.

Tan, K. H. *et al.* (1986) *FEBS Lett.*, **207**, 231–232.

Teebor, G. W. *et al.* (1984) *Proc. Natl. Acad. Sci. USA*, **81**, 318–321.

Walker, G. C. (1985) *Ann. Rev. Bichem.*, **54**, 425–457.

Wang, J. C. (1985) *Ann. Rev. Biochem.*, **54**, 665–729.

Willis, A. E. and Lindahl, T. (1987) *Nature*, **325**, 355–359.

22 Flow Cytometry and Drug Resistance

DAVID W. HEDLEY

The application of flow cytometry to oncology has expanded rapidly over the past two or three years, with the development of sophisticated assays of cell structure and function to complement the more established use of fluorescent antibodies to surface markers, and techniques for measuring DNA content. This recent progress stems largely from cross-fertilisation of ideas and expertise between developers of flow cytometry instrumentation, computing and fluorescent probes on the one hand, and the increasing number of cell biologists, immunologists and clinicians using the technique on the other. Although this chapter will review the principles of flow cytometry and the earlier work related to cancer, emphasis will be placed on these newer developments. It is not intended to give a comprehensive treatise, but rather to inform those unfamiliar with flow cytometry about the many applications to clinical and basic science which are opening up.

FLOW CYTOMETRY

Principles

Analytical cytology is concerned with quantitating structural or functional properties in cell populations. In flow cytometry these measurements are made with the cells in suspension, stained with fluorescent probes for the property of interest. In addition to probes for macromolecules, there is an increasing repertoire of fluorescent probes sensitive to various aspects of cell function, such as concentrations of ions, intracellular pH, membrane potential, oxygen radical generation and enzyme

Genes and Cancer. Edited by D. Carney and K. Sikora
©1990 John Wiley & Sons Ltd

kinetics. In general these stains are designed to be specific and stoichiometric, i.e. with fluorescence intensity directly proportional to concentration of target.

Flow cytometers contain fluidic, optical and electronic systems. The fluidic system uses laminar flow to cause cells in suspension to stream in single file past a light source. Traditionally this source has been a powerful ion laser, requiring its own power source, water cooling system and the replacement of an expensive plasma tube every two or three years. But improvements in machine performance and laser technology are now leading to the age of small 'plug in' air-cooled lasers or arc lamps, which greatly reduces cost. As cells pass through the system they emit pulses of light. By using an appropriate set of optical filters and dichroic mirrors, emissions from up to three different fluorochromes can be separated and their intensity measured using photomultiplier tubes, while additional information about cell size and structure can be obtained by simultaneously measuring narrow angle and orthogonal light scattering (Figure 1). These separate pieces of information about each cell are converted into digital form, and stored for subsequent analysis. Typically cells are examined at rates of several hundred per second, and the number examined per sample ranges from 10 000 to several hundred thousand, depending on the sample's complexity. This huge influx of raw data requires sophisticated computing

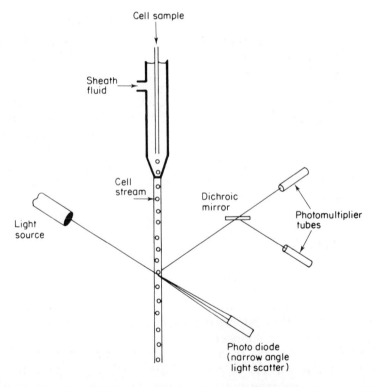

Figure 1. Schematic of the fluidic and optical systems of a flow cytometer. A stable stream of cells is obtained by injecting them into a wider tube where sheath fluid is flowing, and then tapering off. As individual stained cells pass through the light beam they produce narrow angle light scattering, a measure of cell size, and emit pulses of light which are detected by photomultiplier tubes

to acquire, retrieve and analyse, and developments here are progressing as rapidly as in other branches of computer science.

Data displays

The simplest form of flow cytometric analysis measures only one cell property, and the results are displayed as a frequency distribution histogram. Figure 2 shows a typical result measuring cellular DNA content of a human cancer biopsy. Note that cell cycle phase distribution has been approximated using a computer program. The simplest display of two correlated parameters is a dot plot, but computer-drawn contour or isometric displays are generally more informative (Figure 3). Three-parameter analyses can still be displayed in two-dimensional space, but these complex data sets can be more comfortably analysed using recently developed software such as the Becton-Dickinson 'Paint-a-Gate' system, where a population defined by two parameters can then be examined for its other correlates. These sophisticated multicolour flow cytometric analyses have proved particularly useful in cellular immunology, where it is possible to identify lymphocyte subsets which are not demonstrable using any other currently available technology.

Cell sorting

Many flow cytometers are also cell sorters. The cell stream is broken up into droplets, and individual cells identified and sorted electrostatically using deflector plates as

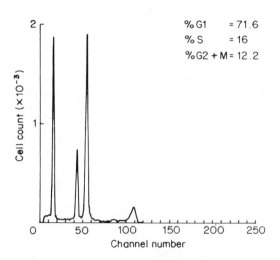

Figure 2. Typical single parameter DNA histogram, obtained from a malignant melanoma. Fluorescence intensity is expressed as arbitrary units (channel numbers), which are directly proportional to DNA content. The extreme lefthand peak is a biological marker (chicken red blood cells). A small peak representing G_1 of normal host cells appears in channel number 43, while to the right in channel number 54 is the G_1 peak of an aneuploid tumour population. The extreme righthand peak consists of tumour cells in G_2 or mitosis, and has twice the DNA content of the G_1 tumour population, while cells in S-phase line between the two peaks. Cell cycle phase distribution of the tumour cells is indicated

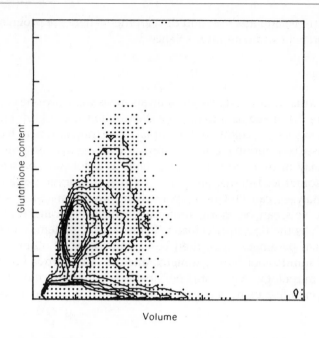

Figure 3. Two parameter analysis of Coulter volume and cellular glutathione content of mouse bone marrow. Glutathione was stained using the probe monochlorobimane, and the results from over 100 000 cells displayed as a contour plot (intervals 20, 50, 100, 150, 200 and 300 cells; dots represent 10 cells). Note that a number of subpopulations are defined by size and glutathione content

they stream through the system. They can then be subjected to further analytical techniques or cultured. Preparative flow cytometry is an extremely powerful technique, capable of sorting particles ranging in size from individual chromosomes up to intact pancreatic islets. Considering the major additional expense compared to purely analytical systems, surprisingly few cell sorters are heavily used as such. Unless you *really* need to sort cells regularly you are probably better off buying a bench-top analysis-only machine, and contracting out the occasional cell sorting experiment.

Basic staining techniques

Most flow cytometry experiments involve staining with fluorescent probes, and despite the rapid expansion of the field most staining methods fall into one of a limited number of basic techniques.

Antibody staining. Surface antigens are readily demonstrated using monoclonal antibodies and fluorescent secondary antibodies. With appropriate techniques up to three separate antigens can be identified simultaneously, which has proved particularly useful in the study of T-cell ontology. Cytoplasmic antigen staining is more difficult, and usually requires prior fixation under often critical conditions. Finally, antibody staining can be combined with DNA content analysis.

DNA staining. A range of fluorochromes bind to DNA with high specificity. All cross-react with RNA to some extent, and resolution is improved by addition of ribonuclease. For routine purposes the intercalating agent propidium iodide is most often used, permeabilisation of the cell membrane being achieved by fixation, or more simply by detergent lysis. Of special interest are the bisbenzimidazole dyes such as Hoechst-33342, which can be used for viable cell DNA staining, and the metachromatic dye acridine orange, which intercalates DNA and dye stacks onto single-stranded RNA. The former has a green fluorescence and the latter red, so that total DNA and RNA contents can be measured simultaneously.

Trapped probes. Trapped probes are increasingly used to study viable cell function. These are loaded into cells as lipid-soluble esters, which are hydrolysed by cellular esterases to membrane-impermeant fluorochromes. The emission spectra of these probes shift following interaction with their specific target. Spectral shift is determined by taking the ratio of fluorescence intensity at two separate wavelengths, which gives an index of target concentration independent of individual cell dye content. Trapped probes have been developed for, e.g. H^+, Na^+, K^+, Ca^{++} and H_2O_2, and their construction is now a precise science. Being on the Molecular Probes mailing list is a good way of keeping in touch with commercial developments in this field.

APPLICATIONS TO CLINICAL ONCOLOGY

Cell structure

DNA analysis. DNA flow cytometry can give two pieces of information. Firstly, by reference to an internal standard the G_1 DNA content gives an indication of modal chromosome number. The majority of human cancers are aneuploid, and flow cytometry is a rapid and reliable method for detecting it, although individual chromosomes are not identified and minor abnormalities are likely to be overlooked. The main interest in aneuploidy is as a possible prognostic indicator. The earlier literature tended to suggest that it could be of major clinical value, but it is now apparent that this is not always the case. Study of the various tumour types and stages has been facilitated by the development of techniques for DNA analysis using archival paraffin-embedded material, because patients whose outcome is already known can be studied retrospectively. By using multivariate analysis, aneuploidy has major and independent prognostic significance in some situations, such as ovarian cancer and operable colorectal cancer, while in other cases an apparent prognostic importance is accounted for by an association between aneuploidy and other, more powerful indicators. Interestingly, some childhood cancers which appear diploid by flow cytometry do worse than those which are aneuploid. In the case of acute leukaemia, parallel cytogenetic studies show that the aneuploid cancers contain multiple copies of intact chromosomes, while the 'diploid' leukaemias in fact show significant translocations. This probably explains why DNA flow cytometry has proved less of a prognostic indicator in adult cancer than was originally predicted; much of the excess DNA in aneuploid tumours is irrelevant so far as biological aggression is concerned.

In addition to giving information about tumour ploidy, DNA flow cytometry also gives an indicator of proliferative activity by allowing an estimate of the percentage of cells in S phase. This is correlated with thymidine labelling index, although it is not the same thing. Figure 2 shows a typical DNA histogram obtained from a fine needle aspirate of malignant melanoma metastatic to axillary lymph nodes. By reference to an internal biological standard (extreme left-hand peak) the tumour is hyperdiploid, and its cell cycle phase distribution is shown. As was the case with labelling index, a high percentage of S phase in tumour biopsies may be an adverse prognostic feature, although there are a number of technical limitations to its routine clinical use.

Chromosome analysis. Individual metaphase chromosomes can be stained for DNA content and examined by flow cytometry. Better resolution is obtained by combined staining with two fluorochromes, one specific for A-T and one for G-C rich regions, individual chromosomes then being readily apparent on a two-dimensional plot. Flow karyotyping is best suited for chromosome sorting; the High Speed Sorter at Los Alamos National Laboratory is capable of achieving 93% purities at flow rates of 3000 events per second.

In situ *hybridisation.* Flow cytometers have a fluorescence detection limit equivalent to several hundred molecules of fluorescein. Specific DNA and RNA sequences have been detected using, for example, biotinylated oligonucleotide probes and streptavidin-FITC, but these sequences have been present in large numbers, for example ribosomal RNA, and it is not certain what the lower limit of detection will be.

Oncogene expression. Proteins are much easier to quantitate in flow cytometry than are specific nucleotide sequences. A standard method is the use of a primary monoclonal antibody and a FITC-conjugated antimouse Ig as the secondary antibody. Because propidium iodide excites at the same wavelength as FITC but has a much more red shifted emission, the two fluorochromes can be combined to correlate antigen expression with DNA content. This approach has been used to study nuclear-associated oncogene products such as *myc* and *fos* proteins, simultaneous DNA measurement allowing an aneuploid tumour cell population to be distinguished from diploid host cells in tumour biopsies, or cell cycle phase distribution to be studied in cell lines. This subject is reviewed elsewhere in this volume.

Proliferation

For many years, cell kinetics has been considered an area where flow cytometry could be particularly useful. In general, results using single parameter DNA analysis have shown poorer prognosis for patients with high percentage S-phase tumours, but the technique has serious limitations, mainly because of admixture with normal host cells, and further progress will require the use of multiparametric flow cytometry. One possibility would be to identify the malignant population using a specific antibody to, for example, an appropriate intermediate filament, and confine the DNA analysis to these cells. Alternatively, S-phase cells contain DNA polymerase α and other replicase-associated enzymes in their nuclei, which can be identified using commercially available monoclonal antibodies.

Sophisticated cell kinetic studies can be performed *in vivo* by treating with the thymidine analogue bromodeoxyuridine (BUdR) prior to tumour excision, and measuring incorporated DNA precursor using antibodies to BUdR. This general approach is considerably more powerful than traditional [^{3}H]-thymidine labelling. For example, intermitotic time of tumours can be approximated using a single two-parameter DNA versus incorporated BUdR plot following a pulse of BUdR. Recently, Frank Dolbeare's group at Lawrence Livermore National Laboratory have described pulse-chase experiments using iododeoxyuridine plus appropriate specific antibody in addition to BUdR incorporation, and this is potentially a very powerful technique. The clinical use of BUdR for cell kinetic studies now has ethical approval in a number of countries.

Assays of cell function

Flow cytometry is now widely used in cell biology to study viable cell function, often by loading cells with trapped probes sensitive to ion concentrations. Interest in other functional aspects such as membrane potential, enzyme kinetics and oxygen radical generation is growing rapidly, while the development of flow cytometry assays of drug resistance is likely to impact on clinical practice in the near future.

Ion concentrations. To date most studies have concentrated on Ca^{++} and H^+ concentrations, because of their obvious relevance to cell function. A wide range of probes of both ions now exists, choice depending on spectral properties required. We have been particularly interested in intracellular pH regulation within solid tumour masses because of indirect evidence that cell acidosis could result in quiescence and therefore resistance to certain types of cancer treatment. The advantage of flow cytometry is that one can measure pH distribution within populations of cells, and sort acidotic cells in order to determine if they are kinetically different.

Oxygen radical production. Generation of reactive oxygen species plays an important role in inflammatory processes, and some anti-cancer agents such as the anthracyclines and bleomycin may cause cell death through a similar mechanism. A number of flow cytometry studies have been published, mainly examining phagocytic cells. The trapped probe dichlorofluorescin is oxidised to the fluorescent dichlorofluorescein by H_2O_2, while superoxide generation can be measured by its oxidation of nitroblue tetrazolium to a black, insoluble formazan. The latter is then semi-quantitated by its absorption of nuclear fluorescence in cells pre-loaded with the vital DNA stain Hoechst-33342.

Functional assays of drug resistance. These promise to be of great use in the day-to-day treatment of individual cancer patients. A number of basic mechanisms for drug or radiation resistance have been recognised. Multidrug resistance, for example, is characterised by failure to concentrate cytotoxic drugs because they are actively extruded by cells. Resistance to agents which act by free radical generation can be achieved by increasing cellular glutathione content or the activity of its related enzymes, and finally, enhanced capacity for DNA repair may salvage cancer cells which sustain damage despite the first two protective mechanisms. These types of resistance are better characterised in experimental systems than in human cancer, but there is an urgent need to determine their clinical relevance because specific methods for circumventing them are being developed. Flow cytometry methods for detecting multidrug and glutathione-mediated resistance are now available.

Multidrug resistance. Multidrug resistance is dependent on a 170 kDa transmembrane ATPase (P-glycoprotein), which actively pumps out a range of agents, including vinca alkaloids and the anthracyclines. The latter are fluorescent, and cellular concentration can be determined by flow cytometry. Because multidrug-resistance phenotype is reversed by calcium channel blockers or calmodulin antagonists, an increase in fluorescence by co-incubating anthracycline-treated cells with, e.g. verapamil, is indicative of functional P-glycoprotein. Development of verapamil-reversible failure to concentrate daunomycin has been observed by flow cytometry in peripheral myeloblasts of patients with anthracycline-resistant acute myeloid leukaemia.

Glutathione content. A number of fluorescent probes bind to sulphydryl groups. Perhaps the best characterised is monochlorobimane, which forms a fluorescent adduct with glutathione under the action of glutathione-S-transferase. Because the catalytic reaction takes place much faster than non-enzymatic binding to thiols, monochlorobimane shows a high specificity for glutathione. Flow cytometric measurement of glutathione in normal tissues and human cancer biopsies shows a very wide range of individual cell values, which is not simply a function of cell size (Figure 3).

Sufficient material for multidrug resistance and glutathione assays can be obtained by 23-gauge needle aspiration biopsy, making flow cytometry ideal for clinical monitoring of these drug resistance phenotypes.

CONCLUSIONS

Flow cytometry has moved from being the preserve of a few instrumentation and computing enthusiasts into the mainstream of cellular and molecular biology. In contrast to other widely used techniques within these disciplines, flow cytometry gives an indication of cellular heterogeneity and allows the cross-correlation of several properties within cell populations. This makes it ideally suited to the study of cancer in the laboratory, and increasingly in the clinic.

FURTHER READING

Shapiro, H. M. (1988) *Practical Flow Cytometry*, 2nd edn. Alan R. Liss, New York.
Various (1989) *Methods in Cell Biology*, vol. 33. Academic Press, Orlando.
Various (1988) Abstracts from Society for Analytical Cytology XIII International Meeting, September 1988. *Cytometry*, (suppl. no. 2).

PART E

Molecular Therapy: Growth Factors and Receptors

23 | Tumour Growth Factors

PAUL STROOBANT

Recent advances in the isolation and structural analysis of tumour growth factors, and in the understanding of the roles of oncogene proteins in tumorigenesis, have led to some unexpected insights into the mechanisms by which at least some types of tumour cell may acquire their characteristics of uncontrolled growth. These advances have now stimulated a variety of experimental strategies designed to clarify the contribution of these growth factors to tumour growth and development, and to develop reagents to inhibit their actions in model systems.

Indications that some tumour cells could produce growth factors which might be associated with their malignant properties came from two commonly reported sets of observations. The first was the general indication that although many cells in culture required whole-blood-derived serum for growth, their counterparts, which had been transformed by viruses or chemicals, were relatively independent of exogenous serum growth factors. The second came from equally widespread reports that the media from many types of transformed cells in culture contained mitogenic material which had apparently been secreted by the cells themselves.

However, the characterisation of the small quantities of putative growth factors present in conditioned medium presented formidable problems of purification and analysis.

ISOLATION AND PROPERTIES

The recent development of more refined purification techniques, in particular, high-performance liquid chromatography, and of more sensitive protein sequence

Genes and Cancer. Edited by D. Carney and K. Sikora.
Published 1990 by John Wiley & Sons Ltd.

analysis, has enabled a number of tumour growth factors to be highly purified and their properties fairly well described. Five classes of factors have been particularly well studied.

Insulin-like growth factor II (IGF-II, originally called multiplication stimulating activity) was first purified from the conditioned medium of a rat liver cell line and later from a human fibrosarcoma line. Types α and β transforming growth factors (TGFα, TGFβ) were originally isolated from virus-transformed cells as a partially purified preparation termed sarcoma growth factor. Both TGFα and TGFβ have now been independently isolated from many cells and many tissues of normal and neoplastic origin. TGFα is a member of the epidermal growth factor (EGF) family, while there is now known to be a TGFβ superfamily, including closely related TGFs β1, 2, 3, 4, and 5. Bombesin-like peptides have been detected in human small cell lung cancer tumours and are produced and secreted by cell lines established from these tumours. A number of mitogens related to platelet-derived growth factor (PDGF) have been identified from spontaneously and virus-transformed cell lines of various kinds.

The biological properties of tumour growth factors are clearly of great interest. In general, these factors bind to specific high-affinity receptors of responsive cells and, under the appropriate conditions, trigger multiple growth and related metabolic processes. It is conceivable that some of these processes, such as the generation of prostaglandins (seen with fibroblasts in the presence of PDGF) which can be released to produce secondary effects on surrounding cells, may be essential for the role of tumour growth factors in addition to their effects on cell proliferation. The observations that the TGFs β can either stimulate or inhibit growth depending on the cell type and the presence of other growth factors emphasise the importance of studying in detail the interactions between tumour growth factors and the cells which are likely to be exposed to them.

The presently known biological properties of the tumour growth factors are consistent with the 'autocrine' hypothesis of Sporn and Todaro, in which the abnormal production and secretion of a growth factor by a cell which has receptors for that factor, transform such a cell into one capable of independent replication. Plausible variations on this theory include paracrine and endocrine effects, and the possibility that the growth factor may not necessarily need to be secreted.

NORMAL ROLES

The production, by some tumour cells, of growth factors with potent biological activities raises the question of whether these factors have evolved independently of 'physiological' growth modulatory polypeptides, or whether they are closely related to normal factors and expressed inappropriately or with aberrant activity. Before considering the properties of these tumour cell derived factors, it is important to summarise some striking findings concerning apparently 'physiological' growth factors.

There are now more than 30 well-characterised and distinct polypeptide growth factors known, and probably many more new factors as yet only partially purified or undiscovered. The well-known factors have been identified from a wide range of sources, including adult tissues, foetal tissues, and conditioned media from cultured cells of continuous lines. An unexpected feature of many of these factors is that they can be grouped into superfamilies of structurally related members. A further surprise has come from the realisation that many so-called polypeptide growth factors exhibit a range of biological activities not necessarily related to growth. These include chemotaxis, differentiation, and cell survival, and effects such as vasodilation, angiogenesis, and inhibition of gastric acid secretion at the level of specific organs. The current consensus is that these factors almost certainly play crucial roles in many biological processes, including development, normal cell and tissue maintenance, wound repair and disease, although their actual functions are still very poorly understood.

Recent studies show clearly that most tumour growth factors for which sufficient structural information is available are closely related, although not necessarily identical, to known growth factors previously isolated from normal tissues. The important question of whether the secretion of such factors by tumour lines is causally related to the characteristics of the tumour tissues from which they were derived, awaits close analysis of the expression of growth factors in a range of tumours at various stages of their development.

ONCOGENES AND CANCER

At least 40 distinct oncogenes have been recognised as primary mediators of cell transformation through their discovery in certain types of acute transforming RNA tumour viruses of animals and from gene transfer experiments. They are now known to be derived from highly conserved genes (proto-oncogenes), normally present in all cells but not necessarily constitutively expressed, which are thought to be involved in key functional roles such as proliferation. While the transfer of an oncogene via a tumour virus or in the form of DNA may be sufficient to produce transformation of cultured cells (as measured from anchorage-independent growth) or tumours in animals, the question of how relevant such a process is to human cancer is controversial, and the subject of intense investigation. It seems possible that while human cancer involves multistep changes in normal cells, the ability of tumour cells to produce a growth factor could give them a selective advantage, important, for example, for their ability to metastasise.

RELATION TO ONCOGENES

The first direct connection between an oncogene protein and a known protein emerged when structural analyses of PDGF revealed that of the homologous A and B chains present in the dimeric growth factor isolated from human platelets, the 109 amino acid residues of the B-chain were essentially identical to the transforming protein of *sis*, the oncogene of simian sarcoma virus. The minor differences in amino acid sequence between the two proteins are consistent with those expected between highly conserved proteins from humans and the woolly monkey from which the virus was isolated. This discovery was of great interest because it dramatically reinforced the autocrine hypothesis from an unexpected direction, and strongly suggested that other oncogene proteins could be involved in growth control.

Evidence from a number of laboratories now suggests that cells transformed with simian sarcoma virus synthesise and secrete a PDGF B-chain homodimer, which has mitogenic activity. The rate of tumour growth in athymic nude mice injected with simian sarcoma virus transformed cells correlates directly with the levels of secreted growth factor activity *in vitro*, reinforcing the notion that the *sis* oncogene protein plays a fundamental role in tumorigenesis.

Since the discovery of the relationship between the *sis* oncogene protein and PDGF, other oncogenes have been linked with various components of the mitogenic signal pathways leading to cell division and which are thus closely implicated in the abnormal growth properties of tumour cells. An additional direct relationship between fibroblast growth factors (FGFs) and four distinct oncogene proteins has been established on the basis of sequence similarities. The *int*-2 oncogene was identified as a transforming gene following the integration of mouse mammary tumour virus into the mouse DNA. Two other oncogenes were then recognised following transfection assays with tumour derived DNA. Thus using DNA from a human stomach tumour, a Kaposi's sarcoma tumour and a human bladder carcinoma, three genes were independently identified (hst, KS and FGF5) which were then found to be identical and are now termed FGF5. A third oncogene, FGF6, was detected following a screen for other hst-related genes. None of these oncogene

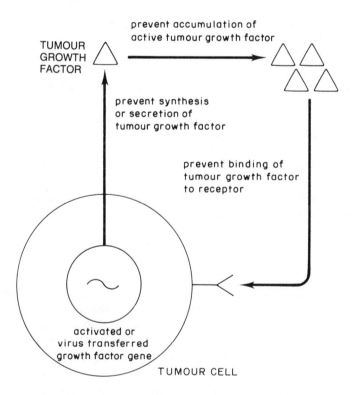

Figure 1. Strategies to inhibit tumour growth factor action

proteins is directly related to known members of the FGF family isolated as proteins. However, all of these related sequences form the members of an FGF superfamily, whose precise relationships have yet to be clarified.

IMPLICATIONS FOR ANTI-CANCER TREATMENT

If tumour growth factors do play an important role in the uncontrolled growth or dissemination of tumour cells, then a number of strategies to inhibit their action can be envisaged (Figure 1). Since the mechanism of action of growth factors, as presently understood, involves the initial binding of the factor to an external cell membrane receptor, then, as well as the possibility of preventing the synthesis or secretion of the factor by the tumour cell, the biological consequences of factor secretion could be prevented by using anti-factor reagents such as antibodies, or reagents which would prevent receptor binding such as competitive-binding inhibitors, or direct anti-receptor reagents. Although there have previously been few experimental opportunities to test such strategies, we are now at the beginning of a range of studies in which the roles of tumour growth factors in tumorigenesis and the possibility of inhibiting tumour growth *in vivo*, using anti-functional tumour growth factor reagents, can now be thoroughly explored.

FURTHER READING

Cuttitta, F., *et al.* (1985) *Nature*, **316**, 823.
Glover, D. M. and Hames, B. D. (eds) (1989) *Oncogenes*. IRL Press.
Huang, J. S., *et al.* (1984) *Cell*, **39**, 79.
Marquardt, H., *et al.* (1981) *J. Biol. Chem.*, **256**, 6859.
Sporn, M. B. and Roberts, A. B. (eds) (1990) *Handbook of Experimental Pharmacology*, Volumes 95/I and 95/II. Springer-Verlag.
Sporn, M. B. and Todaro, G. J. (1980) *New Engl. J. Med.*, **303**, 878.
Stroobant, P., *et al.* (1985) *EMBO J.*, **4**, 1945.
Todaro, G. J. and DeLarco, J. E. (1978) *Cancer Res.*, **38**, 4147.

24 | Bradykinin Receptors

RUTH A. ROBERTS

THE BIOLOGICAL EFFECTS OF BRADYKININ

Polypeptide growth factors play an important role in the growth, development, maturation and normal functioning of many mammalian cell types. It has been suggested that locally produced peptides may also play a role in the control of cell proliferation, and several such peptides have been discovered in neural tissue, where they appear to be acting in a paracrine fashion as local hormones. Recent interest in bradykinin has been generated by suggestions that it may belong to this family of growth modulating peptides. These suggestions have arisen from several lines of evidence. Firstly, bradykinin has recently been implicated as a putative neuro-transmitter, a property shared with other members of the family. Secondly, bradykinin appears to have similar biochemical and physical properties to the peptide bombesin, which has been shown to act as a mitogen in several systems: both peptides are small, positively charged, relatively amphipathic and bind to their specific cell surface receptor with an affinity of around 5 nM. Thirdly and most importantly, bradykinin itself has been shown to act as a mitogen for some cell types under certain experimental conditions.

This emerging role for bradykinin as a modulator of animal cell proliferation must be considered as one of its most important biological effects. However, bradykinin has a host of other biological actions, most of which are less controversial than its putative role in growth regulation. Bradykinin acts to cause a fall in systemic blood pressure through its ability to elevate vascular permeability and induce alterations in the contractile properties of smooth muscle. This latter effect causes vasodilation by relaxing the walls of veins and arteries as well as affecting the muscles of the gut, aorta, uterus and urethra. Bradykinin also mediates prostaglandin release, an

Genes and Cancer. Edited by D. Carney and K. Sikora
©1990 John Wiley & Sons Ltd

effect which serves to perpetuate its vasodilatory and inflammatory activities. These responses to bradykinin have been widely documented in numerous experiments on animals and on isolated organs and have led to the acceptance of the view that bradykinin plays a major role in the regulation of peripheral blood flow and in the primary reaction of tissues to noxious stimuli.

Bradykinin is also thought to play a major role in the initiation of pain perception, since the cascade triggered by its release culminates in the activation of nociceptive neurones. Evidence has also implicated bradykinin as a putative neurotransmitter.

Transduction of signals from bradykinin receptors

Bradykinin interacts with its receptor to induce activation of phospholipase C, leading to changes in intracellular calcium ($[Ca^{2+}]_i$) and inositol polyphosphates. This process is generally thought to involve a pertussis toxin (PTX)-insensitive G-protein and is therefore mediated by a G-protein other than G_i (inhibitory) or G_0, both of which are PTX-sensitive. However, there are reports of a PTX sensitivity of

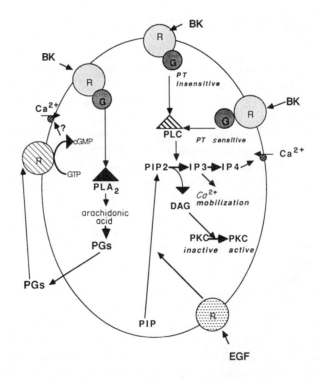

Figure 1. Schematic representation of the receptors and pathways involved in the response to bradykinin. BK = bradykinin; DAG = diacylglycerol; EGF = epidermal growth factor; G = G protein; GTP = guanosine triphosphate; cGMP = cyclic guanosine triphosphate; IP3 = inositol trisphosphate; IP4 = inositol tetrakisphosphate; PGs = prostaglandins; PIP = phosphatidyl inositol phosphate; PIP2 = phosphatidyl inositol bisphosphate; PLA$_2$ = phospholipase A$_2$; PLC = phospholipase C; PKC = protein kinase C; PT = pertussis toxin; R = receptor

phospholipase C activation in MDCK cells and in the elevation of $[Ca^{2+}]_i$ and inositol polyphosphates in NG108-15 (neuronal) cells. These data suggest that a G-protein of the G_i or G_0 type and at least one other G-protein is involved in the transduction of intracellular signals from ligand-stimulated bradykinin receptors.

The interaction of bradykinin with its receptor leads to phospholipase A_2-mediated generation of arachidonic acid (see Figure 1) and subsequent prostaglandin synthesis. This activation of phospholipase A_2 occurs in parallel with the activation of phospholipase C in fibroblasts, but these two events are reported to be independent and non-sequential suggesting that two separate G-proteins are involved. It is therefore unclear how many G-proteins are required for the transmission of signals from activated bradykinin receptors, although current evidence supports the involvement of at least two.

SYNERGY WITH OTHER LIGANDS

A variety of other growth-regulating ligands have been reported to synergize with bradykinin. Epidermal growth factor (EGF) has been demonstrated to synergize with bradykinin to stimulate phosphodiesteric cleavage of phosphatidyl inositol bisphosphate (PIP_2). This effect is thought to be mediated by the kinase activity of the activated EGF receptor protein acting on phosphatidyl inositol kinase to elevate levels of the phosphodiesterase substrate, PIP_2. Some workers have demonstrated that interleukin 1 (IL-1) also synergizes with bradykinin to activate the phospholipase A_2-prostaglandin synthetase pathway, whereas recent reports have indicated that bradykinin stimulates IL-1 as well as tumour necrosis factor (TNF) release from macrophages. Together, these data appear to suggest some sort of sequential or perpetuating interaction. Insulin also possesses the ability to synergize with bradykinin since these two ligands, when added together, can cause mitogenesis in fibroblasts. In summary, it appears that the bradykinin receptor may be involved in a series of inter-receptor and messenger transmodulation events which combine to mediate a cellular response.

BRADYKININ FORMATION AND RELEASE

Bradykinin is formed in biological fluids by the action of members of the kallikrein family of proteolytic enzymes on the precursor kininogen proteins (Figure 2). These kallikreins are themselves produced as inactive precursors (prekallikreins) by the liver and by exocrine glands and are stored in the liver, the pancreas and the intestine. The cascade reaction leading to bradykinin production is thus triggered when prekallikrein in plasma is activated by the Hageman Factor, an enzyme released as part of the clotting mechanism. This mechanism is triggered when blood comes into contact with the negatively charged surface of the basement membrane exposed during damage to the vascular wall. The specificity of the proteolytic cleavage leads to the generation of the naturally occurring kinins Met-Lys-bradykinin, Lys-bradykinin (kallidin) and bradykinin itself (see Figure 3 for structures). These peptides are rapidly degraded at their site of action by kininases I and II, the latter of which is also known as angiotensin I-converting enzyme.

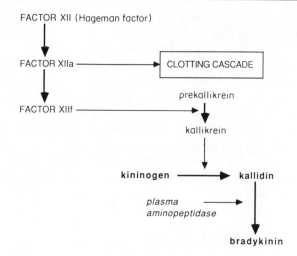

Figure 2. Scheme showing the current hypothesis for the activation of the kinin pathway. Factor XIIa has a major role in initiating the clotting cascade but a minor one in activating prekallikrein. Factor XIIf plays a major role in the prekallikrein to kallikrein conversion. Transformations are depicted as heavy arrows and enzymic actions as light arrows

RECEPTORS FOR BRADYKININ

Bradykinin acts through a specific cell surface receptor(s) to initiate an intracellular response. Receptors for bradykinin have been reported on such tissues as uterus, intestine, aorta, kidney, heart and spinal cord as well as on endothelial, epithelial, fibroblastic and neuronal cells *in vitro*.

Bradykinin receptors are classified as B_1 or B_2 according to the system originally devised by Regoli and Barabé. This system is based on a consideration of (a) the order of potency of receptor agonists; (b) the measurement of the affinity of competitive antagonists; and (c) ligand-induced receptor desensitization. In practical terms, this system applied to bradykinin distinguishes two main receptor types according to their affinity for the bradykinin fragment des-Arg^9-BK and the bradykinin analogue [Tyr-(Me)^8]-BK, both of which are agonists (see Figure 3 for structures). In rabbit aorta, a classic example of a B_1 type receptor, the affinities of the ligands for the receptor are in the order des-Arg^9-BK > BK > > [Tyr-(Me)^8]-BK. However, in rabbit jugular vein and dog carotid artery, the classic examples of a B_2 type receptor, the affinities are [Tyr-(Me)^8]-BK > BK > > des-Arg^9-BK.

Receptors *in vivo*

Bradykinin B_1 receptors appear to be absent *in vivo* under normal conditions but appear after exposure of tissues to such noxious stimuli as lipopolysaccharide or Triton X-100. Another unusual feature of B_1 receptors is that their numbers and apparent sensitivity to ligand stimulation tend to increase as a consequence of ligand exposure. These phenomena appear to be a direct effect of *de novo* synthesis of B_1

NATURAL KININS

			1	2	3	4	5	6	7	8	9
Bradykinin			Arg	Pro	Pro	Gly	Phe	Ser	Pro	Phe	Arg
Lys-bradykinin (kallidin)		Lys	Arg	Pro	Pro	Gly	Phe	Ser	Pro	Phe	Arg
Met-Lys-bradykinin (met-kallidin)	Met	Lys	Arg	Pro	Pro	Gly	Phe	Ser	Pro	Phe	Arg

ARTIFICIAL ANALOGUES AND FRAGMENTS

			1	2	3	4	5	6	7	8	9
Tyr^0-BK		Tyr	Arg	Pro	Pro	Gly	Phe	Ser	Pro	Phe	Arg
Tyr^5-BK			Arg	Pro	Pro	Gly	Tyr	Ser	Pro	Phe	Arg
Tyr^8-BK			Arg	Pro	Pro	Gly	Phe	Ser	Pro	Tyr	Arg
des-Arg^9-BK			Arg	Pro	Pro	Gly	Phe	Ser	Pro	Phe	–
[Tyr(Me)^8]-BK			Arg	Pro	Pro	Gly	Phe	Ser	Pro	TyM	Arg
Thi^{5,8}D-Phe^7-BK			Arg	Pro	Pro	Gly	Thi	Ser	D-Phe–	Thi	Arg
Hyp^{3}D-Phe^7-BK			Arg	Pro	Hyp	Gly	Phe	Ala	Ser	D-Phe	Arg
D-Phe^7-BK			Arg	Pro	Pro	Gly	Phe	Ala	Ser	D-Phe	Arg
D-Arg-[Hyp^3-Thi^{5,8}-D-Phe^7]-BK			D-Arg	Pro	Hyp	Gly	Thi	Ser	D-Phe–	Thi	Arg
Lys-Lys-[Hyp^{2,3}-Thi^{5,8}-D-Phe^7]-BK		Lys	Arg	Hyp	Hyp	Gly	Thi	Ser	D-Phe–	Thi	Arg
D-Nal^{1}Thi^{5,8}			D-Nal	Pro	Pro	Gly	Thi	Ser	D-Phe–	Thi	Arg

Figure 3. Structures of bradykinin analogues and fragments. Me = methyl; TyM = methyl tyrosine; Thi = β-[2-thienyl]alanine; Hyp = 4-hydroxyproline; Nal = β-[2-napthyl]alanine. D- indicates D-isomer

Table 1. Occurrence and affinities of bradykinin receptors measured *in vitro*

Tissue type	Cell type	Ligand used	Affinity	Receptor conc. (receptors/cell)	Comments
Ileum, duodenal and colon membranes	Epithelia	^{3}H-BK	5 nM	25 pmol g^{-1} (15 000)	
Human foreskin fibroblasts	Fibroblasts	^{3}H-BK	4.6 nm	230 fmol mg^{-1} (140 000)	Estimate by competition with ^{125}Tyr-BK
Bovine uterine myometrium membranes	Fibroblasts	BK	0.225 nM	N.D.	
NIE-115 cell line	Neuroblastoma	^{3}H-BK	0.83 pM 0.93 nM 4.9 nM	12 fmol mg^{-1} (8000) 160 fmol mg^{-1} (100 000) 250 fmol mg^{-1} (140 000)	Only report of three receptor types per cell
Primary rat brain cultures	Mainly neurones	^{125}TyrBK	1 nM 16 nM	100 fmol mg^{-1} (80 000) 1000 fmol mg^{-1} (600 000)	
Intestinal membranes	Epithelia	[^{125}Tyr]^8-BK	0.7 nM	332 fmol mg^{-1} (200 000)	
Guinea pig ileum heart and kidney membranes	Epithelia	^{3}H-BK	0.01 nM 0.9 nM	8.3 pmol g^{-1} (5000) 14 pmol g^{-1} (8400)	
Bovine uterine myometrium solution	Epithelia	^{125}Tyr-Lys-BK	0.2–0.35 nm	0.13 pmol mg^{-1} (78 000)	Membranes solubilized in CHAPS
NG108-15 cell line	Neuroblastoma X glioma	^{3}H-BK	0.8 nM 9.3 nM	74% 26%	
Bovine pulmonary artery membranes	Endothelial	^{3}H-BK	1.28 nM 'LOW'	111 fmol mg^{-1} (68 000) ?	Low affinity site non-saturable and is B1 type
Rat1 cell lines transfected with *ras* oncogenes	Fibroblasts	[^{125}Tyr]^8-BK	3.5–5 nM	(220–8000)	*Ras* transfection increases receptor number
Rat13 cells (Rat1 cell line transfected with Ha-*ras*-13)	Fibroblasts	^{3}H-BK	4.9 nM 2.7 pM 75 pM	(51 800) (1000)	
Guinea pig brain	Mainly neurones	^{3}H-BK		4.9 fmol mg^{-1} (3000)	
A431 cell line	Epithelial	^{3}H-BK	7.3 nM	(40 000)	
3T3 cell line	Fibroblasts	^{3}H-BK	3.1 nM	(82 000)	

receptors since this sensitization is completely blocked by cyclohexamide and actinomycin and is not due to indirect effects of prostaglandins and catecholamines. This mechanism might represent receptor regulation during the response of tissues to injury, especially fever, inflammation and allergic reactions. Thus, formation of the B_1 receptor type could mediate some of the effects of kinins such as hypertension and coronary vasodilation seen locally after exposure to noxious stimuli. In contrast to this, work on B_2 bradykinin receptors *in vivo* indicates that they are a stable component of the cell membrane of tissues.

Receptor studies *in vitro*

The majority of *in vitro* studies carried out on bradykinin binding appear to involve the B_2 receptor system. This includes work carried out on epithelial, endothelial, fibroblast and neuronal cell lines, as well as primary rat brain cultures, solubilized preparations of bovine uterus and intestinal epithelial membranes.

Varied reports exist on the number of different B_2 receptor types and their affinities for bradykinin (Table 1). The majority of workers report one class of receptors with a dissociation constant (K_d) of 0.7–5 nM, whether they are working on rat or human fibroblasts, intestinal or renal epithelia, or heart muscle membranes. However, there are reports of two types of receptor on intestinal epithelia, primary rat brain cultures and rat fibroblasts, and three receptor types on a neuroblastomal cell line. These are all reported to be of the B_2 type. In summary, measurements of affinity for bradykinin binding *in vitro* suggest the existence of more than one type of B_2 receptor, with some reports of more than one type of B_2 receptor present on one cell type.

Agonist/antagonist studies of bradykinin receptors

Pharmacological evidence supports the existence of more than one type of B_2 bradykinin receptor. This evidence falls into two main categories: (a) experiments where different biological effects of bradykinin can be shown to be totally independent in the same cell and (b) experiments where specific bradykinin antagonists can be shown to be agonists in some B_2 receptor systems. An example of the first category is provided by findings that bradykinin stimulates inositol-1-phosphate turnover and that prostaglandin synthesis can be dissociated, suggesting that bradykinin receptors are coupled to both phospholipase C and phospholipase A_2 via independent mechanisms. The second category of evidence is typified by work using the compound [Thi^{5,8}-DPhe^7]-BK, which is an antagonist of most B_2 receptors but has unexpected agonist activities in the presynaptic nerves of the vas deferens. Differences in response to the compound [Hyp^3-DPhe^7]-BK have also been seen pre- and post-synaptically in the rat vas deferens, leading to suggestions of a distinct B_2 bradykinin receptor of neuronal location. In addition, biological response studies have indicated that the kinin receptors involved in vascular pain and rat paw hyperalgesia may be distinct ([DNal^1-Thi^{5,8}-DPhe^7]-BK sensitive and insensitive, respectively). Taken together these data suggest the presence of at least two non-neuronal B_2 receptors, together with at least one B_2 receptor unique to the neuronal system. It is possible that these receptor subtypes are represented by one gene product that has been modified (perhaps by differential glycosylation) to obtain different patterns of specificity.

BRADYKININ RECEPTOR REGULATION

In the context of accumulating evidence of a role for phosphorylation in the regulation of many receptor types, it seems likely the bradykinin receptor possesses cytoplasmic sites that may become phosphorylated during receptor occupation. However, there is currently no clear evidence to suggest whether the bradykinin receptor itself possesses tyrosine kinase activity or whether it can be a substrate for specific cytoplasmic receptor kinases. Some data provide evidence for bradykinin receptor desensitization during ligand exposure by a mechanism dependent on active cellular metabolism and co-occurring with the phosphorylation of both membrane and cytoplasmic proteins. Interestingly, a role for phosphorylation in regulation has clearly been demonstrated in work carried out on both the serotonin (5-hydroxy-tryptophan) receptor and the β_2-adrenergic (β_2-A) receptors, both of which have properties possibly similar to those of the bradykinin receptor (see later).

Effects of *ras* and other oncogenes

Recently, there have been several reports of an increase in the number of bradykinin receptors present on the cell surface after transfection of cells with the *ras* oncogene. It appears that the increase in receptor number is a *ras*-specific event (rather than a general effect of transformation) and occurs after over-expression of each of the three normal *ras* gene products (Ha-, Ki- and N-) as well as after expression of the three activated *ras* gene products.

The *ras* protein, p21, is structurally and functionally related to the family of G-proteins and may be involved in receptor-mediated signal transduction. It is thus tempting to speculate that p21^{ras} interacts with bradykinin receptors at the cell surface to alter the mechanisms controlling receptor exposure or availability of cryptic binding sites. This effect is quite distinct from any increase in efficiency of receptor-phospholipase coupling as might be expected with p21^{ras}, by analogy with classical G-protein systems.

A report has recently emerged which argues against the effect of *ras* being mediated by its analogy with G-proteins. In this report, the *dbl* (human diffuse B-cell lymphoma) oncogene is shown to increase the expression of bradykinin receptors in NIH3T3 cells to the same extent as *ras*, whereas other oncogenes (v-*src*, v-*abl*, v-*mos*, v-*raf*, v-*fos*) did not have this effect. This raises the possibility that both p21^{ras} and p66^{dbl} (unrelated in structure to p21^{ras}) are having a direct influence on the regulation of receptor expression at the surface and/or a direct effect on receptor gene expression. A potential mechanism for this latter possibility is provided by recent findings that the c-Ha-*ras* oncogene activates both the transcription factor PEA1/AP1 and the polyoma (Py) virus enhancer. This activation may lead to altered transcription of transformation-related genes and could play a key role in tumori-genesis. Recent demonstrations of bradykinin as a mitogen suggest that the bradykinin receptor gene may be one of the many possible targets for this effect.

THE BRADYKININ RECEPTOR: PART OF A NEW RECEPTOR SUPERFAMILY?

It is becoming apparent that many small peptide ligands belong to a family of structurally related molecules which interact with a family of receptor subtypes. In turn, the members of these receptor families appear to belong to an emerging 'superfamily' of peptide ligand receptors. The cloning of the mammalian adrenergic receptors has so far revealed four subtypes (a_1, a_{2a}, b_1 and b_2), whereas two subtypes of muscarinic receptors have so far been identified (M1 and M2). Similarly, at least six subtypes of receptor for 5-hydroxytryptophan (5-HT—serotonin) have been identified (1A, 1B, 1C, 1D, 2 and 3). This emerging family, dubbed 'The Magnificent Seven', is characterized by receptors possessing seven alpha-helical transmembrane regions and the ability to interact with G-proteins. The possibility that multiple G-protein-linked bradykinin receptors exist, taken together with the known family of bradykinin receptor ligands, suggests that receptors for bradykinin may belong to this family of homologous receptors. Another potential member of this family is the bombesin receptor, by virtue of: (a) its molecular size; (b) the nature of its ligand and (c) its ability to interact with a G-protein. The different subtypes of receptor in each of these families are generally believed to be involved in mediating different cellular responses to the same ligand and/or conferring tissue specificity on these responses.

FUTURE DIRECTIONS

Overall, it appears that multiple bradykinin receptors, each coupled to their own G-proteins or interacting with different G-proteins may be involved in the various bradykinin-mediated responses. An additional complexity arises from the discovery of three more naturally occurring kinins (T-kinin, ornitho-kinin, hyp-kallidin) in addition to the three already discussed (bradykinin, Met-bradykinin [kallidin] and Met-Lys-bradykinin).

Emerging reports linking oncogenic transformation with increases in bradykinin receptor expression are very exciting, especially when taken together with the putative role for bradykinin as a mitogen. Basal levels of bradykinin in the blood of those measured during various models of inflammation (15 pM and 57 pM, respectively) are well below the reported K_d for bradykinin receptor-mediated mitogenesis (5 nM). However, the local concentrations of bradykinin in inflamed tissue (1 nM) are sufficiently high to trigger this response. This raises the possibility that bradykinin released in the reactive inflammation to malignant invasion may stimulate proliferation of some tumour cells (see Figure 4). This may be particularly pertinent in cases where *ras* or *dbl* oncogenes are involved. Many antagonists of bradykinin are available, which may be exploited as specific therapeutic agents in such cases.

A greater understanding of these processes could be gained by a knowledge of the receptor structure. It seems likely that this knowledge may be achieved within the next few years since many groups are currently involved in bradykinin receptor characterization experiments, presumably with the goal of receptor cloning. This

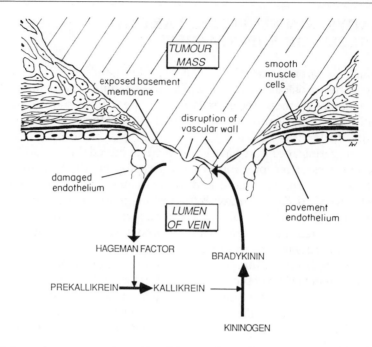

Figure 4. Schematic representation of bradykinin release during malignant invasion of vein. Hageman factor is released when blood comes into contact with the negatively charged surface of the basement membrane exposed during damage to the pavement endothelium of the vein wall

approach may prove difficult due to the absence of a cell line or tissue expressing bradykinin receptors in sufficiently high numbers for receptor purification and sequencing. Cloning could be achieved by inducing receptor expression in oocytes by injection of total messenger RNA, an approach which has recently proved successful for both the muscarinic acetylcholine receptor and the serotonin receptor. Alternatively, an approach based on the polymerase chain reaction may be used to selectively amplify and clone proteins containing consensus sequences found in receptors belonging to the 'Magnificent Seven' receptor family. Such an approach has recently yielded four new clones belonging to this family, two of which are as yet unidentified.

FURTHER READING

Benovic, J. L., DeBlasi, A., Stone, W. C., *et al.* (1989) β-Adrenergic receptor kinase: primary structure delineates a multigene family. *Science,* **246**; 235–246.

Casey, P. J. and Gilman, A. G. (1988) G protein involvement in receptor-effector coupling. *J. Biol. Chem.,* **263**, 2577–2580.

Dohlman, H. G., Caron, M. G. and Lefkowitz, R. J. (1987) A family of receptors coupled to guanine nucleotide regulatory proteins. *Biochemistry,* **26**, 2657–2664.

Downward, J., de Gunzburg, J., Riehl, R. and Weinberg, R. A. (1988) p21^{ras}-induced responsiveness of phosphatidylinositol turnover to bradykinin is a receptor number effect. *Proc. Natl. Acad. Sci. USA,* **85**, 5774–5718.

Regoli, D. and Barabe, J. (1980) Pharmacology of bradykinin and related kinins. *Pharmac. Rev.*, **32**, 1–46.

Roberts, R. A. and Gullick, W. J. (1989) Bradykinin receptor number and sensitivity to ligand stimulation of mitogenesis is increased by expression of a mutant *ras* oncogene. *J. Cell Sci.*, **94**, 527–535.

Roberts, R. A. and Gullick, W. J. (1989) Bradykinin receptors undergo ligand-induced desensitization. *Biochemistry*, **29**, 1975–1979.

Roberts, R. A. and Gullick, W. J. (1989) Bradykinin receptors: characterization, distribution and mechanisms of signal transduction. *Progress in Growth Factor Research*, **1**, 237–252.

Ruggiero, M., Srivastava, S. K., Fleming, T. P., Ron, D. and Eva, A. (1989) NIH3T3 fibroblasts transformed by the *dbl* oncogene show altered expression of bradykinin receptors: effect on inositol lipid turnover. *Oncogene*, **4**, 767–771.

Zachary, I., Woll, P. J. and Rozengurt, E. (1987) A role for neuropeptides in the control of cell proliferation. *Dev. Biol.*, **124**, 295–308.

25 GnRH Agonists: Treatment Paradigm for the Autocrine Hypothesis

JONATHAN WAXMAN

ABDUL QAYUM

It is ten years since the gonadotrophin-releasing hormone agonists were first applied to the treatment of patients with prostatic cancer. These compounds have been found to have an efficacy equivalent to conventional therapies for prostatic cancer. They obviate the need for orchiectomy and are without the cardiovascular toxicities of oestrogen therapy. Initially the agonists were introduced into clinical practice as intranasal or subcutaneous daily treatment. Pharmacological advances have meant that treatment has been refined, such that clinicians will shortly be able to offer patients subcutaneous depot therapies that can be applied once every three months. The use of these compounds has led to an advance in our understanding of the nature of response in prostatic cancer and it has been shown that the basis for response relates to specific receptors within the cell surface of prostatic cancer. It would seem that response is directly mediated through these receptors rather than through down-regulation of the pituitary-gonadal axis. The tumours themselves have been found to produce stimulatory peptides that are structurally similar to gonadotrophin-releasing hormone. This has provided a paradigm for the autocrine hypothesis and has directed research into other peptide antagonists of growth factors, which act, as do the gonadotrophin-releasing hormone agonists, to block specific growth factor receptors.

GONADOTROPHIN-RELEASING HORMONE AND ITS AGONISTS

In 1971 gonadotrophin-releasing hormone (GnRH) was purified and its structure identified. Intravenous injection of micrograms of this decapeptide was found to

Genes and Cancer. Edited by D. Carney and K. Sikora.
©1990 John Wiley & Sons Ltd.

```
      1   2   3   4   5   6   7   8   9   10
```

D-Glu-His-Trp-Ser-Tyr-Gly-Leu-Arg-Pro-Gly   GnRH

D-Glu-His-Trp-Ser-Tyr-D-Ser-Leu-Arg-Pro-EA   Buserelin
                              |
                             TBU

D-Glu-His-Trp-Ser-Tyr-D-Leu-Leu-Arg-Pro-Gly   Leuprolide

D-Glu-His-Trp-Ser-Tyr-D-Trp-Leu-Arg-Pro-Gly   Tryptorelin

D-Glu-His-Trp-Ser-Tyr-D-Ser-Leu-Arg-Pro-Aza-Gly   Zoladex
                              |
                             TBU

Figure 1. Gonadotrophin-releasing hormone and its analogues

lead to the release of luteinizing hormone and follicle-stimulating hormone from the pituitary. Synthetic analogues of the parent decapeptide were synthesized and it was found that those compounds with substitutions at the 6th and 10th amino acid residues were superactive, i.e. a single injection produced supraphysiological release of luteinizing hormone and follicle-stimulating hormone (Figure 1). It was hoped that these compounds would be of use in the management of hypothalamic hypogonadism, but with their repeated administration no such effect was observed. When given repeatedly to laboratory animals these analogues were found to have a paradoxical effect, causing down-regulation of the pituitary-gonadal axis and regression of the animals' secondary sexual characteristics.

As a result of these observations it was initially thought that these compounds would have no practical use and because of this, drug companies shut down their production facilities. However, a few workers exploited the potential of these compounds to limit gonadal function and applied these peptide analogues to situations where gonadal down-regulation was of advantage in gynaecological conditions, endocrine disorders and malignant disease. In malignant disease GnRH agonists have an important role in, premenopausal breast cancer, where they can be applied to perform a medical oophorectomy, which is reversible, in ovarian cancer, where they have a response rate, as second line agents, of approximately 30%, and in prostatic cancer, the second most common malignancy of men in the western world, where they provide a rational treatment without side-effects and one of exact equivalence to conventional therapies.

GnRH AGONISTS IN PROSTATIC CANCER

Clinical studies

Over 2000 structurally different analogues of GnRH have been synthesized. Clinical studies in prostatic cancer are, for the main, limited to the investigation of four different compounds: leuprolide, decapeptyl, buserelin and zoladex. Early work in prostatic cancer using these compounds aimed to establish dosage regimens and response rates. Treatment was given either as intranasal insufflation five or six times daily, or by daily subcutaneous injection. These somewhat inconvenient methods of administration demonstrated that this group of compounds were effective in the treatment of prostatic cancer; in non-randomized studies a response rate was reported equivalent to conventional therapies.

The impetus to explore alternative therapies for prostatic cancer had two sources. The first was the observation, established nearly 20 years previously, that oestrogen therapy had an excessive cardiovascular morbidity and mortality rate associated with its use. The second was that orchiectomy was regarded in a slightly unfavourable light by patients, who felt that it was bad enough to have cancer but it was an additional, rather tiresome burden, to have their testes removed as part of the treatment.

In initial studies of the use of the GnRH agonist for prostatic cancer, enthusiastic reporting, using criteria which are not now considered acceptable definitions of response, led to descriptions of higher response rates than are currently accepted. Following these initial descriptions, randomized studies were instituted comparing orchiectomy and oestrogen therapies with GnRH agonist treatment. The first to be reported and the most meticulous, came from the Leuprolide Study Group. This group compared treatment with leuprolide given as a daily injection to 1 mg thrice daily of diethylstilboestrol and found an identical initial response rate of approximately 50%. A follow-up study described the median duration of response and the median duration of survival of these groups of patients: these were not significantly different, at 1 year and 2½ years respectively for both groups. Much more important, the Leuprolide Study Group specifically examined the incidence of side-effects: gynaecomastia, cardiovascular toxicity and gastrointestinal toxicity were much more commonly seen with oestrogen therapy. Orchiectomy too, has been compared to treatment with one of the analogues, decapeptyl. Again, the same initial order of response was observed in both groups of treated patients. Later studies confirmed these observations regarding initial response rate and median duration of responsiveness comparing zoladex with orchiectomy and zoladex with oestrogen therapy.

In the mid-1980s, when the results of these studies were first reported, controversial claims were being made for the therapeutic advantage of additional anti-androgen therapy. It was argued that in a disease that is androgen responsive, the elimination of all sources of androgen production was important. Adrenal production of androgens is significant and may contribute to 5% of the circulating androgenic steroid levels. The contribution of adrenal androgens to the total level of androgen within the prostate may be much greater than that reflected by simple plasma levels: this is because of the local concentrating mechanisms involving androgen receptors and non-specific binding by sex hormone-binding globulin and albumin. Because of this the concurrent administration of anti-androgens additional to the use of a GnRH agonist was advocated. Such was the force of the argument from the main protagonist of this hypothesis that it was considered that the panoply of the patients' defences against the tumour would be somehow incomplete if an anti-androgen was not added to their treatment regimen.

The initial investigation of the combination of anti-androgen and GnRH agonist was not randomized and was much criticized. However, such was the interest generated by the idea that the National Cancer Institute initiated its own randomized study. A number of different anti-androgens were considered; however, flutamide was thought to be the most advantageous of the group becasue of its lack of inherent androgenicity and minimal side-effects. This anti-androgen was applied in a randomized study with leuprolide to a group of over 600 patients with metastatic prostatic cancer. Although the initial response rate was identical in each of the treatment groups, the median duration of response was significantly longer in the combination therapy arm at 16.5 months as compared to 13.9 months. The median duration of survival was also significantly extended to 35 months, as compared to 28 months. Although this difference is significant, the level of improvement in survival and response duration is effectively minimal in terms of the overall impact of combination therapy upon the disease itself. It may be of interest to investigate whether or not early treatment for a short period with a combination anti-androgen provides the same survival advantage as prolonged therapy.

Tumour flare

One of the disadvantages of gonadotrophin-releasing hormone agonist therapy is the early development of tumour flare. This is the acute exacerbation of the symptoms and signs of the disease that occurs within the first week of treatment. It is thought to relate to an increase in serum testosterone, though as will be discussed below, this phenomenon may be due to a direct effect at the level of the tumour itself rather than through any stimulation of the pituitary-gonadal axis. The syndrome is variably reported as occurring in 5–40% of patients. This variation is probably due to the intensity with which patients are observed in the early phases of treatment. Randomized studies have been initiated comparing the effects of different anti-androgens in abrogating the development of tumour flare. Different dosages of cyproterone acetate and flutamide have been compared, and it has been found that pretreatment with cyproterone acetate at 100 mg thrice daily for one week prior and then for the first month of GnRH agonist therapy prevents any increase in serum testosterone with GnRH agonist therapy and the development of tumour flare. Subsequent to this randomized study our group have seen no cases of tumour flare in nearly 100 patients with prostatic cancer treated in this fashion.

Pharmacological developments

It is obviously less than ideal to treat elderly patients, who tend to be a little forgetful, with daily injections or with five- or six-times daily intranasal spray insufflations, and so depot preparations of GnRH agonists have been developed. Three different types of depot were initially investigated: a microencapsulated form given as a deep intramuscular injection; a subcutaneous polyhydroxybutyric acid tablet implant; and an injectable lactide-glycolide co-polymer rod implant. The microencapsulated preparation is relatively difficult to synthesize and early forms had variable release characteristics. The tablet implant requires a surgical incision and so is impractical in terms of the time it takes to administer. The rod implant has relatively stable and reproducible release characteristics and is easy to administer. It is this implant that has undergone extensive pharmacological development. After initial studies a 1-month depot implant became available. The release characteristics of the implant have been altered by changing the ratio of lactolide and glycolide within the co-polymer base, by experimenting with different surface coatings and by adding different amounts of analogue. By these means very long-acting preparations of GnRH agonist in depot formulation have entered limited clinical trial. A 2-month implant has been shown to be effective in suppressing testosterone for prolonged periods, and more recently a 3-month depot preparation has been shown to be effective in suppressing patients' testicular function for periods of up to 2 years. It would seem that this pharmacological development is the way forward for the patient with cancer, optimally fitting in treatment with clinic visits.

SCIENTIFIC DEVELOPMENTS— A PARADIGM FOR THE AUTOCRINE HYPOTHESIS

The therapeutic effects of GnRH analogues in prostatic cancer have traditionally been thought to be mediated through suppression of the pituitary-gonadal axis, leading to decreased production of testosterone. However, in patients treated with these compounds close observation shows response at a time when serum testosterone, luteinizing hormone and follicle-stimulating hormone are all at pre-treatment levels, with clinical improvement seen generally at the end of the first treatment week. Similarly, the phenomenon of tumour flare does not coincide with the initial rise in serum androgen concentrations. These observations suggest the possibility that GnRH analogues may not be exerting their effect directly through the reduction of circulating androgen levels.

Because of these observations we have investigated the possibility of there being GnRH receptors within human prostatic cancer. Two human cell lines have been investigated: the LNCaP line is a human hormone-responsive line derived from a lymph node metastasis; the DU145 line is a human hormone-responsive line derived from a brain metastasis. Cells were grown in culture and harvested, and from these cells membrane preparations were obtained. Membranes were incubated with labelled buserelin and varying concentrations of unlabelled buserelin. From the displacement of labelled by unlabelled buserelin the binding affinity of the membrane preparations was established. The LNCaP line had high-affinity binding with a K_d of between 5×10^{-8} M and 1×10^{-9} M. This binding was specific in that addition of protease substrate resulted in no significant displacement of the label. In contrast the DU145 line only exhibited low-affinity binding with a K_d of 10^{-5} M (Figure 2) and this, in contrast to the LNCaP line, was virtually completely inhibited by addition of protease substrate. This level of affinity is of interest because it corresponds to the approximate steady-state serum concentrations of buserelin achieved with depot preparations.

Having demonstrated high-affinity binding, we next investigated whether or not a GnRH-like factor was secreted by these cell lines. Culture medium from both cell lines was concentrated and a GnRH-specific radioimmunoassay performed. GnRH-like immunoreactivity, which was directly dependent upon the number of cells in culture, was found in both cell lines, providing supportive evidence for the hypothesis investigated. These biochemical observations taken in isolation might be considered of interest, but could be dismissed as an epiphenomenon, without corroborative evidence of a biological effect. Accordingly, both cell lines were grown in short-term culture with different concentrations of buserelin. In these experiments

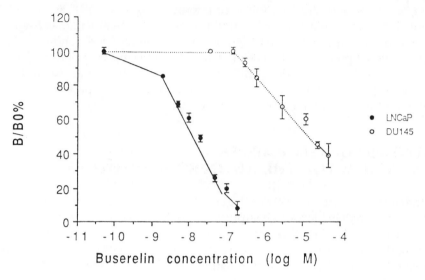

Figure 2. Binding affinity for gonadotrophin-releasing hormone in the LNCaP and DU145 cell lines

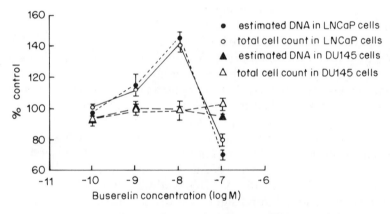

Figure 3. Growth stimulation of LNCaP and DU145 cell lines

it was observed that there was a direct, dose-related stimulation of the hormone-responsive line and that there was no dose-related stimulation of growth of the hormone-independent line (Figure 3), evidence in support of our biochemical observations. This work implies that a locally produced growth factor is stimulating the growth of hormone responsive prostatic cancer through its own surface receptor, GnRH analogues acting by competitively binding with and then down-regulating this receptor.

This work has been extended, and currently we have confirmed the presence of high-affinity GnRH binding in human tumours removed premortem by transurethral resection. This work is at an early stage, and in our patients we will correlate response to GnRH agonist treatment with receptor status. It is of interest to postulate why hormone-unresponsive lines are receptor negative. This may be due to a defect at a number of levels, including the gene or gene transcription, or abnormal processing of the protein product of the gene. In some futuristic scenario it may be possible to insert by transfection experiments the normal gene for GnRH receptor and confer by this means hormone responsiveness in a hormone-unresponsive patient.

CONCLUSIONS

The development of the gonadotrophin-releasing hormone agonists has provided an effective non-invasive treatment for prostatic cancer that is humane and without side-effects. This has led to increased interest in the biochemical basis for response in this disease. It may well be that our new understanding of the controlling processes in prostatic cancer will lead to us solving the major problem in this illness, which remains the treatment of patients in relapse. This requires an evolutionary jump in terms of the development of new therapeutic manoeuvres by means of the application of our new molecular understanding of the biochemical basis of cancer.

FURTHER READING

Crawford, E. D., Eisenberger, M. A., McLeod, D. G., *et al.* (1989) A controlled trial of leuprolide with and without flutamide in prostatic carcinoma. *N. Engl. J. Med.*, **321**, 419–424.

Waxman, J., Man, A., Hendry, W. F., *et al.* (1985) Importance of early tumour exacerbation in patients treated with long acting analogues of gonadotrophin releasing hormone for advanced prostatic cancer. *Br. Med. J.*, **291**, 1387–1388.

Waxman, J., Sandow, J., Abel, P., *et al.* Three-monthly GnRH agonist (buserelin) for prostatic cancer. *British Journal of Urology*, (in press).

26 Inhibitors of Growth Factor Receptors

W. J. GULLICK

Polypeptide growth factors are multi-functional molecules with influences on cell growth, the immune system, wound healing, embryogenesis, differentiation and inflammation. Progress in this field has resulted primarily from the identification and molecular characterisation of these factors and, more recently, from their production by recombinant expression systems in large quantities.

The most well-studied factors are generally members of structurally related protein families (Table 1). The receptors for these factors are of necessity partly on the cell surface since the peptide ligands are not soluble through the plasma membrane. Some receptors bind more than one ligand, sometimes with the same affinity and sometimes differentially. Most receptors for this class of molecules are transmembrane glycoproteins with an extracellular glycosylated domain and an intracellular domain which possesses protein tyrosine kinase activity that is stimulated by ligand binding.

In this chapter I will consider firstly the known examples of aberrant growth factor receptor signalling, and secondly current concepts and approaches towards developing inhibitors of growth factor receptor activity. Such drugs would have potential value in regulating normal systems, such as inflammation, the immune system and some of the mechanisms involved in wound healing, but their greatest potential impact may be in the control and elimination of malignant cells.

MECHANISMS OF ABERRANT SIGNAL TRANSDUCTION

Three classes of change affecting systems conveying growth regulatory signals can be predicted: over-stimulation, qualitatively altered signalling and 'loss of function' mutations.

Genes and Cancer. Edited by D. Carney and K. Sikora
©1990 John Wiley & Sons Ltd

Table 1. Growth factors which bind to receptors
with tyrosine kinase activity

EGF Family
1. Mammalian factors
        EGF
        TGF-alpha
        Amphiregulin
        CRIPTO

2. Viral factors
        Vaccinia virus
        Shope fibroma
        Molluscum contagiosum
        Myxoma virus

FGF Family
        Acidic FGF
        Basic FGF
        int-2
        HST
        FGF.5
        FGF.6

PDGF Family
        PDGF BB
        PDGF AB
        PDGF AA

Insulin Family
        Insulin
        IGF I
        IGF II
        Relaxin

Haemopoietic Growth Factors
        CSF-1

Over-stimulation

Over-stimulation can be achieved in two distinct ways:

Over-expression of normal growth factors or normal growth factor receptors. This
concept originated as the autocrine hypothesis of Todaro and DeLarco, which may
be stated as 'over-expression of a growth factor by a cell that possesses receptors
for that factor may lead to uncontrolled proliferation'. Elevated expression of EGF,
TGF-alpha, PDGF, HST and the CRIPTO gene (which encodes a protein related
in structure to the EGF family, see Table 1) in NIH3T3 fibroblasts is partially
transforming. *In vivo* in human tumours only the HST and *int*-2 growth factor genes
are amplified in breast cancer and oesophageal cancers but paradoxically they are
not expressed, suggesting that an unidentified linked gene is the dominantly selected
locus. Since the elevated levels of growth factor proteins observed in human tumours
are not the result of gene amplification, it is often difficult to determine rigorously
that they represent aberrant events. Perhaps the most convincing example is the
high level of TGF-alpha associated with psoriatic skin. However, this condition of

non-neoplastic hyperplasia emphasizes that simple over-expression of a growth factor in the absence of other genetic changes is unlikely to cause frank malignancy. Despite this the influence of autonomous growth factor production on the biology of some human cancers, for instance of the breast, may be profound and inhibitors of growth factor activity may prove to be valuable clinically.

Central to the strategy of designing growth factor inhibitors is the question of whether growth stimulation can occur intracellularly. Growth factors and their receptors are synthesized and processed along common secretory pathways providing the opportunity for them to interact within this space. Although this compartment is continuous with the extracellular space it is in fact highly secluded and inaccessible to extracellular factors. Evidence in the PDGF/PDGF receptor system is conflicting as to whether ligand receptor interaction is intracellular or extracellular. EGF and TFG-alpha, however, appear to act only after secretion and at the cell surface.

Over-stimulation of growth may also be achieved by elevated levels of expression of normal growth factor receptors. Elevated expression of the c-erbB2 protein or the EGF receptor (in the presence of EGF) will transform cultured cells. Both receptors are frequently over-expressed in a wide range of common solid human tumours (Table 2). EGF receptor over-expression may be either through gene amplification (common in head and neck and glioblastoma multiforme tumours) or by increased transcription (common in breast, bladder and lung tumours). Over-expression of the c-erbB2 protein is generally due to gene amplification (common in breast, stomach, ovary and pancreatic tumours) and occasionally due to increased transcription (approximately 10% of cases of elevated protein expression are due to increased transcription in breast cancer, for example).

Over-stimulation of growth by mutant growth factor receptors. Mutation of the *neu* gene (the rat homologue of the c-erbB2 gene) by chemical carcinogens *in vivo* activates the *neu* protein to transform cells. Introduction of the same mutation into the c-erbB2 gene is also transforming. Truncation of the EGF receptor to remove the extracellular ligand-binding domain is activating and also increases the ability of mutant *neu* to transform cells. In human cancers so far no point mutations have been found in the c-erbB2 gene, although few tumour types have been examined. A single case of a rearranged c-erbB2 gene, capable of expressing a truncated protein, has been reported in a gastric adenocarcinoma. Several instances have been reported in brain tumours of rearranged EGF receptor genes leading to the expression of proteins lacking parts of their extracellular sequences. A single similar example of a rearranged

Table 2. Over-expression of c-erbB2 and EGF receptors in human tumour types

c-erbB2	EGF receptor
Breast (30%)	Astrocytoma grade III and IV (50%)
Stomach (30%)	Breast (30%)
Ovary (10–30%)	Head and neck squamous carcinomas*
Pancreas (10%)	Bladder carcinomas*
Lung NSCLC (3%)	Lung NSCLC*
	Vulval squamous carcinomas*

*Reported incidence variable.

EGF receptor gene has been observed in an adenocarcinoma of the uterine endometrium. In some cases the mutant receptors possessed constitutively activated ligand-independent tyrosine kinase activity. Paradoxically, a glioblastoma cell line has been examined which possessed an amplified EGF receptor gene but the protein product was catalytically inactive and unresponsive to EGF. The explanation for this remains obscure; however, the over-expression of EGF receptors appears to be a selective disadvantage to cultured brain tumour cells, and this may represent an adaptation to tissue culture.

'Loss of function' mutations

Although these are not directly relevant to the design and use of growth factor receptor inhibitors they may be revealing as to the mechanisms by which receptor function can be lost. Two examples of *in vivo* loss of function mutations have been reported, both occurring in the insulin receptor in patients with non-insulin-dependent diabetes with acanthosis nigricans. Cloning and sequencing of the insulin receptor from the patients' somatic DNA revealed that one allele contained a mutant receptor gene. In one case a mutation substituted a valine residue for a critical glycine residue in the receptor's ATP-binding site, leading to the expression of a receptor lacking tyrosine kinase activity. The other patient possessed a receptor gene that had become recombined with an unrelated sequence deleting the majority of its cytoplasmic domain. As discussed below, such mutant receptors may also affect the function of the protein encoded by the normal allele.

GROWTH FACTOR RECEPTOR INHIBITORS

Ligand antagonists

Ligand antagonists exist for many of the peptide growth factor receptors, including bombesin, substance P, bradykinin and LHRH. Several attempts have been reported to produce ligand analogues of the polypeptide growth factors, notably EGF and TGF-alpha, with antagonistic properties. So far these have proved unsuccessful. Two approaches have been employed. Synthetic peptides, usually representing 10–20% of the linear sequence of the natural factor, have been synthesized and tested for their ability to compete with natural ligand binding and thus affect receptor functions. In summary, despite one or two reports of their having weak (1000 times less than the natural ligand) agonistic properties, no antagonism was observed. Although some effort was made to give these a constrained tertiary structure similar to the natural molecule (for instance by disulphide bond peptide cyclization) no systematic study of residue substitutions with natural and unnatural amino acids has been reported. In the light of the almost totally ineffectual nature of the natural short sequences so far tested this is perhaps not surprising.

The second approach involves site-directed mutation of growth factor genes in vitro followed by the expression, purification and characterization of the mutant protein. The main model for this has been TGF-alpha, where several residues have been replaced by conservative or non-conservative substitutions. In summary, alterations of residues homologous in several or all the members of the EGF/TGF-alpha family lead to total or substantial loss of binding affinity for the EGF receptor and consequent low biological activity. Substitution of non-conserved residues generally produce similar but quantitatively less dramatic effects. No antagonism was seen; rather, the molecules were always to some degree weaker agonists due to lower binding affinities. In some cases high concentrations of mutated factors were shown to be complete agonists. Again, so far no non-naturally occurring amino acids have been introduced, largely because of the biological expression systems employed. Both TGF-alpha and EGF have now been totally chemically synthesized, providing the opportunity to test this approach.

Natural growth factors such as TGF-alpha have been produced as fusion proteins with plant toxins such as *Pseudomonas* exotoxin which bind to EGF receptors and are cytotoxic. This is an interesting and promising approach, but since these are not inhibitors of growth factor receptors per se they are not within the scope of this chapter.

Although ligand antagonists have not yet been produced, this will remain an active area of research since the concepts are relatively simple and the possible prizes are large. The availability of the three-dimensional structures of EGF and TGF-alpha, obtained by 2-D nuclear magnetic resonance, and the use of interactive molecular graphics may help to accelerate developments in this field.

Monoclonal antibodies

So many monoclonal antibodies have been produced to growth factors and their receptors that only very general experimental concepts will be discussed here. Firstly, several monoclonal antibodies are available which bind to and neutralize growth factors. These include antibodies to EGF, TGF-alpha, IGF1, acidic FGF, basic FGF, bombesin, TGF-beta and PDGF. Surprisingly, only one report has examined the effect of their *in vivo* applications; it concerned the properties of a monoclonal antibody to bombesin, which was reported to inhibit the growth of a small cell lung cancer cell line in nude mice. This seems an under-represented area of research, either because such experiments have not been done or they have not worked and so have been unreported.

Monoclonal antibodies to growth factor receptors have been studied in much greater detail *in vitro* and *in vivo*. Several antibodies which bind to intracellular determinants have been described which inhibit tyrosine kinase activity using solubilized receptors. These are, however, probably destined to remain research reagents because of the problem of access to their site of action in live cells. Antibodies to the extracellular domain of *neu* and c-*erb*B2 proteins and the EGF receptor have been described which bind to live cells. Various effects have been observed, partly due to the idiosyncratic properties of each reagent and partly due to their different abilities to inhibit ligand binding or promote receptor clustering. Antibodies that prevent ligand binding do so competitively by steric inhibition, and these are so far the only true antagonists of growth factor receptors that have been studied in detail. The most well characterized are monoclonal antibodies 528 and 255, which inhibit EGF-induced receptor autophosphorylation but promote receptor internalization and degradation. They inhibit the growth of some tumour lines *in vitro* and the growth of A431 cells (which have large numbers of EGF receptors) *in vivo*. Most work *in vivo* has centred around tumour imaging using radioisotopically labelled antibodies or antibodies coupled to plant toxins. Some tumour growth inhibitory effects have been reported but these tend to be reductions in tumour incidence when tumour cells are simultaneously injected with antibodies, or decreases in growth rates of small established tumours.

Antibodies to the rat *neu* protein inhibit the growth of NIH3T3 cells transformed by expression of mutant *neu in vitro* and *in vivo* rather efficiently. Pre-immunization of mice with the rat *neu* external domain using a vaccinia virus construct protected the animals against the development of tumours.

Antibodies to the extracellular domain of c-*erb*B2 protein inhibited the growth of a human breast cancer derived cell line (SKBR-3). This is a particularly encouraging result since this line (like breast cancers *in vivo*) possesses other oncogenic mutations (c-*myc* amplification) yet suppression of the influence of high levels of c-*erb*B2 expression still had an appreciable effect on its behaviour. Experiments on the effect of tumour growth in animals have not yet been reported but may be anticipated.

The future of such studies is uncertain since the efficiency of monoclonal antibodies in tumour treatment has been quite variable. The advantage of growth factor receptors as targets of immunotherapy is their high level of cell surface expression and their proposed role in sustaining tumour growth. The problems involved concern tumour penetrance and, in common with all inhibitors of growth factor receptors, the effects on normal tissues (see below).

Dimerization inhibitors

A problem that has intrigued molecular biologists for some years is how the binding of a growth factor to the extracellular domain of a growth factor receptor succeeds in promoting the catalytic activity of the cytoplasmic domain through the single polypeptide chain that connects them. Two models are envisaged (Figure 1). The first, called the intramolecular model, involves the propagation of a conformational change induced by ligand binding across the membrane to alter the shape' and therefore the activity of the cytoplasmic domain. There is generally rather little

INTRAMOLECULAR ACTIVATION

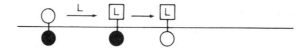

INTERMOLECULAR ACTIVATION

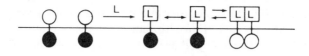

Figure 1. Models of growth factor receptor activation

experimental support for this, but no experiments that exclude it as a potential mechanism. The second hypothesis, called the intermolecular model, involves the promotion of receptor dimerization by ligand binding. More accurately perhaps, ligand binding may remove a negative influence on receptor dimerization since, as discussed above, deletion of the extracellular domain of several growth factor receptors is to a certain extent activating.

The concept of inhibition of growth factor receptors by preventing receptor dimerization has recently been proposed. The observation that mutational changes in *neu* or c-*erb*B2 proteins (or possibly EGF receptor) at a particular position in the transmembrane region leads to receptor dimerization, kinase activation and cell transformation has suggested that receptors may interact (at least in part) by helix-helix packing of specific residues in this region. The introduction of peptides (synthesized chemically and added exogenously) or the expression of short receptor sequences using minigene expression vectors is being examined to determine whether these may form specific non-productive complexes with mutant or normal growth factor receptors thereby limiting their activity. Such peptides, if they were effective, would have the merit of being simple to prepare, possibly poorly immunogenic or non-immunogenic, and have good penetration properties.

Another approach is to utilize extracellular domains of growth factor receptors to promote dimerization of a full-length receptor with only the ligand-binding part of the external sequences. This approach does work, as demonstrated with cells over-expressing EGF receptors, where inhibition of EGF receptor function was observed. Problems still exist as to the size and complexity of such molecules, but the results to date are very encouraging.

Inhibitors of dimerization may become more sophisticated with the determination of growth factor receptor structures. Perhaps the ideal objective would be to target small peptides to the contact regions of the interacting surfaces of the receptor's extracellular domains to prevent dimerization. Such chemicals would have many of the merits and few of the disadvantages of the substances described above, but they cannot be designed without three-dimensional information and knowledge of the receptor-receptor contact surfaces.

Tyrosine kinase inhibitors

The tyrosine kinase domain catalyses the transfer of the terminal phosphate of ATP to the para-hydroxyl group of tyrosine residues at particular sites in substrate proteins. The enzyme reaction is an ordered bi-bi reaction where the peptide or protein is the first substrate to bind and ADP is the last product to be released. Two classes of inhibitors have been examined, those based on ATP and those on substrates.

ATP analogues. Although the three-dimensional structures of growth factor receptors have not been determined, the structure of the ATP-binding site has been examined in detail. By homology with other kinases the sequence Gly-x-Gly-x-x-Gly, followed by a variable length of amino acids (10–20), followed by the sequence Val-Ala-x-Lys forms the ATP-binding site. The ATP analogue 5'-*p*-fluorosulfonylbenzoyl adenosine (FSBA) has been shown directly to react with the conserved lysine residue of the EGF receptor, and a series of 26 ATP analogues have been employed to determine the important regions for recognition and high-affinity binding. A three-dimensional model for the residues involved in ATP binding has been proposed, based upon the known structures of the NAD-binding region of glyceraldehyde-3-phosphate dehydrogenase, lactate dehydrogenase and alcohol dehydrogenase, and the FAD-binding regions of glutathione reductase and *p*-hydroxybenzoate hydroxylase.

In an early report a chloromethyl ketone derivative of lactic acid was shown to inhibit the kinase activity of EGF receptor, but the mechanism involved was not determined. As mentioned above FSBA covalently modifies the EGF receptor and inhibits tyrosine kinase activity, as does a photoaffinity label, arylazido-β-alanyl-ATP, which was employed as a probe of the binding site rather than for its properties as an inhibitor.

Several competitive inhibitors of ATP binding have been developed (Figure 2). The isoflavone compound genistein, isolated from *Pseudomonas*, was found to be a specific inhibitor of tyrosine kinase activity with little effect on serine and threonine kinases. It was, however, a general inhibitor of tyrosine kinase. The compound amiloride—3,5-diamino-N-(aminoiminomethyl)-6-chloropyrazinecarboxamide—which had been employed commonly as an inhibitor of the Na^+/H^+ antiporter, was found also to inhibit growth factor receptor tyrosine kinase activity directly. The inhibition was non-competitive with histone but competitive with ATP. Again, this compound was a general tyrosine kinase inhibitor affecting the activity of EGF receptor, insulin receptor and PDGF receptor.

Tyrosine

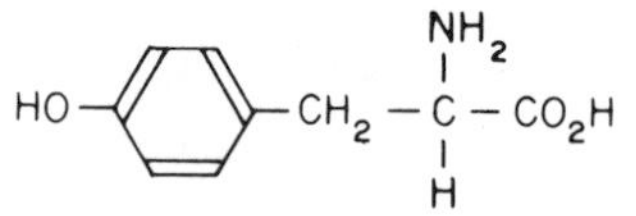

Staurosporine

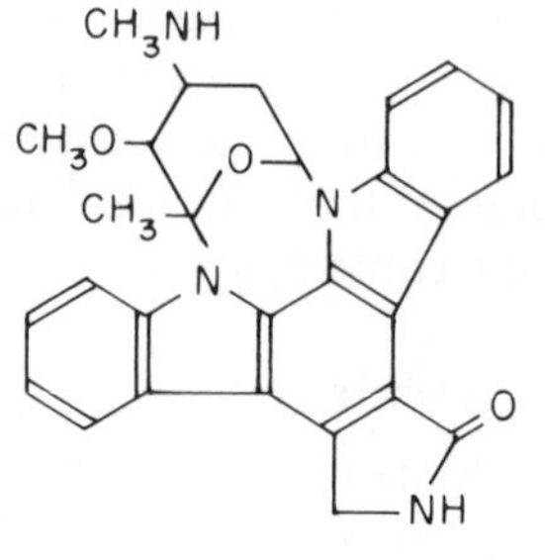

ST 638
(4–Hydroxycinnamide
analogue)

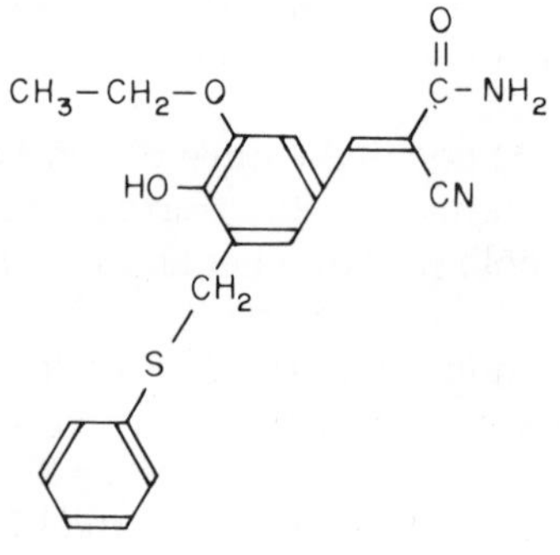

As can be seen from the above one of the disadvantages of ATP analogues is their lack of specificity of action on different growth factor receptors.

Substrate analogues. The tyrosine kinase of growth factor receptors catalyses the transfer of phosphate to tyrosine residues. Thus within the catalytic site all receptors must possess residues which interact specifically with tyrosine. On the other hand each receptor displays a different substrate protein specificity and generally catalyses the phosphorylation of only a few of their available tyrosine residues. Examination

ATP

Genistein

Amiloride

Erbstatin

Tyrphostin 12

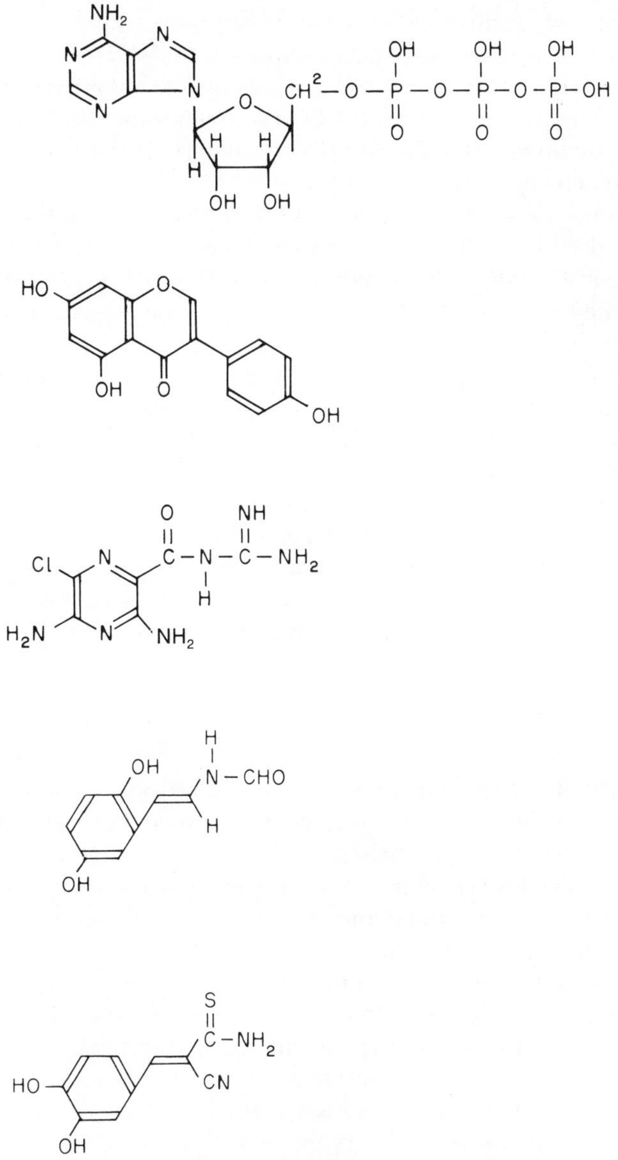

Figure 2. Structures of some inhibitors of tyrosine kinase activity

of the sequences surrounding such sites reveals only that the modified tyrosine is generally preceded by an acidic residue. No motif therefore has reliably been defined which allows prediction of whether a particular tyrosine in a sequence will be modified or not. It seems likely therefore that the three-dimensional shape and the hydrophilicity and ionized groups surrounding a particular tyrosine residue provide the specificity of the interaction.

Substrate-based inhibitors have therefore been prepared, generally with some resemblance to tyrosine but decorated with various functional groups, and their specificity of action on particular growth factor receptors examined (Figure 2). A series of derivatives of 4-hydroxycinnamamide were synthesized and their effects on various tyrosine kinases studied. One, ST638 (α-cyano,3-ethoxy,4-hydroxy, 5-phenylthiomethyl cinnamamide) competitively inhibited the phosphorylation of an exogenous substrate for the EGF receptor with a K_i of 2.1 μM. Its order of efficacy of inhibition was: EGFR > c-*fgr* > c-*src* > c-*fps*. It did not inhibit serine or threonine kinase activity.

Another substrate analogue which has been examined is staurosporine, a microbial alkaloid with antifungal activity. This compound was non-competitive with ATP on the insulin receptor kinase activity and was a better inhibitor of insulin receptor than the EGF receptor and IGF I receptor. The ED_{50} for insulin receptor was 61 nM and for IGF I receptor 6.2 μM.

A compound named erbstatin has been isolated from *Streptomyces neyagawaensis*. This subsequently formed the basis for a series of analogues which inhibit the EGF receptor tyrosine kinase activity by competing with the protein substrate and not with ATP binding. This class of compounds was named 'tyrphostins', members of which display quite varied abilities to differentially inhibit the EGF receptor and insulin receptor tyrosine kinase activities.

Finally, peptide substrates have been developed which inhibit the cAMP-dependent protein kinase A, and such substances may prove useful models for developing effective tyrosine kinase inhibitors in the future.

SUMMARY

This chapter has considered the incidence and various mechanisms of growth factor signalling system abnormalities associated with different types of human cancers. Several approaches have been investigated for producing inhibitors of growth factor receptors with tyrosine kinase activity, based on the premise that these might be developed into clinically useful reagents. The problems encountered are of specificity, access to the receptors and activity of the antagonists. When such substances are developed they will be tested *in vitro* in the first instance. Should they prove sufficiently encouraging the next hurdle will be to address their activity *in vivo*. Growth factor receptors are expressed widely on normal tissues and it is not known presently how best to affect selected tissues and sites in the body without unacceptable pathological consequences to other tissues. Growth factor receptor inhibitors are likely to be more cytostatic rather than cytotoxic in action, but this problem will be the principal challenge of the next decade for this area of research.

FURTHER READING

Akiyama, T., *et al.* (1987) *J. Biol. Chem.*, **262**, 5592–5595.
Basu, A., *et al.* (1989) *Mol. Cell. Biol.*, **9**, 671–677.
Darlak, K., *et al.* (1988) *J. Cell. Biochem.*, **36**, 341–352.
Di Marco, E., *et al.* (1989) *Oncogene*, **4**, 831–838.
Gullick, W. J. and Ventner, D. J. (1989) In: Waxman, J. and Sikora, K. (eds.), *The Molecular Biology of Cancer*. Blackwell Scientific, Oxford, pp. 38–53.
Lazar, E., *et al.* (1988) *Mol. Cell. Biol.*, **8**, 1247–1252.
Masui, H., *et al.* (1986) *Cancer Res.*, **46**, 5592–5598.
Sternberg, M. and Gullick, W. J. (1989) *Nature*, **339**, 587.
Yaish, P., *et al.* (1988) *Science*, **242**, 933–935.

Tumour Biology

27

Gene Rearrangement in B-cell Lymphomas

TAMAS HICKISH
DAVID CUNNINGHAM

Cytogenetic studies first indicated that chromosomal translocations were common in B-cell lymphomas. It is now clear that specific chromosomal translocations result in rearrangement of established or presumptive oncogenes. Although these genes are implicated in the development of B-cell malignancies, their precise role in tumorigenesis and the manner in which rearrangement perturbs their function is still not completely understood. Nevertheless, their presence at or near the translocation breakpoints has provided insights into the natural history of the malignancies in which they occur, and will increasingly help the clinician in diagnosis, in defining the extent of disease and in prognosis.

IMMUNOGLOBULIN GENES—WILLING PARTNERS FOR TRANSLOCATION

Immunoglobulin genes are rearranged in the process of normal B-cell differentiation and the reciprocal translocation present in many B-cell malignancies (Table 1) occurs at one of the sites of rearrangement. The resulting translocation creates a chromosome on which an immunoglobulin gene is inappropriately adjacent to a gene from another chromosome. The heavy-chain variable locus, located at 14q32.3, is frequently involved (Figure 1).

The probable explanation for this lies with the process that produces functional immunoglobulin heavy-chain genes. As the progenitor B-cell matures into a pre-B-cell the heavy chain variable region is assembled. This region is encoded by an exon generated by the union of a variable (V), diversity (D) and junctional (J) exon, each

Genes and Cancer. Edited by D. Carney and K. Sikora.
©1990 by John Wiley & Sons Ltd.

Table 1. Examples of reciprocal chromosomal translocations present in B-cell malignancies

Tumour type	Chromosomal translocation	Genes rearranged	
		Proto-oncogene	Immunoglobulin
80% follicle centre cell 20% diffuse follicle centre cell	t(14;18) (q32.3;q21.3)	bcl-2	J_H
Diffuse follicle centre cell (infrequent)	t(3;14) (p21;q32.3)	?	J_H
	t(3;14) (q27;q32.3)	?	J_H
	t(5;14) (q11;q32.3)	?	J_H
	t(1;14) (q41;q32.3)	?	J_H
	t(8;14) (q24.1;q32.3)	c-myc	J_H
Diffuse small-cell lymphoma, myeloma (uncommon)	t(11;14) (q13.3;q32.3)	bcl-1	J_H
Burkitt's	80% t(8;14) (q24.1;q32.3)	c-myc	J_H
	15% t(8;22) (q24.1;q11.2)		C_λ
	5% t(2;8) (p11.2;q24.1)		C_x
L3 ALL	(8;14) (q24.1;q32.3)		J_H

selected apparently at random from the heavy-chain multigene family. DNA recombination first joins a D and J exon, and these are then joined to a V exon. The assembly process is mediated by the VDJ recombinase enzyme system. The rules governing the activity of this system are only just being discovered. This system appears to catalyse recombination only when specific signals, consisting of two paired heptamer/nonamer sequences, one pair containing a 12-base spacer and the other a 23-base spacer, are apposed in the recombining exons (V_H, D_H, J_H) (Figure 2). The system is error prone—deletions, substitutions and the addition of extra nucleotides (N regions) commonly occur. In many B-cell malignancies these hallmarks of VDJ recombinase activity are found in the joining regions on the 14q+ and reciprocal translocations, implying VDJ recombinase has incorrectly recognised a signal on another chromosome, e.g. 8, 11 or 18, during VDJ recombination and thereby produced a translocation.

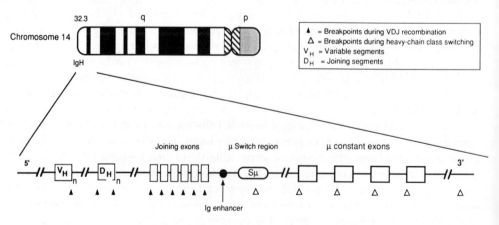

Figure 1. The heavy chain variable locus

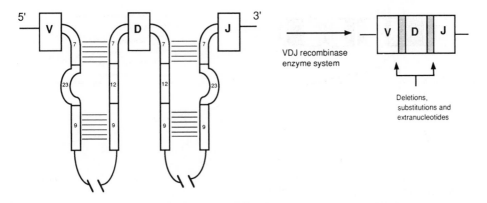

Figure 2. The VDJ joining system

DNA recombination occurs again later in B-cell differentiation; next during immunoglobulin light chain rearrangement (VJ joining) in the pre-B-cell, and then during heavy chain class switching in cells destined to become memory or plasma cells. An error during DNA recombination at these stages may lead to a translocation.

In a minority of cases, features of VDJ recombinase activity are absent at the breakpoint, indicating that more than one mechanism may produce translocations at the 14q32.3 locus.

The *bcl*-1 sequence

The translocation t(11;14) (q13;q32.3) occurs in cases of diffuse small-cell lymphoma, CLL, follicular lymphoma and myeloma. The complete genomic detail at band 11q13 has yet to be characterised but the term *bcl*-1 (B-cell leukaemia/lymphoma 1) has been coined for this putative oncogene. Most translocation breaks in *bcl*-1 occur in a 1000 base pair region. The translocation related breaks in the immunoglobulin heavy chain locus can occur outside the joining region.

The role of *bcl*-1 in tumorigensis is unknown and the *bcl*-1 product has not been isolated. The translocation may result in inappropriate expression of *bcl*-1. It is of note that the *bcl*-1 transcript is over-expressed in breast and head and neck cancer without an associated chromosomal rearrangement.

The *bcl*-2 gene: a presumptive oncogene

Approximately 90% of follicular lymphomas, a low-grade non-Hodgkin's lymphoma (NHL), and 20% of diffuse lymphomas (an intermediate-grade NHL) carry the translocation t(14;18) (q32.3;q21). The gene translocated from chromosome 18 and juxtaposed to the heavy chain junctional locus has been termed *bcl*-2 (B-cell leukaemia/lymphoma 2). The *bcl*-2 gene consists of three exons (Figure 3). There are two alternate promoters (P1 and P2) located upstream of either exon 1 or exon 2. Transcripts initiated at P2 are spliced together to include the whole of exon 2 and exon 3. Transcription from P1 results in the splicing of exon 1, the 3' portion of exon 2 and the whole of exon 3. The coding portion of the mRNA is split between exons 2 and 3. Exons 2 and 3 are separated by an intron of approximately 60 kb. There are

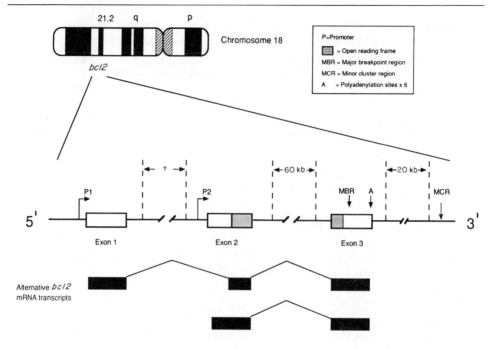

Figure 3. The *bcl2* gene

two tightly clustered regions through which the translocations occur. Approximately 70% occur in the 2.8 kb untranslated AT-rich 3′portion of exon 3, mostly within a 150-base pair major breakpoint region (MBR). The remainder of the translocations occur in a region 20 kb downstream of the gene termed the minor cluster region (MCR). A breakpoint region upstream of exon 2 (possibly through exon 1) has also been described. The (14;18) (q32.3;q21) translocation joins the truncated *bcl*-2 gene to the 5′ end of the J_H gene on chromosome 14+ (Figure 4). The Ig enhancer lying 3′ to J_H is always preserved in the translocation. The resulting *bcl*-2-*Ig* fusion gene spans the derived chromosome 14+ breakpoint and produces chimaeric *bcl*-2-*Ig* RNAs.

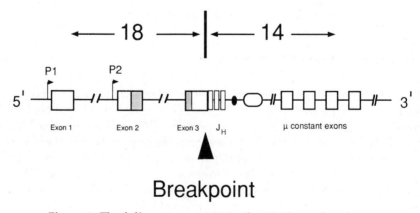

Figure 4. The *bcl2* rearrangement in the 14:18 translocation

Normally *bcl*-2 expression depends on the stage of B-cell maturation. It is expressed in pre-B-cells and proliferating B-cells, but not in resting and differentiated B-cells. The *bcl*-2 gene codes for two proteins—α (239 amino acids long, 26 kDa) and β (205 amino acids long, 22 kDa), which differ at the carboxy terminus as a result of alternative splice site selection. In general, *bcl*-2 rearrangement does not appear to alter the coding sequence; however, recently, somatic mutations have been found in the coding sequence of a NHL cell line. In NHL in which the B-cells have reached an advanced stage of maturation, the t(14;18) translocation is associated with *bcl*-2 over-expression. For example, in one study an anti-*bcl*-2 antibody detected *bcl*-2 protein in histopathology sections of NHL but not in non-neoplastic lymphoid disorders. Similarly in t(14;18)-bearing cells, the steady-state level of *bcl*-2 mRNA is raised.

The likely explanation for *bcl*-2 over-expression is the proximity of the IgH enhancer, although this is at least 60 kb from the promoters associated with exons 1 and 2. Alternatively, the translocation may perturb post-transcriptional regulation by disrupting the AT-rich 3′ untranslated portion of the mature mRNA. As yet the biological function(s) of the *bcl*-2 gene is unknown. The *bcl*-2α protein is associated with the inner surface of the cell membrane and recently it has been reported to have GTP binding activity. Furthermore, there is weak homology with the small molecular weight GTP binding protein family. Homology also exists with a protein encoded by the Epstein–Barr virus; this protein is encoded by a viral early gene (BHRF1) of unknown function.

There is direct evidence that the *bcl*-2 gene has a role in oncogenesis. In one gene transfer study, plasmids encoding either the *bcl*-2α or *bcl*-2β protein were introduced into NIH3T3 cells by transfection. These cells were not transformed *in vitro*, but when injected into nude mice they produced lethal tumours. Cells isolated from the tumours displayed a transformed morphology. Analysis of the tumours by Southern blotting showed they were of oligoclonal origin, and Northern blotting showed the level of the recombinant *bcl*-2 transcripts was higher than in the original NIH3T3 transfectants. There was no difference in the tumorigenicity of the *bcl*-2α and *bcl*-2β expressing cells.

It seems, in this system at least, that expression of *bcl*-2 provides a growth advantage. This property has been demonstrated in B-cells. For example, transfecting the *bcl*-2 gene into an interleukin-3 (IL-3)-requiring lymphoid cell line which had been deprived of IL-3, resulted in survival rather than proliferation of the cell line.

The functional effect of *bcl*-2 over-expression may act to promote survival. Inappropriate expression during B-cell maturation may underlie the oncogenic potential displayed by *bcl*-2. There is support for this idea in a study of transgenic mice in which the *bcl*-2 and immunoglobulin genes were linked. As a result their lymphoid cells constitutively expressed *bcl*-2. These mice developed lymphadenopathy with an expanded follicle compartment. Unlike follicular NHL these cells were polyclonal: this was predictable since all the maturing B-cells expressed *bcl*-2. However, these cells had reached an advanced stage of differentiation (IgM/IgD positive) similar to that seen in follicular NHL. Analyses of these mice correlated well with follicular NHL in terms of histology, stage of differentation and natural history. Follicular NHL is a low-grade malignancy characterized by its indolent progression. In this context *bcl*-2 over-expression may be enhancing survival of a clone of B-cells which have reached an advanced stage of maturation. As mentioned the t(14;18) translocation also occurs in intermediate- and high-grade NHL. In these cases the malignancy may have started as a follicular NHL and progressed to a higher grade due to a further event. What might the nature of such an event be?

A partial answer comes from an experiment in which plasmids containing *bcl*-2 were transfected into pre-B-lymphocytes taken from transgenic mice which constitutively express high levels of c-*myc* in cells of the lymphoid lineage. These cells proliferated *in vitro* and some clones were tumorigenic in mice. This study shows how a further event, in this case over-expression of *myc* in the presence of *bcl*-2 expression, is associated with the development of a lymphoid malignancy. As will be discussed, other chromosomal abnormalities are found in NHL and these may promote malignant expansion of a clone in which *bcl*-2 has been rearranged.

Translocations involving c-*myc*

Burkitt's lymphoma (BL) is a high-grade malignancy with two distinct epidemiological forms, African and sporadic BL. These are characterised by translocations involving the c-*myc* oncogene (see Chapter 4) located on chromosome 8 at position q24.1. The breakpoint on chromosome 8 varies from far 5' to far 3' of c-*myc*. Typically in African BL the breakpoint is approximately 50 kb upstream of c-*myc*, whereas in sporadic BL the breakpoint is usually immediately 5' or 3' of c-*myc*. Eighty-five percent of translocations move c-*myc* to 5'of either the heavy-chain joining or constant segments on chromosome 14. In the remainder, the light-chain constant segments, on C_λ or C_x on chromosomes 22 and 2 respectively, translocate downstream of c-*myc*. The clinical course of the malignancy appears to be independent of the form of the translocation.

The molecular features at the breakpoint indicate that in many cases the translocations have arisen during VDJ recombination or heavy-chain class switching. On this basis African (predominantly VDJ recombination) and sporadic BL (heavy-chain class switching) can be further distinguished.

The role played by c-*myc* in BL is unknown and clearly complex. Generally, only the translocated c-*myc* allele is expressed, the c-*myc* product is usually normal and the level of expression may be normal, raised or low. The mechanism(s) underlying deregulation of the translocated allele present a conundrum. Different translocations result in a range of alterations to the presumed regulatory region of c-*myc* from none to many. Translocation to the active Ig loci may result in deregulation in some cases by virtue of the proximity of the Ig enhancer. However the Ig enhancer is lost in some translocations. With this in mind it has been proposed that c-*myc* has a secondary role in BL, with the altered expression resulting from mechanisms that follow tumour development.

bcl-2, c-*myc* and the evolution of B-cell malignancies

African BL typically affects children and is endemic to regions where malaria is common; unlike sporadic BL there is a strong association with Epstein–Barr virus (EBV). One model for the evolution of African BL relates EBV infection to c-*myc* rearrangement. Malaria immunocompromises its sufferers and this results in an antigenic load leading to a high rate of B-cell blastogenesis. Infection by EBV promotes polyclonal B-cell proliferation. In these circumstances there is a high level of DNA recombination and hence a translocation is likely. If c-*myc* is translocated then a malignant oligoclonal proliferation of B-cells follows. It is of considerable interest that an essentially identical tumour occurs in AIDS patients who are only moderately immunocompromised, indicating a difference only in the cause of the immuno-deficiency.

B-cell surface marker studies have revealed phenotypic similarity between BL and follicular NHL, thereby indicating a common cell lineage. This relates well to cases of B-cell malignancy in which both t(14;18) and t(8;14) occur. In one example an analysis was made of the molecular genetics of an acute pre-B-cell leukaemia which developed in a patient who had a history of a follicular lymphoma. The lymphoma carried the t(14;18) translocation with the *bcl*-2 gene juxtaposed to J_H4. The leukaemia contained both the t(14;18) and a t(8;14), in which *myc* was juxtaposed to $C_\gamma2$ on the other chromosome 14. The evolution of the B-cell malignancies in this case may be considered as follows: a pre-B-cell acquired the t(14;18) during heavy chain rearrangement and so survived either as a single progenitor cell or as a clone due to *bcl*-2 expression. Subsequently this clone gave rise to the follicular lymphoma. At some time later a cell derived from this clone also acquired the t(8;14) translocation and the altered c-*myc* expression in these cells then produced an aggressive pre-B-cell malignancy.

Other gene rearrangements and chromosomal abnormalities in B-cell lymphomas

The 14q32 locus participates in other reciprocal chromosome translocations (Table 1). The genes involved have yet to be characterised.

It is interesting that genes on several chromosomes are associated with both diffuse and follicular NHL. It is unlikely their effects are a result of disturbing IgH function itself since the immunoglobulin genes have not been shown to be oncogenic. It is more probable that they are either homologous to each other and perform similar functions or they act at different points on the same pathway controlling B-cell growth and differentiation.

In addition to the reciprocal translocations, a variety of chromosome duplications and deletions are commonly found in all types of NHL. These abnormalities are associated with tumour histology and prognosis. Deletions are thought to be tumorigenic due to the loss of a suppressor gene. In the case of NHL, duplications may promote tumour development by adding an extra copy of an oncogene or growth factor (e.g. epidermal growth factor in duplication 7p).

GENE REARRANGEMENT IN B-CELL LYMPHOMA AND THE CLINICAL SETTING

The study of gene rearrangements in B-cell malignancy is becoming increasingly important in the clinical setting. They have been used in diagnosis, staging and assessment of prognosis.

The advent of the polymerase chain reaction (PCR) has enabled the presence of a gene rearrangement to serve as a marker for disease. The unique segment of DNA created by gene rearrangement can be used as a target for PCR (Figure 5). The sensitivity of PCR is such that one target cell in 10^5 normal cells can be detected—exceeding the sensitivity of routine cytology and immunocytochemistry—and so it is capable of detecting micrometastatic disease. In this way the extent of spread or stage of disease can be determined more precisely and treatment planned accordingly.

In follicular lymphoma, 80% of which have *bcl*-2 rearrangement, PCR has been used to reveal micrometastatic disease from blood and marrow in patients considered by routine assessment to be in complete remission. Similarly, in cases of B-cell malignancy in which *myc* has been rearranged, malignant cells can be detected in blood and marrow. At present, we are studying PCR as a means of staging NHL; preliminary results so far indicate PCR can alter the staging for a significant proportion of patients. In a case of non-Hodgkin's gastric lymphoma (for which the incidence of *bcl*-2 rearrangement is unknown) we have used PCR to detect malignant cells in the peritoneum and marrow when conventional staging localised disease to the resected gastric specimen alone. After intraperitoneal cytotoxic chemotherapy, PCR no longer detected disease at these sites. PCR has also been used to detect follicular lymphoma cells in pleural fluid when cytology was normal.

In addition to serving as a target for determining the extent of spread of a B-cell malignancy, gene rearrangements and/or chromosome abnormalities have implications for prognosis. For example, in one study *bcl*-2 rearrangements identified by Southern analysis in cases of follicular and diffuse lymphoma were associated with a decreased likelihood of complete remission (7/23) compared to cases without the rearrangement (21/26). In diffuse large cell NHL presence of chromosome 14+ was associated with a better prognosis. Multiple non-specific chromosome abnormalities also contributed to prognosis (Table 2). In follicular lymphoma, five out of five patients with duplication of chromosome 3 had a complete remission compared to only one of

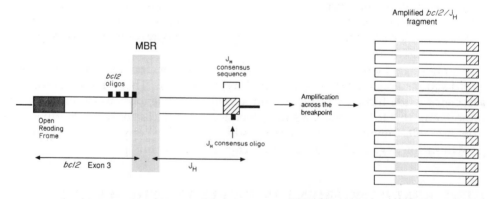

Figure 5. The polymerase chain reaction (PCR) can be used to detect *bcl2* rearrangement when the position of the breakpoint is unknown. In this example the breakpoint is in the MBR. The J_H oligonucleotide is directed at the J_H consensus sequence (the sequence shared by the six J_H exons). The *bcl2* directed oligonucleotides span the MBR. Parameters for PCR are optimised. If *bcl2* is rearranged then the *bcl2* oligonucleotide(s) directed to the left of the breakpoint will participate in specific amplification

four patients with duplication of chromosome 2. This type of study requires relatively large amounts of high-grade material (5 μg DNA is required for Southern analysis). However, the quality of DNA isolated from paraffin-embedded sections is sufficient for PCR. By using PCR it may be possible to analyse pathological specimens stored in tissue banks and so retrospectively relate the contribution of a particular gene rearrangement to clinical outcome.

CONCLUSIONS

Translocations are common in B-cell lymphomas and generally follow mistakes in DNA recombination during immunoglobulin gene rearrangement. A given translocation introduces one of a number of genes, including bcl-2 and myc, into the immunoglobulin gene family. The presence of these translocations has provided insights into the evolution of B-cell lymphomas. They have prognostic significance and are useful as markers of disease, particularly when used in conjunction with PCR.

FURTHER READING

Crescenzi, M., Seto, M., Herzig, G., et al. (1988) Thermostable DNA polymerase chain amplification of t(14;18) chromosome break points and detection of minimal residual disease. *Proc. Natl. Acad. Sci. USA*, **85**, 4960–4973.

Cunningham, D., Hickish, T., Rosin, R., et al. (1989) Polymerase chain reaction for detection of dissemination in gastric lymphoma. *Lancet*, i, 695–697.

Haldar, S., Beatty, C., Tsujimoto, Y. and Croce, C. M. (1989). The bcl-2 gene encodes a novel G protein. *Nature*, **342**, 195–198.

Haluska, F., Tsujimoto, Y. and Croce, C. (1988) The t(8;14) breakpoint of the EW 36 undifferentiated lymphoma cell line lies 5' of MYC in a region prone to involvement in endemic Burkitt's lymphoma. *Nuc. Acid Res.*, **16**, 2077–2085.

Hua, C., Zorn, S., Jensen, J., et al. (1988) Consequences of the t(14;18) chromosomal translocation in follicular lymphoma: deregulated expression of a chimeric and mutated bcl-2 gene. *Oncogene Res.*, **2**, 263–275.

Magrath, I. T. (ed.) (1990) *The Non-Hodgkin's Lymphomas*. Edward Arnold, London.

Magrath, I., Barriga, F., McManaway, M. and Shiramizu, B. (1988) The molecular analysis of chromosomal translocations as a diagnostic epidemiological and potentially prognostic tool in lymphoid neoplasia. *J. Virol. Methods*, **21**, 275–289.

McDonnell, T., Deane, N., Platt, F., et al. (1989) bcl2 Immunoglobulin transgenic mice demonstrate extended B cell survival and follicular lymphoproliferation. *Cell*, **57**, 860–864.

Tsujimoto, Y., Ikogki, N. and Croce, C. M. (1987) Characterisation of the protein product of bcl2, the gene involved in human follicular lymphoma. *Oncogene*, **2**, 3–7.

Yunis, J., Mayer, M., Arnesen, M., et al. (1989) bcl-2 and other genomic alterations in the prognosis of large-cell lymphoma. *N. Eng. J. Med.*, **320**, 1047–1054.

28

Clinical Application of Gene Rearrangement Studies in Lymphoma

M. BRADA

Somatic rearrangement of immunoglobulin (Ig) and T-cell receptor (TCR) genes is a mechanism for generating antibody and T-cell receptor diversity. In the investigation of lymphoid malignancy a specific gene rearrangement can be used as a clonal marker, and its application is of direct relevance to patient management: it is useful in the diagnosis and staging of patients with lymphoma, and it can help to follow the evolution of lymphoid malignancy.

IMMUNOGLOBULIN GENE REARRANGEMENT

The variable parts of the light and heavy chains of immunoglobulins are coded by two or three gene families represented by multiple germline DNA segments. These are assembled during the early stages of B-cell maturation to act as a functional template for mRNA transcription and subsequent translation into an immunoglobulin chain.

The variable region of a heavy chain is coded by three DNA segments described as V_H (variable), D (diversity) and J_H (joining) genes. Each segment is present in a number of variants: six J_H segments, 20 or more D genes and 50 or more V_H genes. These are located on chromosome 14 and each exon is separated by intervening non-coding stretches of DNA (introns) (Figure 1).

Genes and Cancer. Edited by D. Carney and K. Sikora

HEAVY CHAIN GENE SEGMENTS

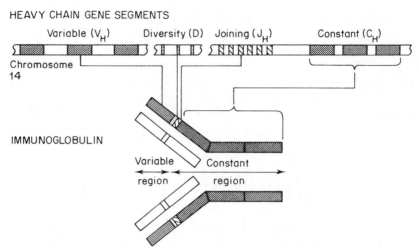

Figure 1. Diagramatic representation of immunoglobulin and Ig heavy (H) chain gene on chromosome 14. The variable region of Ig heavy chain consists of three segments (V_H, D, J_H) which are represented by a number of variants in the Ig H chain gene

During B-cell maturation the recombination of the variable region genes follows a defined sequence. The initial step is the joining of D and J_H genes with deletion of the intervening sequence; and this is followed by joining of a V_H gene to form a $V_H D J_H$ sequence (Figure 2). This gene complex encodes the entire variable region of the heavy chain. The diversity of gene sequences encoding the variable portion of Ig is generated by recombination of different V_H, D and J_H genes, and by additional mechanisms which include the addition of nucleotides at the recombination site (N regions), mistakes in joining and somatic mutations.

The recombination between the germline elements is mediated by a putative recombinase enzyme. It recognises conserved recombination sequences, which consist

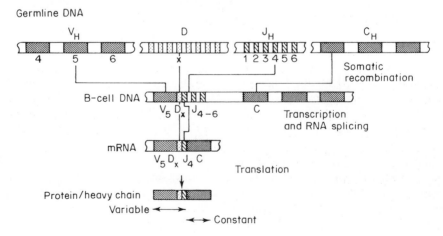

Figure 2. Sequence of Ig gene rearrangement followed by transcription and translation into functional Ig chain

of a heptamer and a nonamer separated by a spacer of 12 or 23 base pairs (bp). 5' to each *J* segment is a recognition sequence with a 23 bp spacer, and 3' to each *D* segment is a flanking 12 bp spacer recognition sequence. The assembly of *DJ* and subsequently *VDJ* elements is mediated through the recognition of nonamer-spacer-heptamer sequences where a 12 bp spacer is brought to proximity with a 23 bp spacer sequence (the 12/23 rule).

The light chain variable region is present on chromosome 2 for kappa and chromosome 22 for lambda chain. The mechanism of assembly of variable gene segments is similar to that of heavy chain, except the variable region is encoded by only two germline elements, V_L and J_L. The assembly through a common recombinase also follows the recognition of conserved sequences and the 12/23 spacer rule.

The rearrangement of Ig genes follows a sequence of heavy chain recombination followed by kappa light chain rearrangement. Only a defective kappa rearrangement allows the recombination of lambda chain genes. In most B-cells both Ig heavy chain alleles are rearranged. The process of recombination is prone to error, but once a recombined functional allele is obtained, further rearrangement ceases.

Subsequent Ig production can be switched from IgM to other isotypes which retain the same antigen-binding specificity. At DNA level this is achieved through the switching of constant region genes. The appropriate heavy chain genes lie downstream from the C_μ constant region.

The specific $V_H DJ_H$ and $V_L J_L$ sequence of heavy and light chain genes is unique for each B-cell and its clone, and the configuration provides an individual fingerprint, which is the basis for clinical application. However, the Ig genes of mature B-cells can undergo further recombination events by insertion of new upstream *V* genes. In addition, a *V* gene is susceptible to mutations, particularly in the hypervariable segments of complementarity-determining regions. Consequently the recognition of new rearrangements does not necessarily imply an emergence of a new clone and may represent mutations or new rearrangements within the existing clone.

T-CELL RECEPTOR GENE REARRANGEMENT

A T-cell receptor (TCR) is involved in the recognition of antigen in a manner similar to Ig. It is attached to the T-cell membrane and contains both intracellular and extracellular components. It is a heterodimer molecule composed of either alpha/beta or gamma/delta chains. The alpha/beta receptor molecules are expressed mainly on CD4+, CD8− and CD4−, CD8+ T-cells. The gamma/delta receptor molecules are expressed mainly in CD4−, CD8− T-cells. The majority of peripheral blood T-cells express alpha/beta chains, with gamma/delta cells constituting only a minor fraction of T-lymphocytes.

The variable portion of each TCR chain is represented by variants of *V*, *D* and *J* gene segments. The beta chain locus is present on chromosome 7 and the sequence is shown in Figure 3. The gene segments recombine during T-cell maturation to produce a functional mRNA template for a specific T-cell receptor chain. The sequence of rearrangement is similar to that of Ig, with *DJ* followed by *VDJ* recombination. As in the case of Ig, each cell generates a specific rearrangement

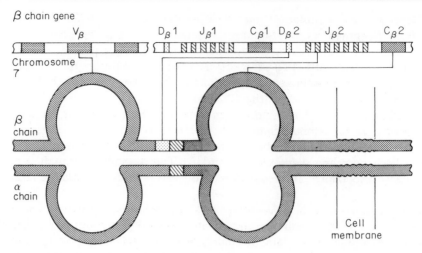

Figure 3. T-cell receptor and gene for beta chain of TCR present on chromosome 7. In a T-cell V, D and J segments rearrange to produce a specific TCR

of the TCR gene, which is unique to the cell and its clone, and this can also be exploited as a specific clonal marker of T-cells. Alpha, gamma and delta chains also undergo a sequence of rearrangements. Although gamma and delta heterodimers may not be expressed on T4+ and T8+ lymphocytes the rearrangement of gamma and delta chains may precede those of alpha and beta chains.

GENE REARRANGEMENT IN LYMPHOID MALIGNANCY

Gene rearrangement can be detected with DNA hybridisation techniques as a change in the position of restriction enzyme sites, demonstrated as a change in the size of DNA fragments on a Southern blot hybridized with an Ig or TCR gene probe. B-cell non-Hodgkin's lymphoma (NHL) is a clonal expansion of B-lymphocytes as detected by Ig gene rearrangement in the DNA from lymphoma tissue. An example of the results of DNA hybridisation is shown in Figure 4. Each electrophoretic strip is an autoradiograph of a Southern blot of DNA from lymphoma tissue from one patient hybridised with Ig gene probe (J_H). The rearranged bands (one or two) represent rearranged alleles of a clonal population of cells assumed to be tumour cells, and the germline band represents cells in the tumour biopsy which are not of B-cell lineage, such as stromal tissue, T-lymphocytes and endothelial cells. The detection of clonality in lymphoma tissue merely describes an expansion of the identified clone of cells, and does not in itself indicate neoplasia.

Clonal rearrangement of T-cell receptor gene has been demonstrated in tumour tissue from T-cell lymphoma and leukaemia, with Ig gene usually in germline configuration. Although in the majority of lymphomas the specificity of T- and B-cell lineage is reflected by TCR and Ig gene rearrangement respectively, a small proportion of T-cell lymphomas demonstrate an Ig gene rearrangement, and vice versa. This phenomenon, which was demonstrated initially in acute lymphatic leukaemia, is described as lineage infidelity. In the majority of cases appropriate

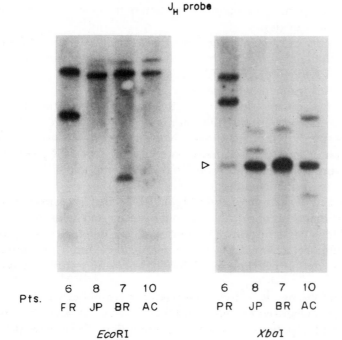

Figure 4. Autoradiograph of DNA analysis obtained from lymphoma tissue from four patients. Each DNA was digested with two enzymes (*Eco*RI and *Xba*I) and hybridised with J_H probe. Open triangle indicates the position of germline band

lineage can be assigned, as the rearrangement of Ig gene in T-cell malignancy is commonly restricted to heavy chain alone.

Technical aspects

Successful DNA hybridisation studies usually require fresh or frozen tissue material for analysis. Electrophoresis demands 5–10 μg of DNA, an amount equivalent to a minimum of 10^6 cells. A sufficient number of cells can be obtained by needle aspirate and this obviates the need for more invasive biopsy procedures. It is also possible to extract DNA from paraffin-embedded material, although the quality of the result depends on the degree of DNA degradation during initial specimen handling.

As an initial screening test a DNA sample from a suspected lymphoma should be digested by at least two enzymes. Hybridisation with heavy chain probe (usually J_H) is diagnostic in over 85% of B-cell NHL. The sensitivity is increased to >90% with additional hybridisation with light chain probes. The detection of one or two rearranged bands on a single restriction enzyme digest is insufficient for diagnosis, and a third enzyme digest is mandatory.

Diagnostic application

Ig or TCR gene rearrangement is found in most lymphoma tissue samples and should be considered as diagnostic of NHL. False negative results may occur and are most likely due to sampling error where the portion of the biopsy specimen analysed does not contain tumour tissue.

In the majority of cases of Hodgkin's disease (HD), Ig and TCR genes can only be detected in their germline form. However, in biopsy material containing a large proportion of Reed–Sternberg (RS) cells and in cell suspensions enriched for RS cells, Ig gene is frequently rearranged.

In cases of diagnostic difficulty on the basis of conventional histological and immunohistochemical criteria, the finding of gene rearrangement may assign the tumour to a specific lymphoid lineage. None of the tumour tissue of non-lymphoid lineage so far examined has demonstrated either Ig or TCR gene rearrangement. In benign lymphoid proliferation and in reactive lymphoid tissue Ig and TCR genes also remain in germline configuration.

The detection of rearrangement of Ig or TCR genes in suspected NHL therefore confirms the diagnosis of clonal lymphoid disorder and helps in cases of diagnostic difficulty. However, a negative result does not exclude the presence of lymphoma. Where immunocytochemistry with conventional B- and T-cell-specific antibodies is unable to define cell lineage, DNA hybridisation studies may provide the answer.

'Pseudolymphoma' is a term reserved for lymphoid proliferation mostly at extranodal sites where conventional histology and immunocytochemistry are unable to distinguish lymphoma from benign proliferation. The clinical behaviour is that of low-grade lymphoma and the finding of Ig gene rearrangement in such lymphoid aggregates in the orbit and in salivary glands in association with Sjögren's syndrome suggest that 'pseudolymphoma' is a misnomer better described as low-grade NHL.

A majority of cases of pure 'histiocytic' lymphoma and Ki-1 positive NHL have demonstrated rearrangement, as did two cell lines of suspected 'histiocytic' lineage. This suggests that the majority of 'histiocytic' lymphomas represent a lymphoid malignancy of either B or T lineage.

The clonal nature of T-cell disorders has been confirmed in cases of adult T-cell leukaemia/lymphoma (ATL), Sezary syndrome, mycosis fungoides, T-gamma lymphocytosis and in a proportion of cases of angioimmunoblastic lymphadenopathy. TCR gene rearrangement has also been detected in cases of lymphoid proliferation in the bowel associated with coeliac disease.

Detection of minimal disease

DNA hybridisation with Ig and TCR gene probes detects clones of neoplastic cells with 1–5% sensitivity. With this technique lymphoma cells have been demonstrated in peripheral blood and bone marrow when not detectable by conventional means. A third of patients with active NHL may have circulating lymphoma cells, and the peripheral blood involvement appears to be related to the extent of disease, although lymphoma cells can be detected in a proportion of patients with clinical stage I and II disease and in patients with normal bone marrow. These findings may have important clinical implications but at present their prognostic significance is not clear. A sensitive method of detecting lymphoma cells in bone marrow and peripheral blood may also help in assessing remission status and may have an important role in bone marrow transplantation, particularly if autologous marrow is used.

Oligoclonality

Immunosuppressed patients, such as recipients of organ transplants may develop lymphoproliferative lesions akin to lymphoma. Their clonal nature was demonstrated by Ig gene rearrangement. However, lesions at several sites from the same patient exhibited different rearrangements, suggesting the presence of different clones. The individual clonal nature of lymphoid proliferations in organ transplant patients has also been confirmed by demonstrating clonality of inserted episomal EBV genome. Similar findings of 'multiclonality' were seen in a 12-year-old boy with combined immune deficiency who died following bone marrow transplantation and severe EB virus infection. A number of lymphoid lesions were noted at autopsy and each contained a different clonal B-cell proliferation. These findings are in keeping with the hypothesis of EBV-induced clonal B-cell proliferation in immunosuppressed patients as a stage in lymphoma genesis.

Apparent biclonality of lymphoma has been demonstrated in approximately 10% of lymphomas by kappa/lambda staining and by gene rearrangement criteria. However, cells of phenotypic diversity observed at different tumour sites and progression of nodular to diffuse histology may involve the same clone. Using gene rearrangement criteria alone in the assessment of clonality of lymphoid tissue is complicated by the finding of further recombination events and frequent mutations within the hypervariable region of *V* genes in mature B-cells. To overcome this, studies of clonality should include the use of more stable markers such as the t(14;18) chromosomal translocation found in the majority of cases of nodular lymphoma (see Chapter 27). More detailed analysis of translocation sites and sequencing of Ig gene recombination sites suggests that the apparent biclonality reflects the development of a subclone rather than the presence of two independent clones.

CONCLUSION

Gene rearrangement studies help in the diagnosis of lymphoma and in assigning cell lineage in cases of diagnostic difficulty. The sensitivity of hybridisation techniques also allows for detection of minimal disease in peripheral blood and bone marrow at different stages of disease. With the advent of gene amplification by polymerase chain reaction it may be possible to detect tumour cells with considerably higher sensitivity.

FURTHER READING

Brada, M., Mizutani, S., Molgaard, H., *et al.* (1987) Circulating lymphoma cells in patients with B and T non-Hodgkin's lymphoma detected by immunoglobulin and T-cell receptor gene rearrangement. *Br. J. Cancer*, **56**, 147–152.

Cleary, M. L., Galili, N., Trela, M., *et al.* (1988) Single cell origin of bigenotypic and bi-phenotypic B cell proliferations in human follicular lymphomas. *J. Exp. Med.*, **167**, 582–597.

Cleary, M. L. and Sklar, J. (1985) DNA rearrangements in non-Hodgkin's lymphomas. *Cancer Surveys*, **4**, 331–348.

Davis, M. M. and Bjorkman, P. J. (1988) T-cell antigen receptor genes and T-cell recognition. *Nature*, **334**, 395–402.

Marrack, P. and Kappler, J. (1987) The T cell receptor. *Science*, **238**, 1073–1079.

O'Connor, N. T. J., Gatter, K. C., Wainscoat, J. S., *et al.* (1987) Practical value of genotypic analysis for diagnosing lymphoproliferative disorders. *J. Clin. Pathol.*, **40**, 147–150.

Rosen, N. and Israel, M. A. (1987) Genetic abnormalities as biological tumor markers. *Seminars in Oncology*, **14**, 213–231.

Urba, W. J. and Longo, D. L. (1985) Cytologic, immunologic, and clinical diversity in non-Hodgkin's lymphoma: therapeutic implications. *Seminars in Oncology*, **12**, 250–267.

Waldmann, T. A. (1987) The arrangement of immunoglobulin and T cell receptor genes in human lymphoproliferative disorders. *Advances in Immunology*, **40**, 247–321.

29 Molecular Genetics of Colon Cancer

NIGEL K. SPURR

Colorectal cancer kills about 19 000 people a year in the UK and is the second most common cancer after lung cancer. Many factors have been suggested for the high incidence of this cancer in Western populations, including low dietary fibre intake, vitamin A deficiency and changes in gut flora. None of these factors has been fully substantiated by epidemiological studies.

The formation of colon tumours is an ideal system for studying the multistage process of carcinogenesis. At least three pathological stages have been identified (Figure 1). Normal colon epithelium is smooth and flat; this progresses through a preneoplastic stage involving hyperplastic growth of epithelium and leading to the formation of polyps or adenomas which are outgrowths into the lumen of the colon. They are varied in shape and size from large pedunculated growths to small flat lesions. These adenomas do not necessarily progress to form tumours but it is thought that all tumours arise from adenomas. The final pathological stage is the formation of adenocarcinomas which if left untreated will invade into the muscle layers of the colon and metastasise into the bloodstream.

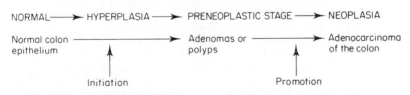

Figure 1. The colon cancer progression

Genes and Cancer. Edited by D. Carney and K. Sikora
©1990 John Wiley & Sons Ltd

Table 1. Genetically inherited colon cancer syndromes

Syndrome	Clinical and pathological characteristics	Comments
Familial adenomatous polyposis (FAP)	Autosomal dominant disease characterised by multiple adenomatous polyps in the colon during childhood and early adulthood. If left untreated adenomas progress to adenocarcinomas	It is now accepted that these conditions are caused by the same genetic defect
Gardner's syndrome	The same as FAP, but with extra-colonic manifestations, e.g. multiple osteomas and epidermoid cysts. Fibrous desmoid tumours seen in 4–10% of individuals	
Turcot's syndrome	This is a rare condition which appears to be autosomal recessive. Adenomatous polyps occur in large bowel but fewer than in FAP. Syndrome is associated with tumours of the central nervous system (mainly astrocytomas), focal nodular hyperplasia of the liver and multiple skin lesions, including café au lait spots and basal cell naevi and carcinomas	
Cancer family syndrome (CFS)	Autosomal dominant condition in which there is a high incidence of adenocarcinomas, mainly in the colon but also uterus, breast, ovary and rarely other sites	Average age of onset 45 years
Muir–Torre syndrome	Autosomal dominant condition with multiple carcinomas of the large bowel, duodenum, larynx, multiple skin tumours (e.g. sebaceous adenomas, keratoacanthomas, basal cell carcinomas)	High survival rate suggesting low malignancy. May be similar to CFS suggesting same gene defect
Site-specific colon cancer	Autosomal dominant inheritance of site-specific colorectal cancer with adenocarcinomas in other tissues absent. Less polyps than FAP often associated with solitary adenomas	Age of onset 36–53 years
Juvenile polyposis	Autosomal dominant condition with hamartomatous polyps in the large colon, occasionally in stomach and small bowel. Associated with congenital malformations, mental retardation	
Gorlin syndrome	Autosomal dominant condition with juvenile polyps mainly associated with bone abnormalities and skin lesions such as basal cell naevi developing into carcinomas	
Peutz-Jegher's syndrome	Autosomal dominant condition with hamartomas of the bowel, particularly the small colon. Main characteristic of this syndrome is mucocutaneous pigmentation. Adenocarcinomas at other sites may be seen, e.g. stomach, pancreas, ovary and fallopians	
Cowden's syndrome (multiple hamartoma syndrome)	Autosomal dominant condition with juvenile polyps and colorectal cancer associated with mucocutaneous lesions. Increased risk of malignancies of breast and thyroid; also CNS abnormalities and skin lesions such as lipomas and sebaceous cysts may be seen	Closely related to symptoms of Muir's syndrome
Mixed adenomas and hamartomatous polyps	A very rare autosomal dominant condition; juvenile polyps associated with site-specific colon cancer	This may be a variant of juvenile polyposis of site-specific colon cancers

The average age of onset of colon tumours is 65 years and they appear to arise sporadically in the population. However, a proportion of colon cancers do not arise sporadically but are inherited. These genetic diseases which predispose to colon cancer have been reported to account for from 5% up to 26% of the total incidence. A number of different inherited syndromes have been identified on the basis of their different clinical and pathological characteristics and these are listed with key diagnostic features in Table 1.

This chapter will discuss how molecular genetics has been used to locate the chromosome and region in which the gene responsible for one of these inherited conditions, familial adenomatous polyposis (FAP), is to be found. How this work may lead to a greater understanding of the pathogenesis of colon cancers in the general population will also be discussed.

FAMILIAL ADENOMATOUS POLYPOSIS (FAMILIAL POLYPOSIS COLI)—FAP

FAP was first clinically described in 1882 by Harrison-Cripps and in the 1920s it was recognised as being inherited in an autosomal dominant manner. FAP is characterised by the development of multiple colorectal adenomas during childhood and adolescence. If left untreated these adenomas may progress to adenocarcinomas, usually seen in adults in middle age (30–50). The average age of onset of colon tumours in non-inherited cases is 60–70 years.

In the 1950s Gardner reported a number of extracolonic symptoms. In these cases patients had adenomatous polyps, multiple osteomas and epidermoid cysts. It was originally suggested that this was a different syndrome from FAP. However, it is currently thought that these are probably more severe symptoms of the same disease, and individuals in the same family can be seen with both types of condition. There is no clear definition or grading of the severity of symptoms and this still leads to some problems in diagnosis.

The adenomas are a precancerous lesion and the standard method of treatment is to remove most of the large bowel and then to annually check by sigmoidoscopy for any further adenoma development. The age of appearance of the multiple polyps is variable and annual sigmoidoscopy of all first-degree relatives of the patients is essential as there is a 50% risk of a positive diagnosis. This form of screening is expensive, time-consuming and unpleasant for the patients, who may require this form of screening from early teens until mid-twenties. About six years ago we set out to find the chromosomal location of the gene which causes these changes in normal cells, causing them to convert to tumour cells. To achieve this, DNA markers detecting restriction fragment length polymorphisms (RFLPs) were used to look for markers closely linked to the disease locus. This would enable a simple diagnostic test to be developed to screen all at-risk individuals and reduce the amount of expensive screening required. Also the eventual identification of the gene involved should lead to a greater understanding of the colorectal cancer process.

Search for the FAP gene

In FAP and many other genetic disorders the mode of inheritance is known but the gene responsible for the disease phenotype is unknown. In these cases genetic linkage analysis can be used in family studies to look for DNA polymorphisms which segregate with the disease phenotype. The major problem in an autosomal inherited condition is that the disease gene may be on any of the 22 chromosome pairs and it has been estimated that at least 150–200 evenly spaced markers would have to be screened to cover the human genome. This assumes that all markers are equally informative and that at least one of the parents in each family is heterozygous with each marker.

To reduce the number of markers that have to be screened a number of approaches have been used. These include the cytogenetic analysis of cells from tumours and precancerous polyps from patients with FAP or non-familial colon cancer. This type of analysis using tumour cells from patients with retinoblastoma revealed deletions of a portion of chromosome 13 within which the gene responsible for this tumour has been recently identified. The cytogenetic analysis of FAP tumours has been a relatively unproductive area of research. The majority of the adenocarcinomas examined from FAP patients showed many karyotypic rearrangements; however, no consistent pattern of changes could be distinguished. An examination of the precancerous adenomas was more informative, and an excess of changes involving chromosomes 12 and 17 was seen. The rearrangements of chromosome 17 were observed consistently and initial studies concentrated by testing for linkage with polymorphic markers on these two chromosomes.

In 1986 a report of a single patient with mental retardation and FAP phenotype was described. Cytogenetic analysis of the patient's cells showed a constitutive interstitial deletion of the long arm of chromosome 5, i.e. 5q13→15 or 5q15→22. This paper stimulated testing for linkage using DNA markers which had been assigned to chromosome 5 by other techniques, e.g. mapping using somatic cell hybrids or *in situ* hybridisation. One of these markers called c11p11 was shown to be closely linked to FAP. Six informative families including 79 individuals gave a combined maximum lod score of 3.26 at a recombination fraction of $\theta = 0$. Using *in situ* hybridisation the probe c11p11 was assigned to the region 5q21→q22. Since this initial report of close linkage, a number of other groups have confirmed the assignment and localised it to band q21 on chromosome 5. A number of new markers have been isolated which flank both sides of the FAP gene and position it within a region of DNA approximately 3–5 million base pairs long (Figure 2).

Having located the FAP gene in the human genome the task is now to identify the gene and determine its function in colon epithelial cells. This is, however, an exceedingly difficult task as there are no clues to the gene function. At present researchers are narrowing down the possible region in which this gene may lie. Once this region is defined it will be necessary to identify the defective gene, which in normal colon may not be expressed usually but is expressed in the mutated state in polyps and tumour cells, or vice versa.

The pathogenesis of allele loss

Having determined the position of the gene causing the genetic defect leading to colorectal tumours in patients with FAP the question arises as to the possible role

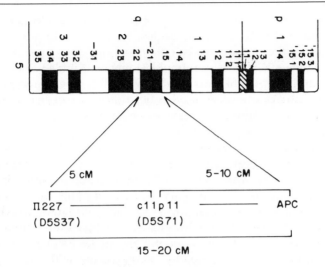

Figure 2. Ideogram of chromosome 5 showing the position of the APC gene. This figure shows the position of the APC gene in the region 5q21 and the two markers first used to confirm linkage. The order and distances between the markers are summarised from published data. Since these initial markers were used a number of new probes have been isolated which are more tightly linked and one YN5.48 (D5S81) is thought to flank the APC gene

of this gene in other forms of colon cancer. In particular the commonest type—the sporadic tumour with late age of onset and not familial.

Knudson in 1971 postulated a two hit model to explain the mutations in the same gene occurring in both sporadic and inherited forms of cancer. Tumour cells lose first one allele and then a second allele at a locus coding for a potential tumour suppressor gene or an anti-oncogene. In inherited cancers the first mutation will occur in the germ line and the second mutation will occur in the somatic tissue, e.g. in the case of colon tumours in the colonic epithelium. In the histologically indistinguishable tumours arising in sporadic cases, both mutations must occur in the same somatic cell. The second mutation in either inherited or sporadic cells can result in large chromosome rearrangements or deletions. By comparing DNA prepared from tumour tissue with normal tissue from the same patient it has been possible to show that this mechanism of allele loss occurs in a number of tumours, including retinoblastoma, Wilm's tumour, acoustic neuroma or NFI (neurofibromatosis type I) and MENI (multiple endocrine neoplasia type I). Allele loss associated with the genetic mutation responsible for these diseases was found on chromosomes 13, 11, 22 and 11 respectively.

Testing for such allele loss in FAP and sporadic colorectal tumours has produced an enormous amount of data and uncovered a number of regions of the genome which are consistently altered during the development of colon tumours. A number of groups have reported such studies, including ones concerning allele loss on the long arm of chromosome 5. Up to 25% of colorectal tumour samples show loss of sequences on 5q, the chromosome to which the FAP gene is assigned. About 20–36% of tumours studied from sporadic colorectal carcinomas show allele loss; up to 75% of tumours in one study showed loss of markers on chromosomes 17 and 18, and up to 50% of tumours showed mutation of one of the *ras* oncogenes, in particular Ki-*ras* on chromosome 12.

It is thus apparent that in colonic tumours the loss of alleles is not monochromosome-specific, as in retinoblastoma or Wilm's tumour, but is seen at a number of sites. These data are consistent with the cytogenic analysis of colorectal rearrangements and deletions. A number of studies have been conducted to explain how allele loss can account for the stages of initiation and development of colon tumours in familial cases or otherwise.

One study has tried to correlate the appearance of allele loss with the size of adenomas and the appearance of carcinomas. This group found that loss of chromosome 18 alleles was seen at 73% in carcinomas and 43% in advanced adenomas, but only at 12% in early adenomas. The chromosome 17 losses were usually only seen in carcinomas. *ras* gene mutations were seen in 58% of adenomas larger than 1 cm. Chromosome 5 losses associated with the FAP gene were not seen in adenomas of patients with FAP but were detected in 29–35% of adenomas and carcinomas from patients with other forms of colon cancer.

More recently Vogelstein and co-workers in two large studies have analysed in greater detail the extent of allele loss in colorectal tumours in general and shown how one gene may act as a tumour suppressor in colon neoplasia. Initially they screened a number of paired colon samples from normal and tumour epithelium with polymorphic DNA markers from each arm of the human autosomes. They found that allele losses were very common and one of the alleles from each polymorphic marker tested was missing in at least one of the tumours tested. Again consistent losses of alleles on chromosome 17p and 18q were seen in 75% of tumours studied. Losses of alleles from other chromosomes were seen although these were inconsistent and not seen in all tumour cells. However, recently a group in Japan have reported consistent loss of alleles on chromosome 22 in their population. As well as allele losses new DNA fragments were seen in some tumours which were not present in normal colon epithelium. These new fragments were generated at regions of hypervariability and these regions of DNA may be recombinational hot-spots giving rise to the generation of new alleles.

The second study by Vogelstein's group used 20 RFLP markers localised to chromosome 17 to define the region of allele loss; this was narrowed to the region 17p12→17p13.3. This region contains the gene for the transformation associated protein p53. No gross rearrangements of the p53 gene were detected but in a more detailed study of p53, mRNA levels in some tumours showed that the p53 gene had been deleted. They found two cases where there was a marked increase in mRNA from the remaining allele.

In both cases the p53 gene product was mutated with an alanine substituted for a valine at codon 143 in one tumour and a histidine substituted for an arginine at codon 175 in the second tumour. It is thought that the normal p53 gene acts as a tumour suppressor and only acts as an oncogene when it is in the mutated form. The normal protein may bind to either DNA or protein to inhibit uncontrolled growth of colon epithelium. If one normal copy is deleted and the second becomes mutated this form may no longer be expressed or becomes unable to act as a tumour suppressor, allowing the tumour to proliferate. The loss of alleles on chromosome

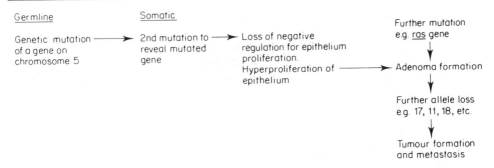

Figure 3. Possible mechanisms for APC tumour formation

17 is thought to occur late in the cancer process and may occur during the adenoma-carcinoma transition.

From these studies it is clear that a large number of changes occur in colon tumours as they proliferate and metastasise, and a possible mechanism for progression to tumour formation is shown in Figure 3. However, ascertaining the role of the gene product of the FAP locus will be important in the understanding of the carcinogenesis process. It has been hypothesised that the FAP gene product acts as a negative regulator of epithelial proliferation. It may act by inhibiting the production of growth factors. Recently, evidence has been presented for a potential role of the FAP gene in a subset of colorectal tumours. Erisman and colleagues looked at the regulation of RNA from the c-*myc* oncogene. Over 70% of colorectal carcinomas have been shown to have increased levels (5–40 times higher) of c-*myc* RNA and its gene product. They found that c-*myc* is controlled by a trans-acting regulator, the loss of which is responsible for deregulation of c-*myc* expression in the majority of colorectal tumours. An allele loss study showed that there was a strong correlation with the loss of markers on the long arm of chromosome 5 and deregulation of c-*myc* expression. In tumours showing normal levels of c-*myc* RNA, allele loss on chromosome 5q was not seen. In conclusion the FAP gene product may act as an anti-oncogene and the loss or mutation of both copies may lead to cellular proliferation and tumour formation. The c-*myc* gene has been shown to be important in cell division, and so the deregulation of c-*myc* expression in a subset of colon cells may lead to uncontrolled cell growth. If one copy of this gene is mutated or deleted then the remaining allele may be insufficient to prevent the proliferation of epithelium giving rise to discontinuous areas of growth or polyps. This hyperplastic proliferation of epithelial cells may increase the chances for second and subsequent events to occur. These second events causing the transition from areas of abnormal growth to adenomas and carcinoma need not be the same. They may involve a variety of changes, including *ras* mutations or allele loss on chromosomes 17 or 18.

CONCLUSIONS

Using molecular analysis and reverse genetics it has been possible to locate the FAP gene responsible for one form of inherited colon cancer. Similarly a number of secondary changes have been identified in colon tumours, including the loss of genes or mutations which may cause the cancer to progress by growing in an uncontrolled fashion, eventually leading to metastasis.

The eventual identification of the gene causing the primary defect in FAP and the other genes involved in the secondary evolution of tumour growth should lead to an understanding of the pathogenesis of colon cancer.

FURTHER READING

Antonarakis, S. E. (1989) Diagnosis of genetic disorders at the DNA level. *New Engl. J. Med.*, **320**, 153–163.

Baker, S. J., Fearon, E. R., Nigro, J. M., *et al.* (1989) Chromosome 17 deletions and p53 gene mutations in colorectal carcinomas. *Science*, **244**, 217–221.

Bodmer, W. F., Bailey, C. J., Bodmer, J., *et al.* (1987) Localization of the gene for familial adenomatous polyposis on chromosome 5. *Nature*, **328**, 614–619.

Dukes, C. (1930) The hereditary factor in polyposis intestini, or multiple adenomata. *The Cancer Review*, **5**, 241–251.

Erisman, M. D., Scott, J. K. and Astrin, S. M. (1989) Evidence that the familial adenomatous polyposis gene is involved in a subset of colon cancers with a complementable defect in c-*myc* regulation. *Proc. Natl. Acad. Sci. USA*, **86**, 4624–4628.

Nakamura, Y., Lathrop, M., Leppert, M. *et al.* (1988) Localization of the genetic defect in familial adenomatous polyposis within a small region of chromosome 5. *Am. J. Hum. Genet.*, **43**, 638–644.

Okamoto, M., Sasaki, M., Sugio, K., *et al.* (1988) Loss of constitutional heterozygosity in colon carcinoma from patients with familial polyposis coli. *Nature*, **331**, 273–277.

Vogelstein, B., Fearon, E. R., Hamilton, S. R., *et al.* (1988) Genetic alterations during colorectal-tumor development. *New Engl. J. Med.*, **319**, 525–532.

Vogelstein, B., Fearon, E. R., Kern, S. E., *et al.* (1989) Allelotype of colorectal carcinomas. *Science*, **244**, 207–211.

30 Molecular Genetics of Lung Cancer

DESMOND N. CARNEY
AMANDA McCANN
NIAMH CORBALLY

In spite of improvements in the diagnosis, staging and identification of prognostic factors of lung cancer over the past two decades, there has not been any significant increase in overall survival from this disease. Currently, the 5-year survival rate of newly diagnosed patients with lung cancer ranges between 5 and 7%, and associated with these findings is the recognition that the incidence of lung cancer continues to rise. Thus it is anticipated that this year there will be approximately 156 000 new cases in the United States and 135 000 deaths. Lung cancer accounts for 35% of all cancer deaths in males and almost 20% of cancer deaths in females. Indeed, female lung cancer deaths have now exceeded deaths from breast cancer.

There are four major histological subtypes of lung cancer: small cell lung cancer (SCLC), which accounts for 25% of all new cases; squamous cell carcinoma; adenocarcinoma; and large cell carcinoma (the latter three types are collectively referred to as non-small cell lung cancer—NSCLC). For patients with SCLC hope for survival is directly related to the sensitivity of this tumour type to chemotherapy ± radiation therapy. With combination chemotherapy between 5 and 10% of all patients with SCLC may now be cured of their disease. For patients with NSCLC hope for long-term survival is directly related to the surgical resection of this tumour type. Chemotherapy and/or radiation therapy have contributed little to improving the overall survival of patients with NSCLC. For all the above reasons, therefore, there is a need to currently identify new therapeutic modalities for the management of patients with these diseases.

In contrast to the above, major advances have been made in our understanding of the biological properties of lung cancer cells. These advances have been brought about by our ability to establish with relative ease continuous cell lines of both SCLC and NSCLC. These cell lines have served as a model for the identification of different

Genes and Cancer. Edited by D. Carney and K. Sikora
©1990 John Wiley & Sons Ltd

biological characteristics associated with individual tumour types, and allow the identification of biomarkers which can be applied clinically in the management of patients with these diseases. Studies of large numbers of cell lines have clearly demonstrated the extreme heterogeneity that exists within these tumour types with respect to a range of biological markers. In addition we have developed a better understanding of the molecular events which take place in this disease, including both specific and non-specific chromosomal abnormalities, DNA content changes and alteration in the expression of a range of oncogenes. These changes include chromosomal rearrangement and deletions, point mutations, gene amplification and altered gene expression. The application to clinical practice of our understanding of the molecular events taking place in lung cancer may allow us to better define prognostic subgroups within a given tumour type and establish different therapeutic modalities for the management of patients with these diseases.

CELL LINES AND BIOLOGICAL CHARACTERISTICS IN LUNG CANCER

Over the past decade considerable success has been achieved in establishing permanent cell lines of both SCLC and NSCLC. This success was achieved primarily through the identification and characterization of serum-free chemically defined medium which would selectively support the growth of SCLC and NSCLC cell lines. With such media cell lines can now be established in 70–80% of all tumour specimens obtained from patients containing viable tumour cells. These cell lines have been established both from primary lung cancer biopsy specimens and from a range of metastatic sites, including bone marrow, pleural effusions, lymph node biopsies and surgically resected tumour masses.

SCLC cell lines in general grow as floating aggregates of tightly-to-loosely packed cells, form colonies in soft agarose and are tumorigenic when injected into athymic nude mice. In contrast NSCLC cell lines grow as adherent monolayer cultures and will also form tumours in athymic nude mice. In contrast to SCLC cell lines, cell lines of NSCLC origin can be more readily established from metastatic lesions when compared with the primary lesions, suggesting that the metastatic deposits may be of a more malignant behaviour than the primary lesion. For most lung cancer cell lines, once established as permanent cultures the cells retain the morphology of the original tumour type both *in vivo* and when forming tumours in athymic nude mice.

A range of biochemical and biological properties have been identified which can clearly distinguish SCLC from NSCLC cell lines (Table 1). In addition among cell lines established from patients with SCLC considerable heterogeneity has been demonstrated, allowing sub-classification of these cell lines into two major divisions, namely classic and variant SCLC. Classic cell lines express a range of neuroendocrine properties, including high levels of neurone-specific enolase (NSE), creatine kinase BB (CK-BB), L-dopa decarboxylase (DDC) and the peptide hormone bombesin/gastrin releasing peptide (BLI/GRP). In contrast, among variant cultures there is a selective loss of some of these neuroendocrine properties, including DDC and BLI/GRP. In addition variant cell lines are associated with more aggressive tumours with a more rapid doubling time and a shorter latent time to tumour formation in athymic nude

Table 1. Biological properties of lung cancer cell lines

Characteristic	SCLC		NSCLC
	Classic	Variant	
Growth morphology	Suspension	Suspension	Attached
Cytology	SCLC	SCLC	NSCLC
Colony forming efficiency	2%	13%	6%
Doubling time	72 hr	32 hr	40 hr
Dense core granules	+	−	−
DDC	+ +	−	−
BLI/GRP	+ +	−	−
NSE	+ +	+	−
CK-BB	+ +	+ +	−
Neurotensin	+ +	−	−
Peptide hormones	+ +	+ / −	−
BLI receptors	+	−	−
EGF receptors	−	−	+
HLA/B$_2$ microglobulin	Low/Absent	Low/Absent	Present
Chromosome 3p del	+	+	+
Intermediate cell filaments	Cytokeratins	Cytokeratins	Cytokeratins
Leu-7 antigen	+	+	−
Radiation sensitivity	'Sensitive'	'Resistant'	'Resistant'
c-*myc* amplification	−	+	+ / −
n-*myc* amplification	+ / −	+ / −	−
l-*myc* amplification	+ / −	−	−

mice compared to classic cell lines. In addition, as will be noted, both classic and variant cultures demonstrate different oncogene abnormalities when analysed.

In general NSCLC cultures do not express neuroendocrine properties. However, it should be noted that up to 20% of cell lines established from patients with adenocarcinoma will express a range of neuroendocrine properties, including high levels of DDC and NSE. While currently the significance of these neuroendocrine properties in adenocarcinoma remains unclear, preliminary data suggest that these tumours may be much more chemosensitive than other NSCLC specimens.

While prospective studies of the biological properties of established cell lines have not been carried out, in a study of the clinical behaviour of SCLC patients from whom cell lines were established the median survival of 19 newly diagnosed untreated patients was 14 weeks. In contrast the median survival of 123 extensive stage patients from whom cell lines were not established was significantly longer (48 weeks). It is clear, however, that much work needs to be done on the importance of the biological characteristics in tumour cells and that future clinical trials of lung cancer should assess the clinical relevance of these markers in predicting response to therapy and survival.

DNA ABNORMALITIES IN LUNG CANCER CELLS

Much work has been carried out on determining the prognostic significance of the DNA content of lung cancer cells determined by flow cytometry. For a variety of different tumours, including breast cancer and lymphomas, a significant correlation exists between the degree of aneuploidy and survival. In flow cytometry studies (FCM) of tumours from lung cancer patients approximately 85% of tumours have an aneuploid DNA content, ranging from hypodiploid to tetraploid. In addition stem cell lines are observed in 10–20% of such specimens. In studies of lung cancer patients correlations have been evaluated between the total DNA content, the proliferative characteristics and the number of stem cell lines present, with the overall survival and outcome of the patients treated. In SCLC patients little correlation has been demonstrated between the DNA content and proliferative characteristics of the patients with patient survival. In contrast several studies have demonstrated that patients with multiple stem cell lines have an overall poorer survival. In patients with NSCLC a DNA index in the tetraploid or greater range has been observed more frequently than among patients with SCLC. In addition it has been shown that those patients whose tumours have a low G_0-G_1 cell proportion or a high proliferation fraction have a shorter survival time and poorer response to cytotoxic chemotherapy, suggesting that the analysis of the DNA content of NSCLC tumours may be of prognostic value and should be considered in the evaluation of cytotoxic responses in clinical trials.

PROTO-ONCOGENE AMPLIFICATION AND EXPRESSION IN LUNG CANCER CELLS

The availability of a large number of cell lines of both small cell and non-small cell carcinoma obtained from primary and metastatic sites and from treated and untreated patients formed a pool from which studies of oncogene derangements in lung cancer cells were initially carried out. Early studies were carried out on both classic and variant cell lines to determine if differences exist between these two subtypes of small cell but more recently have been extended to all cell types of NSCLC. As noted, variant cell lines had a more aggressive growth behaviour *in vitro* and *in vivo*, had a selective loss of neuroendocrine markers and were relatively radioresistant; cytogenetic studies revealed both double minute chromosomes or one or more homogeneously staining regions (HSRs). Initial studies of these variant cell lines revealed up to 76-fold amplification of c-*myc* compared to classical small cell cultures. Over-expression of c-*myc* was noted in most amplified cell lines. While one or more HSRs were noted in these variant subtypes, HSRs were not associated with chromosome 8, the location of the proto-oncogene c-*myc*. The importance of amplification of c-*myc* in variant SCLC was suggested by the recognition that the median survival of patients from whom variant cell lines with c-*myc* DNA amplification were derived was shorter (33 weeks) than patients whose cell lines did not have c-*myc* amplification (53 weeks). These studies and other studies of *in vitro* transfection suggested that in SCLC c-*myc* was important in growth regulation and in the expression of the variant morphology.

More detailed studies on extended panels of both SCLC and NSCLC carried out in several institutions have revealed that other members of the *myc* family of oncogenes, namely, N-*myc* and L-*myc*, may be important in the biology of SCLC. As with c-*myc*, in most specimens where N-*myc* amplification has been

Table 2. SCLC: oncogene DNA amplification*

Specimen	c-*myc*	N-*myc*	L-*myc*	Total
Cell lines	14/83	6/83	6/67	26/83 (25%)
Tumours	2/83	7/83	2/38	11/83 (13%)

*5 studies

Table 3. Small cell lung cancer: *myc* oncogene amplification*

	Cell lines	Tumours
Amplification	26/83 (25%)	11/83 (13%)
Prior therapy*	15/35 (43%)	6/32 (19%)
No prior therapy*	3/31 (10%)	0/32 (0%)

*Including c-*myc*, N-*myc*, L-*myc*. Therapy status not available on all specimens

demonstrated, over-expression of N-*myc* messenger RNA has been noted. In contrast, expression of L-*myc* has been found to occur in the absence of gene amplification in SCLC cell lines. No SCLC cell lines have been identified that predominantly express c-*myc*, N-*myc* or L-*myc* together. In addition several examples of c-*myc* and L-*myc* amplification in NSCLC cultures have been demonstrated.

What is the clinical significance of amplification or over-expression of members of the *myc* family of oncogenes in the clinical behaviour of SCLC? As seen in Table 2, a variety of different centres have clearly indicated that amplification of one or more of these oncogenes may occur in up to 25% of specimens of cell lines obtained from patients with SCLC. However, several important factors have emerged from these studies:

1. *myc* amplification is more readily detected in established cell lines than in fresh biopsy specimens of patients with SCLC.

2. Amplification is rarely observed in specimens obtained from previously untreated newly diagnosed patients with SCLC compared to patients heavily pre-treated (Table 3). While amplification of both N-*myc* and L-*myc* has been observed in fresh biopsy specimens of SCLC, amplification of c-*myc* is a much less common event in these fresh specimens.

All of these data suggest that the oncogene abnormalities of the *myc* family are relatively late events in the pathogenesis and biology of SCLC and therefore are more likely to contribute to the more aggressive behaviour frequently observed in these tumours following relapse.

Table 4. Oncogenes in SCLC

Oncogene	Mechanism of activation
c-*myc*	Amplification/over-expression
N-*myc*	Amplification/over-expression
L-*myc*	Amplification/over-expression
c	Amplification/over-expression
L-*raf*-1	Over-expression
p53	Over-expression
jun	Expression
Ki-*ras*	Point mutation

Table 5. Ki-*ras* in lung adenocarcinomas

1. Mutational *ras* activation in 10/34 Ts
2. All mutations in codon 12 of the gene
3. No correlation with survival
4. ?? Association with cigarette smoking

A variety of other oncogenes have been noted in SCLC specimens (Table 4). Again, their finding in only a small percentage of cell lines and/or fresh specimens questions their importance in all SCLC patients.

Detailed studies have been carried out on primary specimens of NSCLC in addition to cell lines of this cell type. Among these tumours the *ras* family of oncogenes has been implicated, particularly in adenocarcinoma specimens. In one study mutational *ras* activation was noted in a third of fresh biopsy specimens, the majority involving the Ki-*ras* oncogene, with all mutations taking place in codon 12 of the gene (Table 5). No clinical correlation was noted with this oncogene abnormality. In addition to the *ras* family of oncogenes a range of other oncogenes have been identified in NSCLC specimens (Tables 6 and 7), but their clinical significance remains unclear.

CYTOGENETIC ABNORMALITIES IN LUNG CANCER CELLS

A range of chromosomal abnormalities have been demonstrated in both cell lines and fresh specimens of lung cancer, in particular SCLC. A specific cytogenetic abnormality involving a deletion in the short arm of chromosome 3 (3p14→23), initially identified in SCLC, has now been identified in all lung cancer specimens using restriction fragment length polymorphism probes (RFLPs) known to map chromosome 3. This deletion has been noted in all cell lines of SCLC and NSCLC.

Table 6. Oncogenes in NSCLC

Oncogene	Mechanism of action
Ki-*ras*	Point mutation
Ha-*ras*	Point mutation
c-*myc*	Over-expression
L-*myc*	Over-expression
p53	Over-expression

Table 7. Oncogene amplification in NSCLC

Oncogene	Incidence of amplification
Ki-*ras*	0/58
c-*myc*	2/58
N-*myc*	0/58
L-*myc*	0/58
c-*erb*B	0/58
neu	0/57
c-*fms*	0/58

Table 8. Expression of retinoblastoma (Rb) gene in lung cancer

Cell type	No.	Rb mRNA expression		
		None detected	Trace	+ +
SCLC	26	15 (60%)	5	6
Carcinoid	4	3	–	1
NSCLC	19	2	2	15 (90%)

It is interesting to note, however, that this deletion is not found in extrapulmonary SCLC. The finding of this deletion in all lung cancer specimens suggests that it is an important early event in the pathogenesis of lung cancer and that the deleted region contains an anti-oncogene, the loss of which uncovers an otherwise recessive mutation on the cytogenetically normal chromosome 3. More recently a second cytogenetic defect including an abnormality in both structure and expression of the human retinoblastoma gene has been detected in SCLC but not in NSCLC specimens (Table 8). The gene determining susceptibility to retinoblastoma has been mapped to chromosome 13q14. In studies of SCLC cell lines chromosome 13 was absent or hypodiploid in 17/21 specimens evaluated. In addition using retinoblastoma (Rb) complementary DNA probes, structural abnormality of the gene was noted in up to 25% of SCLC specimens. In contrast no abnormalities were detected in other cell types of lung cancer. Thus these findings suggest an important role for the Rb gene in the pathogenesis of SCLC but not of NSCLC. The abnormalities of the Rb gene can be found in a variety of other tumours, and the data suggest that this gene may be important in the biology of a wide range of common tumours of different cell type.

DRUG RESISTANCE IN SCLC CELLS

Pleiotropic drug resistance has been noted among cell lines of SCLC (Tables 9 and 10). Studies of the mechanisms of drug resistance have been carried out by evaluating the properties of cell lines from treated and untreated patients and fresh biopsy specimens in addition to the development of drug-resistant mutants *in vitro*. While a variety of specific mechanisms of drug resistance have been noted among individual cell types, much work has been carried out on evaluation of these tumour types for the expression of P-glycoprotein, a membrane glycoprotein of relative molecular mass approximately 170 000, which has been demonstrated to be important in the pleiotropic drug resistance of a variety of other tumour types. In a recent study of a large number of fresh specimens in cell lines of SCLC and using immuno-blocking techniques and enzyme-linked immunosorbent assay, P-glycoprotein was not detected among the majority of tumour specimens evaluated. However, it was of interest to note that among NSCLC with neuroendocrine properties P-glycoprotein was detected among this subtype. In general, however, it can be stated that factors other than the P-glycoprotein may account for the development of multidrug resistance in SCLC. Nonetheless, the development of resistant cell lines should provide a model for evaluating other mechanisms of drug resistance in these tumours and identifying means of reversing such resistance.

Table 9. Multiple drug resistance (MDR1) gene expression in lung cancer*

Cell type	% Positive
Non-tumour lung	7/10 (70%)
Lung Cancer	
SCLC	3/6
NSCLC	8/13
NSCLC-NE	1/2
Carcinoid	2/3
Total	14/24 (58%)
Cell lines	
SCLC*	4/14
SCLC**	0/9
Expul. SCLC	0/4
NSCLC	11/29
NSCLC-NE	5/6
Carcinoid	2/5
Total	22/67 (33%)

*noRx; **prior Rx

Table 10. MDR1 gene expression in lung cancer

1. All tumours, non-tumorous lung and cell lines express low levels of MDR1 RNA
2. No correlation between MDR1 gene expression in cell lines and:
    In vitro chemosensitivity
    Prior therapy status
    Clinical response to therapy

SUMMARY

A range of molecular and oncogene abnormalities have been identified in both fresh specimens and cell lines of SCLC. While a specific cytogenic abnormality is common to all cell types of lung carcinoma, oncogene abnormalities including amplification and over-expression do not appear to be unique to any specific cell type. The finding of a low frequency of many of these oncogene abnormalities in lung cancer cells questions their importance in the early pathogenesis of this disease. Further studies are required to determine earlier molecular events in the biology of lung cancer tumours.

FURTHER READING

Birrer, M. J. and Minna, J. D. (1988) Molecular genetics of lung cancer. *Semin. Oncol.*, **15**, 226–235.
Brauch, H., Johnson, B., Hovis, J., *et al.* (1987) Molecular analysis of the short arm of chromosome 3 in small-cell and non-small-cell carcinoma of the lung. *N. Eng. J. Med.*, **317**, 1109–1113.

Carney, D. N. and De Leij, L. (1988) Lung cancer biology. *Semin. Oncol.*, **15**, 199–214.

Cline, M. J. and Battifora, H. (1987) Abnormalities of proto-oncogenes in non-small cell lung cancer: correlations with tumor type and clinical characteristics. *Cancer*, **60**, 2669–2674.

Harbour, J. W., Lai, S. L., Whang-Peng, J., *et al.* (1988) Abnormalities in structure and expression of the human retinoblastoma gene in SCLC. *Science*, **241**, 353–357.

Johnson, B. E., Battey, J., Linnoila, I., *et al.* (1986) Changes in the phenotype of human small cell lung cancer cell lines following transfection and expression of the c-*myc* proto-oncogene. *J. Clin. Invest.*, **78**, 525.

Johnson, B. E., Idhe, D. C., Makuch, R. W., *et al.* (1987) *Myc* family oncogene amplification in tumor cell lines established from small cell lung cancer patient and its relationship to clinical status and course. *J. Clin. Invest.*, **79**, 1629–1638.

Kok, K., Osinga, J., Carritt, B., *et al.* (1987) Deletion of a DNA sequence at the chromosome 3p21 in all major types of lung cancer. *Nature*, **330**, 578–581.

Little, C. D., Nau, M., Carney, D. N., *et al.* (1983) Amplification and expression of the c-*myc* oncogene in human lung cancer cell lines. *Nature*, **306**, 194–196.

Nau, M. M., Brooks, B. J., Battey, J., *et al.* (1985) L-*myc* a new *myc*-related gene amplified and expressed in human small cell lung cancer. *Nature*, **318**, 69–75.

Nau, M. M., Brooks, B. J. Jr., Carney, D. N., *et al.* (1986) Human small cell lung cancer shows amplification and expression of N-*myc* gene. *PNAS.*, **83**, 1092.

Rodenhuis, S., Van De Wetering, M. L., Mooi, W. J., *et al.* (1987) Mutational activation of the K-*ras* oncogene: a possible pathogenetic factor in adenocarcinoma of the lung. *N. Engl. J. Med.*, **317**, 929–935.

31 The Biology of Metastases

PETER ALEXANDER

There is abundant evidence to show that the vast majority of malignant cells which are released from tumours and shed into the blood or intercellular fluid (and thence into afferent lymph) do not give rise to metastatic lesions but die, differentiate or lie dormant. The mechanisms by which cancer cells in the circulation are eliminated are discussed below. I will first consider the question whether the cancer cells that initiate a metastatic lesion are random survivors of shed cancer cells or whether they derive predominantly (or even exclusively) from pre-existing variants with heritable physiological properties that favour dissemination. Whether metastasis is random or is a selective process from a distinct sub-population within a primary tumour is of more than academic interest as it will greatly affect therapeutic strategies. The fact that in the natural history of some malignant neoplasms there is evidence of progression towards more malignant behaviour does not necessarily imply that such variants, as they arise, become the preferential source of cells from which metastases are drawn.

Quite apart from the phenomenon of tumour progression there is abundant evidence that the malignant cells which make up both human and experimental animal tumours are not all alike, even if the tumour is of monoclonal origin. Several investigators have succumbed to the seductive logic that, because variants are present, metastases derive selectively from them and the earlier view that metastases occur following rare and chance events which permit a shed cell to survive has been challenged.

A TUMOUR IS A MICROCOSM

Heterogeneity of cells within a malignant tumour occurs at several levels and it is self-evident, though often forgotten, that all the cells in a tumour are not tumour

Genes and Cancer. Edited by D. Carney and K. Sikora.
Published 1990 by John Wiley & Sons Ltd.

cells. There are the cells making up the stroma and, particularly, the endothelial cells necessary to establish the micro-circulation, without which a tumour cannot grow beyond a fraction of a millimetre in diameter. In addition, all tumours are infiltrated by leucocytes, and surface markers show that mononuclear phagocytes sometimes make up more than a quarter of all the cells within a tumour, although in normal histological sections they may not be prominent. Variability amongst the malignant cells is frequently evident at the level of the light microscope and pleiomorphism is for pathologists an important diagnostic feature of cancer. In part, variability must arise from differences in metabolism caused by spatial factors in relation to blood vessels; additional variables are the stage of the cell cycle and the degree of differentiation. Many types of malignant cells have retained the capacity to undergo limited differentiation, but the extent to which they do this is not uniform within a tumour and is probably determined both by environmental and genetic factors. Clearly, cancer cells that have become terminally differentiated cannot give rise to a metastasis, but partial differentiation does not preclude successful dissemination and there is at best only a weak correlation between anaplasia and metastasis.

At first sight, one might expect variability at the genetic level to be minimal for a malignant disease which stems from a single cell which has become transformed. Monoclonality has been demonstrated for almost all leukaemias and lymphomas for which there were suitable markers, such as immunoglobulin class (or idiotype) or an X-linked polyallelic enzyme. Indeed, monoclonality is an important criterion for the diagnosis of malignant lymphomas. Monoclonal origin is not universal and in some patients carcinomas have been demonstrated to be polyclonal; similar findings have been made for chemically induced rodent cancers. The frequency of polyclonality in carcinomas and sarcomas is not known because, in the majority of cases, this cannot as yet be determined with the markers that are available.

However, genetic variability within the cancer cells of a tumour is not dependent on polyclonal origin since the karyotype of cancer cells within a tumour is often highly variable. It has long been known that the number of chromosomes in different cancer cells of the same tumour frequently vary widely and that the two daughter cells from a cancer quite commonly may have a different chromosome make up. Perhaps the most characteristic feature of cancer is that malignant cells are karyotypically unstable. The mechanism of sharing the genetic material equally between the two daughters at mitosis which works so perfectly in normal cells frequently fails in cancer and to a lesser extent in the leukaemias. The biochemical basis for this defect, which is only associated with malignant cells, is not yet known, but the result is that even when cancer is of monoclonal origin the individual cells arising from the single clone exhibit a degree of genetic variability which is orders of magnitude greater than that produced in normal cells by 'background' or spontaneous mutations.

Recent developments in the methods of studying chromosomes have made it possible to classify chromosome variations in cancer into primary and secondary. The primary lesion is a change which involves a given chromosome at a specific location and tends to be characteristic of a particular tumour type and is present in every one of the malignant cells of that tumour (or leukaemia). Superimposed on this specific chromosome alteration, which is probably related to the sub-cellular lesions which result in the transformation of a normal cell to one of malignant phenotype, there are variable and sequential changes in chromosomes. The latter are a consequence of karyotypic instability, and must be reflected sometimes in the phenotype and thus give rise to a high frequency of variants. Consequently, it is usually possible to isolate from a given animal, tumour cells which give rise when cloned *in vivo* or *in vitro* to a number of populations with different properties, some of which will have a selective growth advantage in particular environments. Progression, when it occurs, can be viewed as a change in the incidence of the various sub-populations of cancer cells within a tumour leading to overall increased malignant behaviour.

SUB-POPULATIONS OF CELLS IN TUMOURS WHICH ARE MORE METASTATIC

A decisive test to show that metastases originate from a sub-population within a primary would be to compare the biological properties of individual tumour cells in the primary and the secondary lesions. Because of the wide heterogeneity of cells within a tumour, such comparisons would require the analysis of a large number of cells to determine the distribution pattern of the property under investigation. Moreover, isolated examples in which the malignant cells in a metastasis are demonstrably different from the majority of the cells in the primary are not helpful, since selection could have occurred by chance and not be an essential component of the metastatic process. These technical difficulties explain why there is no information from human data which bears decisively on this point. In a critical review of the clinical literature, Weiss failed to find evidence for consistent differences between the cancer cells of primary cancers and their metastases in respect to cytogenetics, immunology or drug sensitivity.

The sub-population hypothesis rests, therefore, essentially on experiments with animal tumours. By complex manoeuvres, which generally involved repeated *in vitro* culture and passage and selection *in vivo*, many investigators have been able to establish from a given tumour a series of sub-lines which varied in their capacity to metastasize when inoculated into animals. There are, however, two major uncertainties in the interpretation of such findings. Firstly, in view of the inherent instability of the phenotype of malignant cells, do the variants isolated after repeated *in vitro* cloning and/or transplantation really represent pre-existing sub-clones, or are they an artefact of the selection techniques? Thus, highly metastatic variants have by such means been obtained from adenocarcinomas that did not metastasize and which evidently did not normally contain cells with metastatic capability. The introduction of *in vitro* culture when dealing with malignant cells is hazardous since phenotypic variability can arise more readily *in vitro* than *in vivo*; the development of heterogeneity in clones cultured from a single malignant cell is often overlooked. Secondly, even when highly metastatic variants are present in the primary, are they in fact selected for in the processes that eliminate the majority of shed cells?

COMPARISON OF METASTATIC POTENTIAL OF TUMOUR CELLS IN THE PRIMARY AND THE METASTASES

If the cells forming the metastases were derived from a sub-population with properties which facilitate metastasis, then the cancer cells taken from the metastases should on average be more metastatic than the cells from the primary tumour. Many investigators have tested this proposition with a variety of transplantable animal tumours and in no instance has this been observed. The metastatic potential of cells from the metastasis is sometimes greater, sometimes less and, most commonly, indistinguishable from that produced by cancer cells taken from the primary. Figures 1 and 2 illustrate two experiments of our own which are representative not only of our studies but those of others. The only apparent exception is an investigation by Talmadge and Fidler which alleges to show a consistent selection of cells with a higher propensity to metastasize within metastatic lesions. This investigation differed, however, from the others by introducing the confounding factors of growing the cells from the metastases *in vitro* prior to testing their capacity to metastasize *in vivo*.

Experiments comparing the metastatic potential of cells in metastases with those of the primary are of direct clinical interest, since studies of human tumours have shown that an important factor in the pattern of dissemination is the metastasis of metastases. From the selection hypothesis, one would be led to the erroneous conclusion that the local treatment of metastases would inevitably be without value since the cells in a metastasis would have a high metastatic capacity and already have brought about further spread.

Tumour	Deaths with spontaneous metastasis -					Total	Host cells	TD_{50}
HSBPA ↓				∗ ■		1/8	41-46	2.4×10^6
LM			■			1/8	40	1.8×10^6
HSN ↓		∗ ●	■			2/8	28-33	3.2×10^5
LNM		● ■		■		3/8	28	2.9×10^5
MC28 ↓	∗ ● ●	● ■	■			5/8	18-22	9.0×10^4
LNM		● ■	■			3/8	24	3.0×10^5

40   80   120   160   365

Days post tumour excision

Figure 1. Comparison of biological properties (i.e. capacity to metastasize, host cell infiltrate (%) and number of cells needed to effect a transplant, TD_{50}) of cells from a metastasis with those from the locally growing tumour for three sarcomas which varied in their capacity to give rise to distant metastases. In these experiments the tumour was implanted i.m., allowed to grow for two weeks and then surgically excised. The animals were then followed for a year for the appearance of metastases. The top line shows the incidence of metastasis from transplants of locally growing tumours and the bottom line the incidence of metastasis when cells derived from the metastasis marked* were transplanted. The tumours which developed from either lung (LM) or lymph node (LNM) metastases showed no trend towards increased metastatic efficiency, and cells which had disseminated to lymph nodes were equally able to metastasize in the lung and vice versa. Also, the spontaneous metastases shown here yielded tumours with host cell infiltration and immunogenicity broadly comparable to that of the parent tumours. (■ lung metastasis; ● lymph node metastasis)

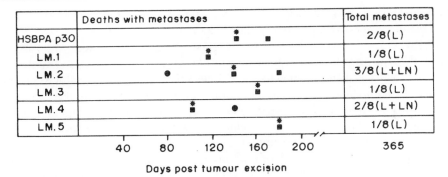

	Deaths with metastases						Total metastases
HSBPA p30							2/8(L)
LM.1							1/8(L)
LM.2							3/8(L+LN)
LM.3							1/8(L)
LM.4							2/8(L+LN)
LM.5							1/8(L)

Days post tumour excision

Figure 2. Repeated transplantation of lung metastases (LM): inability to demonstrate that the cells which comprise distant metastases are inherently more highly metastatic. A tumour with low spontaneous incidence of metastasis in normal rats was implanted and one of the distant metastases was then transplanted successively. It is clear that the transplants from the metastasis behave no differently from the transplants of the locally growing tumour. As in Figure 1 tumours cells were implanted i.m., allowed to grow for two weeks and then surgically excised. The animals were followed for a year to record metastases, the incidence of which is expressed as, for example, 1/8, i.e. one in a group of eight similarly treated rats. (■ lung metastasis; ● lymph node metastasis)

BLOOD-BORNE METASTASES

Cancer cells gain access to the blood via the venous circulation which in general follows the invasion of veins. But there are situations in which the cancer cells have direct access to the blood through the lymph or a defective endothelium in the tumour. The first capillary bed that is encountered by cancer cells disseminated into the blood, except when the primary cancer is in the lung, will be either that of the lung or the liver, depending on whether the blood supply of the tumour is to the vena caval or portal system. The spread of blood-borne metastases to other organs requires that cancer cells pass from the lung into the arterial circulation via the pulmonary vein and the left side of the heart. For this to occur, cancer emboli need either to pass through the capillaries in the lung with their reproductive capacity intact or to stem from metastases within the lung (i.e. metastasis from a metastasis).

Perhaps the most striking aspect of the metastatic process is its inefficiency. Such inefficiency is brought about both by the death of circulating cancer cells before they have succeeded in extravasating, as well as by the inability to proliferate at extravascular sites unless the environment is right.

Destruction of cancer cells arrested within the microvasculature

Post-mortem studies indicate that cancerous invasion of veins is common and that the shedding of cancer cells and their subsequent arrest in small blood vessels, either singly or as clusters, is much more frequent than the incidence of progressively growing metastases. There have been several reports in which circulating tumour cells were detected in patients without metastases. In experimental animals, direct evidence for this comes from three types of experiment:

1. Identification with an antiserum of large numbers of cancer cells in the efferent blood from a tumour that rarely metastasizes.

2. The presence of viable tumour cells in cell suspensions prepared from the lungs of animals bearing subcutaneous tumours that would not be expected to give rise to lung metastases. The cancer cells were detected by a bioassay in which cells from the lung were transplanted into another animal. A bioassay frequently does not reveal cancer cells within the blood since they are trapped in the first passage through the lung and, as a result, the number of cells in the circulation will represent less than one minute's output of cancer emboli.

3. The rapid autolysis of cancer cells arrested in the lung has been demonstrated by the intravenous injection of cancer cells, the DNA of which was radioactively labelled. In mice, more than 90% of cancer cells introduced in this way autolyse completely within 24 hours. That the cancer cells have died and have been broken down in the lung is proven by the disappearance of DNA-associated radioactivity in the lung and its eventual appearance in the urine as low molecular weight breakdown products. Massive destruction of blood-borne cancer cells is also indicated in patients in whom malignant ascites have been drained by a surgically introduced peritoneovenous shunt. As a result of this procedure, millions of cancer cells will be delivered to the lung. Yet in a carefully studied series, no indications could be found that lung metastasis was induced.

Role of immunity. The fact that specific T-cell-dependent immunity to antigenic tumours makes an important contribution to the destruction of tumour emboli from some, but by no means all, cancers has been demonstrated in experimental systems in which immunosuppression was found to facilitate metastasis. In our experiments rodent tumours were grown locally for two to four weeks after which they, and their draining nodes, were surgically removed and the animals kept for a year to allow the detection of distant metastases. (see Table 1 and Figure 3).

There are many sarcomas and some lymphomas where between 80 to 100% of the animals can be 'cured' by surgery, yet almost all will die of distant metastases if

Table 1. Effect of immunosuppression on development of distant metastases of a transplanted rat sarcoma

Immunosuppressive treatment given during period of tumour growth	Number of rats			
	Surviving at 60 weeks	Dead with no tumour	Dead with lung tumour	Dead with only lymph node tumour
None	50/60	2	4	4
Thoracic duct lymph drainage	8/40	11*	11	10
Sham cannulation	16/20	1	2	1
Thymectomy and irradiation	3/20	3	9	5
Sham thymectomy	15/20	1	3	1

Experimental protocol: tumour implanted day 0; tumour+draining nodes excised day 14; animals followed for 60 weeks.
*All the deaths occurred soon after prolonged draining, which is very traumatic

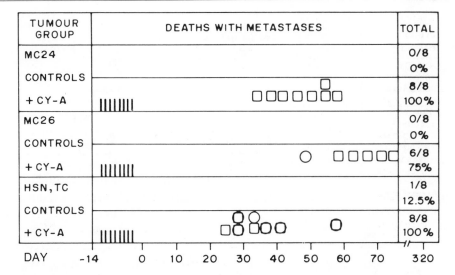

Figure 3. Effect of s.c. inoculation of cyclosporin A given repeatedly between Days − 14 and 0, as indicated on metastasis of rat sarcomas MC24, MC26 and HSN. TC. Tumours inoculated i.m. on Day − 14 and excised on Day 0. Metastases in lung (□) and lymph nodes (○)

the animals are immunosuppressed. That the facilitation of metastasis is caused by impairment of T-cell function and is not the result of other changes induced by the immunosuppressive regimen (e.g. anti-coagulation or leucopenia) was demonstrated by the fact that quite different procedures, which only shared the capacity to prevent T-cell-dependent immunity, all promoted metastasis. These procedures included the drainage of thoracic duct lymph, thymectomy plus total body irradiation and bone marrow graft, and the administration of immunosuppressive drugs, such as cyclosporin A, 1-asparaginase, cytoleucine and desoxycoformycin. All these procedures cause immunosuppression by quite different mechanisms. Moreover, sarcomas which did not metastasize in normal syngeneic rats did so in genetically athymic 'nude' rats (Figure 4). Our data suggest that an important effector mechanism in the immunological control of metastasis is the production of an antibody presumably directed against an antigen which requires the participation of T-lymphocytes for its recognition. The failure of most human tumours to metastasize when grown in 'nude' rodents may be caused by antibodies that are produced by the athymic hosts against antigens on xenografts which are independent of T-cells.

Immune control of dissemination is not a universal phenomenon and there are experimental tumours, particularly carcinomas, in which immunosuppression does not facilitate metastatic spread. In any case, even for tumours in which metastasis is determined by specific immunity, this can play no part in the destruction within the lung of cancer cells injected intravenously into normal (i.e. non-tumour bearing) animals, as this occurs much more rapidly than the induction of immunity.

Non-specific destruction by leucocytes. In vitro granulocytes, monocytes, mitogen-stimulated lymphocytes, and NK cells from normal animals that have not been

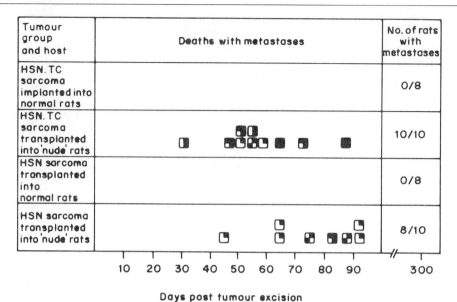

Figure 4. Occurrence of distant metastases from HSN fibrosarcoma in rats which are genetically athymic and immunodeficient (nudes). Tumours which do not metastasize in the normal rats do so in rats which have this genetic defect. Key: Deaths with metastases in lung (▣), lymph node (▣), viscera (▣), and subcutaneously (▣)

exposed to tumours, can all be shown to kill cancer cells in a selective, but immunologically non-specific way. In such a test, the susceptibility of different cancer cells varies and the order of sensitivity of a range of tumour cells is different for different leucocytes. While there is some evidence that killing by granulocytes and monocytes contributes to the intravascular lysis of cancer cells, claims that NK cells play a role have not been supported. At best, however, non-specific destruction by leucocytes can only make a minor contribution to the killing of emboli arrested in capillaries as this phenomenon occurs to nearly the same extent, and nearly at the same rate, in normal rodents as in rodents that have been rendered grossly leucopenic following total body irradiation.

Mechanical trauma. Weiss considers that a major factor in the death of circulating cancer cells is the irreversible mechanical damage sustained from the shearing forces in narrow capillaries. This has been demonstrated directly in elegant experiments with ascites tumour of rats. But the most compelling evidence for this mechanism is the low (frequently zero) capacity of cells to metastasize after having traversed a capillary bed. The damaging effect of transcapillary passage has been clearly evidenced for a variety of rat tumours by my colleague, Paul Murphy, who has injected different cancer cells into the left side of the heart of rats. Experiments with radioactive microspheres confirmed that the proportion of the cardiac output that went to the lung via the bronchial circulation was less than 2%, but when radioactively-labelled cancer cells were given intra-arterially, some 15% were detected in the lung within five minutes. These cancer cells had reached the lung as a result of passing through the major capillary beds, notably skeletal muscle, but they did not give rise to lung tumours, even when more than a million cells had reached the lung. On the other hand, less than 10 000 cells from these tumours were needed to produce lung lesions when they were injected intravenously, thus gaining access to the lung directly. The same applies to the liver: tumour cells which have entered via mesenteric capillary beds are much less tumorigenic than those injected directly into the portal vein.

Oxygen toxicity. The oxygen concentration in fully oxygenated arterial blood is three to four times higher than that in extracellular fluid, the normal milieu for mammalian cells other than those lining blood vessels. We have been testing the hypothesis that toxicity of oxygen at concentrations attained at equilibrium with the air is another factor which contributes to the death of tumour cells trapped in the microvasculature. At first sight, this suggestion would appear to be completely at variance with normal tissue culture experience where mammalian cells are routinely grown in atmospheres containing 18% oxygen. While there can be no doubt that many long established cell lines that grow *in vivo* from low numbers of cells are not inhibited by oxygen at normal concentrations, the evaluation of the optimum oxygen concentration for the *in vitro* growth of cells which require large inocula of cells is complicated. The actual oxygen concentration to which the cells are exposed *in vitro* is, in general, very much lower than that which corresponds to the atmosphere to which the cultures are exposed. This is caused by the consumption of oxygen which is not compensated for by the slow diffusion which occurs in the tissue culture vessels. The magnitude of this effect depends on the seeding density and the metabolic rate of the cells.

In a detailed study using oxygen microelectrodes and liver cells exposed in petri dishes with 0.5 cm fluid overlay, the oxygen concentration in contact with the cells was found to be equivalent to an atmosphere of 1% O_2 for 1.6×10^6 cells cm^{-2}, 5% for 1.0×10^6 cells cm^{-2}, and 8% for 0.5×10^6 cells cm^{-2}. To determine the effect of oxygen tension on growth, therefore, cells need to be seeded at low densities to minimise oxygen depletion. Indeed, at high *in vitro* cell densities, the oxygen concentration may be below that needed for optimum growth even when the culture is exposed to the atmosphere. There have been several reports, notably from the laboratory of Dr Sanford at the National Cancer Institute that some cells isolated directly from animals grow better in cultures exposed to atmospheres containing 5% oxygen than they do in air.

We have investigated the effect of oxygen concentration on the rate of proliferation of sarcoma and carcinoma cells taken from mice and rats with tumours. Most of the cancers studied show the pattern illustrated in Figure 5. That is, at low seeding densities the cells grow only in atmospheres at low oxygen concentrations, but this toxic effect of atmospheres rich in oxygen is lost as the initial seeding density is increased. Indeed, at the highest seeding densities, cells do not grow in atmospheres of low oxygen concentration because the depletion of oxygen in the medium by metabolism is so great that the oxygen concentration becomes insufficient for optimal growth. Although much work remains to be done, it would appear that many cancer cells taken from an animal proliferate optimally at oxygen concentrations equivalent to atmospheres of 2% to 5% and die at concentrations greater than 10% (Figure 6). This optimum range is similar to that found in extracellular fluid where cells, other than those of the vascular endothelium, exist and divide. *In vitro* cells seem to divide

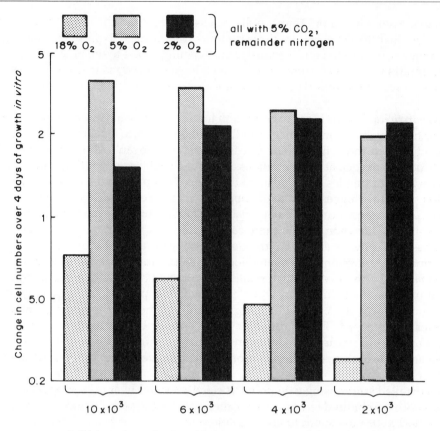

Figure 5. Effect of oxygen concentration in atmosphere on growth *in vitro* of murine sarcoma cells obtained directly from a tumour

less than maximally at oxygen concentrations less than 1%. In preliminary studies, we have noted that cancer cells adapt rapidly to oxygen when grown *in vitro* and that sometimes after a few passages *in vitro* the cells grow equally well at 18% as they do at 5% oxygen, even at low densities. Sometimes when cells that have 'adapted' to oxygen are grown *in vivo*, they again show sensitivity to oxygen on being returned to culture.

In the pulmonary microcirculation, cancer cells will only be exposed to high (i.e. approaching atmospheric) concentrations of oxygen if they have been trapped at the tips of the capillaries where the blood is reoxygenated. If they are arrested in small arteries they will be in an oxygen-depleted environment. Accordingly, if high oxygen concentrations kill trapped cancer cells, metastases will arise more commonly from cancer cells that have been held up within the arterioles than from those arrested in the capillaries. This hypothesis would explain why emboli containing a cluster of cancer cells give rise to lung metastases more frequently than do single cancer cells. This would also explain why an admixture of small microspheres of synthetic polymers and cancer cells increases the numbers of lung colonies produced by a given intravenous inoculation of cancer cells by a factor of 10 to 100.

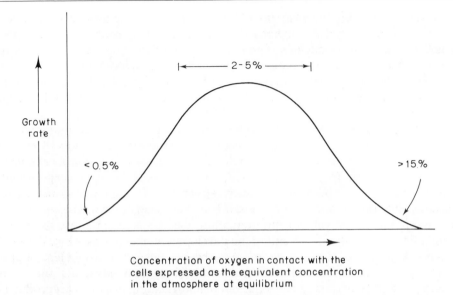

Growth rate

2-5%

<0.5%

>15%

Concentration of oxygen in contact with the cells expressed as the equivalent concentration in the atmosphere at equilibrium

Figure 6. Diagrammatic representation of the effect of oxygen concentration on growth *in vitro* of sarcoma cells obtained directly from a tumour

Protection by anticoagulation. Thrombocytopenia reduces the incidence of pulmonary metastasis in some experimental systems, as does prostacyclin which inhibits the association of platelets with tumour cells. A good case can now be made that in some situations aggregation of platelets to circulating tumour cells facilitates their growth within the lung. This would be consistent with the hypothesis that large aggregates will be trapped in vessels in the lung where the oxygen concentration is low. But it must be mentioned that the results of anticoagulant therapy on metastasis, using coumarin derivatives or heparin, are ambiguous. This could possibly be because fibrin clots around tumour emboli resolve within a few hours and before extravasation or cell death has occurred.

The fate after extravasation

While there have been isolated reports in which cell division has been observed within a large cluster of tumour cells in the vascular space, the general pattern is that blood-borne cancer cells have to extravasate before cell proliferation occurs. Initially, the fate of a cancer embolus is decided by two competing and opposed processes; namely, the rate of intravascular cell death and the rate of extravasation. Alteration of either process will alter the incidence of metastases. There is now much evidence to suggest that for the cancer emboli to extravasate, cells need to bind to the basement membrane. It has been proposed that receptors for intercellular macromolecules effect such an attachment via specific receptors. There is no evidence that cancer cells interact directly with the endothelial cells; exposed basement membrane seems to be necessary if extravasation is to occur. This would explain why metastasis is facilitated by processes which damage the endothelium and expose basement membrane. A striking demonstration of this phenomenon has been observed in mice where the incidence of lung lesions following intravenous injection of tumour cells was greatly increased if the mouse had been exposed to local irradiation of the lungs a day or so before the introduction of the tumour cells. Lung irradiation does not appear to reduce the rate of intravascular cell death, so the most likely explanation is that extravasation is facilitated and a greater, though still small, proportion of the cancer cells trapped within lung capillaries is enabled to avoid destruction.

Growth of a cancer cell that has successfully extravasated is not guaranteed. A clinical metastasis may not develop because the extravasated cancer cell remains dormant while retaining the capacity to divide. Outgrowth of dormant cells seems to be determined by the environment. Changes in host factors in experimental systems have led to the outgrowth of such cells and the formation of a macroscopic metastasis after long periods of quiescence. There has been much discussion recently about the possibility of cellular differentiation, which results in a loss of capacity for unlimited proliferation, preventing the development of metastases by cancer cells that have extravasated. While there are some observations which would lend support to such a process in the case of neuroblastoma and myeloid leukaemia, there is no evidence in the case of carcinomas for differentiation leading to a loss of reproductive integrity nor for such a process being induced by substances such as retinoids or phorbolesters.

Role of growth factors. The failure of a cancer cell to grow once it has extravasated and escaped from the hostile environment of the blood may result from the requirement by cancer cells for growth factors. The evidence is now overwhelming that the division of normal cells requires specific growth factors which bind to receptors on the plasma membrane. One of the processes that ensures the physiological control of the division of normal cells within an organism is the production by one type of cell of the growth factors to which another type of cell responds. The difference between cancer and normal cells is not that the cancer cells do not require such growth factors but that they derive their autonomy by producing growth factors for which they have their own membrane receptors, i.e. autocrine stimulation—an hypothesis first put forward by Sporn and Todaro. These autocrine factors appear to be released from cancer cells into the surrounding medium whence they bind to the cells that produce them. This self stimulation is an essential component of the uncontrolled growth of cancer cells. An attractive, but as yet unproven, possibility is that after extravasation cancer cells remain quiescent or die because the local concentration of a diffusible growth factor released by an isolated cell is too low to initiate its own mitosis.

Elaboration by normal tissues of growth factors that can be used by single cancer cells which would otherwise remain dormant may contribute to the preferential occurrence of blood-borne metastases in certain organs (see below).

ORGAN DISTRIBUTION OF BLOOD-BORNE METASTASES

The discussion of this question has frequently been polarised by the assumption that one of two theories is adequate to explain the peculiarities of the distribution of metastasis. There is Ewing's opinion that 'the mechanism of the circulation will doubtlessly explain most of these peculiarities', and there is the concept of Paget who likened tumour emboli to seeds which need to fall into a suitable soil if they are to grow. Not surprisingly, a synthesis of these viewpoints is possible and both mechanisms contribute.

Metastases to lung and liver

Haemodynamic considerations dictate the first organ which the embolus encounters and this is the organ in which metastases are most common. Indeed, further arterial dissemination may stem from cells which have detached from a metastasis growing within the organ of first encounter. Careful analyses of post-mortems on a larger series of cancer patients have consistently shown that lung metastases are the most common when the blood of the primary cancer drains into the vena caval system, whereas liver metastases predominate for tumours draining into the portal system. A particularly elegant demonstration by Weiss of this phenomenon came from comparing the site of metastases from tumours which have arisen in the upper third of the rectum and the lower third of the oesophagus: for both these sites the principal venous drainage is to the portal system. In contrast, for tumours in the lower third of the rectum and the upper third of the oesophagus the initial venous drainage is into the systemic circulation via the inferior vena cava (Table 2). Haemodynamic considerations also explain why, for tumours that drain into the portal system, the lung is the second most common site for metastasis, after the liver. The lung is the second capillary bed which will be encountered by tumour cells which have passed through, or derive from, the liver.

Metastases from cells that have gained access to the arterial circulation

While the whole of the venous blood traverses the lung and the whole of the portal blood traverses the liver, only a fraction of the arterial blood traverses any one organ or tissue. If mechanical factors of the circulation were the sole determinant of the distribution of metastases, then the incidence of metastases deriving from the arterial

Table 2. Incidence of metastasis in organ of first encounter

Primary tumour	% Incidence of metastases in:	
	Liver	Lung
Draining to portal vein (Organ of first encounter—liver)		
Upper rectum	61	40
Lower oesophagus	50	25
Draining to vena cava (Organ of first encounter—lung)		
Lower rectum	41	46
Upper oesophagus	13	29
Head and neck	21	31
Breast	46	62

circulation should be proportional to the fraction of the cardiac output received by the different organs. The facts are, of course, the opposite. Blood-borne metastases are rare in muscle and gut, which between them take more than half of the cardiac output, but occur predominantly in organs such as liver and adrenal which receive a very small fraction of the cardiac output. The high frequency of liver metastases from primary cancers with initial drainage into the caval system was considered by Willis to provide a striking illustration of the discordance between cardiac output and incidence of metastases. In this situation the cancer emboli reach the liver via the hepatic artery which only receives a few per cent of the arterial blood.

The remarkable site selectivity of metastases stemming from cells in the arterial circulation can be investigated experimentally by injecting tumour cells directly into the left side of the heart. The few studies that have been performed show that the relative incidence of metastases in different organs bears no relationship to cardiac output. At Southampton, Paul Murphy has introduced a variety of different rat cancer cells into the left side of the heart of conscious rats via a cannula introduced into the carotid. The distribution of cardiac output to the different organs was determined by the injection of radioactive plastic microspheres with a diameter of 15 μm which ensures complete trapping in all capillary beds. The proportion of cancer cells arrested at different sites was determined by injecting radiolabelled cancer cells. As mentioned previously, a small proportion of these traversed the capillary beds supplied by the arterial circulation, but the majority were arrested in different organs in the same relative proportion as the plastic microspheres. Finally, different numbers of unlabelled viable cancer cells were inoculated and the sites of metastases determined.

The probability of an arrested cancer cell causing a metastasis could be estimated from the proportion of cells arrested in a particular organ and the number of metastatic lesions detected by post-mortem. The values obtained are imprecise, but as they differ for different organs by several orders of magnitude their biological significance seems real. Thus, 10 sarcoma cells deposited in the microvasculature of an adrenal were sufficient to produce a metastatic deposit, whereas a metastasis in muscle occurred only when more than 10^5 sarcoma cells had been arrested in the animal's skeletal muscles. The number of cells needed to produce a tumour in lung or liver following intravenous or intraportal injection, respectively, was between 1000 and 10 000 cells. With each of the tumours studied (a carcinoma, sarcoma and a hepatoma) the adrenal was always the organ which was most susceptible to metastasis from arterial emboli. Other organs in which tumours developed fairly frequently were the ovary, brown fat, and bone, although the relative susceptibility varied with the different tumours (Table 3).

Clearly, there is a very pronounced 'soil phenomenon', but the reasons for it remain to be elucidated. As early as 1934, Haddow suggested that local growth promoting substances might be involved. Recent discoveries have shown that the growth of tumour cells requires growth factors which may stem both from the tumour cells themselves and from normal tissues. The contribution of growth factors, released locally by normal tissues, to the growth of cancer cells is likely to be particularly important when the cancer cells are delivered via the arterial blood. Since they are dispersed throughout the different organs as single cells, the distance between individual cancer cells may be too great to achieve a build-up of cancer-derived

Table 3. Sites of tumour growth following left ventricular injection of tumour cells

	Sarcoma* $(10^4-2\times 10^6$ cells)	Hepatoma $(3\times 10^5-10^6$ cells)	Breast carcinoma $(10^6$ cells)
Adrenals	96%	100%	100%
Bone	54%	27%	33%
Lung	12%	9%	61%
Brown fat	85%	0%	6%
Kidney	0%	9%	0%
Heart	2%	0%	0%
Liver	2%	0%	0%
Ovaries	81%	100%	94%

*84 rats were given $\geq 10^4$ tumour cells and only 3 of these failed to develop tumours. In this group, 38 of 81 rats were female.

growth factors and the local concentrations of autocrine growth factors would therefore be insufficient to be mitogenic. Consequently, a blood-borne cancer cell that has succeeded in extravasating may not grow autonomously initially, but must rely for its mitogenic stimuli on factors released by the cells which surround it. If the tissue environment does not provide the needed stimuli, the cancer cell may lie dormant and its outgrowth depend on changes in the host. Once the isolated cancer cell has started to divide it creates its own environment in which tumour-derived growth factors are adequate for it to grow independently of the host.

A 'soil effect' need not, however, be related only to promoting successful growth at extravascular sites. It is quite conceivable that anatomical and physiological factors in different capillary beds may alter both the rate of intravascular death (which is multifactorial) and the rate of extravasation. Thus, a good 'soil' would be one in which the rate of extravascular death is slow but where the rate of extravasation is high. The oxygen concentration at the site where the emboli are arrested will vary in different organs and we have speculated that this could contribute to the site selectively of metastases. For example, in organs with a very high metabolic rate the gradient of oxygen concentration between the arterial and venous end of a capillary will be steep and the exact location in the microcirculation at which the tumour emboli are arrested will be critical.

Metastases from metastases

Experimental data using radiolabelled cancer cells show that while lymphoma cells and leukaemic cells can traverse the lung, transpulmonary passage of sarcoma, carcinoma and melanoma cells probably does not occur. Initially, if the preparation of the radiolabelled carcinoma or sarcoma cells is satisfactory, all the radioactivity following intravenous injection is associated with the lung. With time, radioactivity disappears from the lung and in the first hour activity builds up preferentially in the liver. This is most unlikely to be due to transpulmonary passage of intact cancer cells as these would enter the arterial circulation and be trapped in all the organs and tissues in proportion to the cardiac output. The concentration within the liver of radioactivity lost from the lung suggests that the radioactivity is associated with cell destruction in the lung. This releases the radiolabel in a form of debris which is cleared by the reticulo-endothelial system and hence is found in the liver. As has been mentioned already some cancer cells can pass through some capillary beds, such as muscle, though they are damaged during the process. Transcapillary passage probably depends on the anatomy of the microvasculature and occurs in those tissues (like muscle) which have large capillaries, referred to as preferred channels, and not in the lung where there are no such channels.

In man, there is also little evidence for unarrested passage of intact cancer cells through pulmonary capillaries. Willis was of the opinion that entry of cancer emboli into the arterial circulation usually arose from cancer cells that stemmed from metastases and not from cells released from the primary tumour. Willis wrote: 'In the total absence of tumour deposits in the lungs, it is very unusual to see widespread systemic secondary growths. In cases with such growths, and with the lungs seemingly unaffected, adequate microscopic search will almost invariably reveal either microscopic pulmonary metastases or neoplastic thrombi in the arterioles, and in the rare instances where such lesions are not found, it is always possible that these are present but have escaped discovery owing to the impracticability of making a complete microscopic search of the whole of the lungs.' More recently, the importance of metastases arising from metastases has also been stressed following an intricate mathematical analysis of psot-mortem findings. It is clearly important in devising strategies for the eradication of disseminated cancer cells that metastasis should not be regarded as an 'all or none' phenomenon.

FURTHER READING

Day, Myers, Stansley, *et al.* (eds) (1977) *Cancer Invasion and Metastasis*. Raven Press, New York.
Hellmann and Eccles (eds) (1985) *Treatment of Metastasis: Problems and Prospects*. Taylor and Francis, London.
Honn, Powers and Sloane (eds) (1986) *Mechanisms of Cancer Metastasis*. Nijhoff, Boston.
Murphy, P., *et al.* (1988) *Br. J. Cancer*, **57**, 564–568.
Nicolson and Milas (1984) *Cancer Invasion and Metastasis*. Raven Press, New York.
Prodi and Liotta (eds) (1988) *Cancer Metastasis*. Plenum Press, New York.
Skipper, D., *et al.* (1988) *Br. J. Cancer*, **57**, 564–568.
Weiss, L. (1990) *Adv. Cancer Res.*, **54**, 159–211.
Willis, R. A. (1973) *The Spread of Tumours in the Human Body*. Butterworths, London.

32 Bone Marrow Transplantation

NICHOLAS D. JAMES

Experiments in the 1950s first established that, in animal models, bone marrow could be ablated and the animal rescued by infusion of marrow from their genetically identical litter mates. In a series of classical experiments, Billingham, Brent and Medawar showed that if the experiment was performed on young animals using marrow from non-identical donors, the subsequent development of the recipients was impaired—'runt disease'. If the same experiments were performed with immunologically intact adult animals and non-syngeneic donors, the infused marrow was rejected. This work foreshadowed the development of bone marrow transplantation (BMT) as a therapeutic modality and also indicated the likely areas of trouble—rejection and graft-versus-host disease (GVHD)—which needed to be overcome in order to carry out a successful transplant. Initial attempts at BMT in man were uniformly unsuccessful with the exception of transplants from identical twins. Since the 1970s, however, BMT has become established as an important therapeutic tool in a variety of diseases.

The initial use of BMT was in diseases of the bone marrow, the rationale being to ablate the abnormal bone marrow and to replace it with normal marrow from a healthy donor. This has subsequently been extended to non-haematological malignant disorders such as lymphomas, in which therapy is limited by the tolerance of normal bone marrow to chemotherapy and radiotherapy, the donor marrow being used to 'rescue' the patient from the treatment rather than to replace diseased marrow. In this context, the donor marrow can be harvested from the patient and subsequently reinfused as an autologous transplant. The third group of diseases that can be treated are genetic diseases in which the transplanted marrow restores a missing enzyme, correcting the disorder. Examples of such diseases are Hurler's syndrome, osteopetrosis and severe combined immunodeficiency. Of recent topical interest have been the attempts to save victims of the Chernobyl disaster with allogeneic BMT. A list of the diseases for which BMT, either allogeneic or autologous, have been tried is shown in Table 1.

Genes and Cancer. Edited by D. Carney and K. Sikora
©1990 John Wiley & Sons Ltd

Table 1. Diseases in which bone marrow transplantation
has been investigated

AML/ALL
CML
Aplastic anaemia
  Idiopathic
  Fanconi's
Other blood disorders
  Thalassaemia major
  Congenital immunodeficiencies
Glycogen storage diseases
Lymphomas
  NHL
  HD
Other malignancies
  Oat cell Ca
  Breast cancer
  Others
AIDS
Radiation accidents—the Chernobyl experience

TECHNIQUE

The problems to be overcome for successful BMT are four-fold:
  1. The elimination of all malignant cells.
  2. The suppression of graft rejection.
  3. The avoidance of graft-versus-host disease (GVHD).
  4. The support of the patient through the post-transplant period in which marrow function is deficient.
Most conditioning regimens employ a combination of radiotherapy, chemotherapy and immune manipulation to achieve these aims.

Conditioning regimens

The first two objectives are achieved by a combination of high-dose chemotherapy and total body irradiation (TBI). This has the aim of ablating the host marrow, both normal and abnormal, and causes profound immunosuppression allowing the donor marrow to 'take'. In the case of transplants for the aplastic anaemias, this latter aspect of immunosuppression is of overriding importance as graft rejection is a major problem post-transplant, such that heavily transfused patients have a high probability of graft rejection and consequent poor prognosis. Graft rejection also assumes increased importance where the donor is unrelated to the host (see below).

The chemotherapy employed may be either single agent, such as high-dose cyclophosphamide, or combinations of alkylating agents and anthracyclines, such as daunorubicin, the drugs used being tailored to the disease being treated. The chemotherapy is given as a single dose in the immediate pre-transplant period with the intention of achieving ablation of all marrow, both normal and abnormal.

In conjunction with high-dose chemotherapy, most conditioning regimens utilise TBI as an additional ablative and immunosuppressive therapy. Some autologous

BMT regimens omit TBI in favour of more intensive chemotherapy as the problems of immune rejection do not arise and the radiation doses employed (9–12 Gy according to fractionation) are subtherapeutic compared to those given when radiotherapy is the primary treatment (e.g. 40 Gy to treat Hodgkin's disease). The reason for this is that at doses much in excess of 10 Gy the incidence of pulmonary and gastrointestinal problems increases steeply, precluding significant dose escalation. Conversely, the chemotherapy doses can be more easily escalated once the constraint of myelotoxicity is removed. Given the above, and the observation that radiation kills lymphocytes directly (unlike most cells in which the effect is delayed), the main contribution of TBI is likely to be immunosuppressive rather than ablative.

The original TBI technique for BMT was developed in Seattle and utilised a specially designed opposed double cobalt-60 source. The patients were treated using simultaneous antero-posterior then lateral fields to deliver a total dose of 10 Gy as a single treatment. This mode of treatment has two main disadvantages. Firstly, it requires a purpose-built treatment machine. Secondly, giving TBI as a single fraction at low dose rate (as in the Seattle technique) results in prolonged treatment times and considerable subjective toxicity for the patient. The technique employed at Hammersmith Hospital, illustrated in Figure 1, utilises five or six fractions given over three days. There appears to be no difference in overall toxicity or antileukaemic effect between single and fractionated dose schedules, but acute toxicity is diminished.

Toxicity. Bone marrow transplantation is a toxic procedure. It is difficult to disentangle the regimen-related toxicity from other causes of morbidity, such as disease relapse, GVHD and the consequences of pancytopenia such as infection and haemorrhage. The principal acute toxicities are nausea and vomiting, diarrhoea, mucositis and erythema. Pneumonitis is a major cause of morbidity and mortality

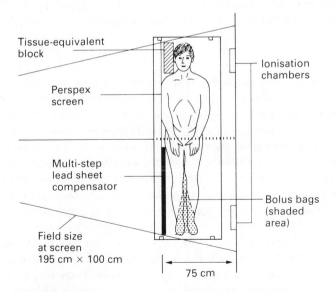

Figure 1. Details of the field set-up for TBI. Parallel opposed lateral fields. FSD 5 m

after BMT and is of multifactorial origin. Contributing causes include TBI dose (see above), infections and GVHD.

Graft-versus-host-disease (GVHD)

GVHD is a major cause of morbidity following transplants of allogeneic marrow and is caused by immunocompetent donor cells attacking targets in the marrow recipient. Three main strategies have been employed to minimise its effects: (a) HLA matching donor and recipient as exactly as possible; (b) post-transplant immunosuppression and (c) T-cell depletion of donor marrow.

Initial attempts at BMT were only successful between identical twins. Subsequently, transplants between HLA-matched siblings also became possible using appropriate conditioning and immunosuppressive regimens. Donors and recipients must match at HLA-A, -B and -C loci. In addition a mixed lymphocyte reaction is performed to test HLA-D compatibility. If an exact match is not obtained, the chances of severe GVHD increase significantly.

The majority of candidates for BMT do not have a suitable sibling donor, necessitating the use of haploidentical family members or matched unrelated donors if BMT is to be undertaken. Recipients of marrow from unrelated or mismatched donors pose a particular problem because of the increased incidence of graft rejection and severe GVHD. In an effort to decrease the incidence and severity of GVHD, T-cell depletion of donor marrow has been introduced into conditioning regimens. The rationale for this manoeuvre is that the putative marrow stem cell does not appear to express T-cell markers, whereas the effector cell for GVHD is the T-cell and thus depletion of donor T-cells may be expected to reduce GVHD. T-cell depletion does indeed reduce GVHD but at the price of an increase in graft failure and delayed engraftment. It is thought that this increased difficulty with engraftment is a host-mediated immune process.

Various methods have been used to increase immunosuppression in the early post-transplant period. These include intravenous anti-T-cell monoclonal antibodies given pre-transplant (producing, as it were, *in vivo* host T-cell depletion) and total lymphoid irradiation (TLI). TLI has been shown to produce profound suppression of T-cell mediated immune function in animal transplant models as well as in patients receiving total nodal irradiation for Hodgkin's disease. TLI, at a dose of 6–8 Gy in 3–4 fractions, was introduced into the pre-transplant conditioning at the Hammersmith Hospital in 1985. Since its introduction, TLI, with or without intravenous anti-T-cell monoclonal antibodies, has proved valuable in preventing graft rejection in patients receiving T-cell depleted marrow from unrelated donors who would otherwise be at high risk of rejection. This allows transplants to be carried out with a good chance of prompt engraftment and an acceptable morbidity from GVHD in this group of patients who would otherwise not be suitable for BMT.

Unfortunately, the use of T-cell depletion of donor marrow in BMT for leukaemia, in addition to the problems of engraftment described above, also carries an increased risk of leukaemic relapse. This raises the possibility that freedom from relapse may depend on a graft-versus-leukaemia effect, which, if suppressed too vigorously, may decrease the chance of eventual cure of the primary disease.

An alternative approach to the problem of GVHD in transplants from matched unrelated donors is to maintain the post-transplant immunosuppression with drugs such as cyclosporin A or methotrexate in an effort to suppress GVHD to acceptable levels without abrogating totally the putative graft-versus-leukaemia effect. This approach is currently under evaluation.

SUPPORTIVE CARE

A major cause of mortality and morbidity attached to BMT is the period of pancytopenia that follows the conditioning treatment. The problems can be broadly grouped into two categories—control of infection and blood product support.

Blood product support

Patients receive blood transfusions according to their clinical needs. Platelet transfusions are generally given when the platelet count is below $20 \times 10^9/l$ or to cover bleeding or invasive procedures. Transfused blood products are an important source of CMV infection post-transplant so CMV-negative patients must receive CMV-negative blood products unless dire need supervenes, as CMV infection is a major cause of post-BMT mortality and morbidity (see below).

Control of infection

Infective problems may be subdivided into early infections arising as a consequence of neutropenia and late infections, usually viral, due to impaired cell-mediated immunity.

Neutropenia-related sepsis. The patient is at high risk of neutropenia-related sepsis whilst the neutrophil count remains below $0.5 \times 10^9/l$ and relatively at risk until the count rises above $1.0 \times 10^9/l$, which is normally when reverse barrier nursing can be discontinued. The control of infection in this early post-BMT period is two-pronged: firstly attempts are made to minimise the contact of the patient with potential pathogens; secondly, any infection is treated promptly with broad-spectrum intravenous antibiotics, changing the antibiotics in the light of microbiological findings or clinical need.

Prophylactic treatment includes the use of oral antimicrobials such as co-trimoxazole, nystatin, and amphoteracin plus regular antiseptic mouthwashes (e.g. corsodyl). In cases heavily pre-treated with antibiotics (e.g. aplastic anaemics) a non-absorbable antibiotic such as colistin may be added to the regimen. Regular cultures should be made from throat swabs, urine and faeces to get advance warning of colonisation with potentially dangerous pathogens to allow appropriate antibiotics to be started in the event of deterioration. Concurrently, to minimise contact with extrinsic pathogens the patient is reverse-barrier nursed in a specialist unit, with strict adherence to hand-washing, gloves, gowns and masks. In the majority of septic episodes, no pathogen is isolated; however, where a pathogen is isolated, most prove to be intrinsically rather than extrinsically acquired, emphasising the importance of prophylaxis and surveillance.

The best prophylactic treatments still do not prevent the inevitable pyrexial episodes that occur in the early weeks following the transplant. As indicated above, following clinical examination, chest X-ray, blood cultures from both Hickman and peripheral sources, plus other cultures as indicated, treatment must be started promptly with broad-spectrum antibiotics. The spectrum chosen should cover both Gram-positive and Gram-negative organisms, including *Pseudomonas*, plus anaerobes. Many combinations may be suitable but a consistent policy is important; examples include single agent ceftazidime and piperacillin with an aminoglycoside such as amikacin. Subsequently, antibiotics may be changed in the light of clinical progress or microbiological findings.

Late infections. The risk of severe infection persists for at least a year after BMT, even when the acute risk from neutropenia has abated. Infections include mycobacterial, fungal and viral, of which CMV infection is probably the most important in terms of mortality. In the presence of a suspected infection, strenuous efforts should be made to isolate and treat the pathogen.

Herpesvirus infections pose a particular problem in view of their ubiquity and potential severity. Infections with herpes simplex will normally respond to treatment with acyclovir, as will herpes zoster infections with an appropriate dose escalation. CMV infections, however, are relatively resistant to acyclovir and are a major cause of death post-transplant. As with acute bacterial infections, a two-pronged approach is used to minimise the risk from CMV. A major source of CMV infection is transfused blood products; thus patients who are serologically CMV-negative at presentation should receive CMV-negative blood products as far as possible post-BMT. Although acyclovir is relatively ineffective in established infections, it does appear to be of value as prophylaxis and studies are underway to evaluate this. Recently, a new antiviral agent, ganciclovir, with increased anti-CMV activity has become available. Unfortunately, this agent is myelotoxic, precluding its use in prophylaxis; however, its increased efficacy compared with acyclovir probably does give it a role in the management of life-threatening infections.

FUTURE DEVELOPMENTS

Who should be transplanted?

Acute leukaemia. Approximately 70% of patients with acute leukaemia aged under 60 years can be expected to achieve complete remission with conventional treatment. With the most intensive current regimens, 4-year disease-free survival rates of 38–55% can be achieved. However 35–60% of the patients experience leukaemic relapse. Allogeneic BMT lowers the leukaemic relapse rate appreciably to 15–20% but at a high cost in BMT-related mortality and morbidity—about 30–40% of BMT recipients die in the first year post-transplant from causes such as GVHD, interstitial pneumonitis and CMV infection. Furthermore, some of these deaths will occur in patients who, had they not been transplanted, would have remained disease-free.

Overall, the addition of allogeneic BMT to the treatment of acute leukaemia in first remission probably does not confer a survival advantage. For patients in relapse or second remission, the likelihood of further disease relapse is much greater with conventional chemotherapy, and for these patients allogeneic BMT from a sibling donor probably does carry a survival advantage. Unfortunately, only about one in three people have a suitable sibling donor and, as discussed above, the risks of transplants from haploidentical relatives or matched unrelated donors are increased. Patients receiving intensive chemotherapy or high-dose chemo-radiotherapy plus autologous marrow grafting (or a graft from an identical twin) have a lower morbidity but a higher relapse rate, supporting the concept of a graft-versus-leukaemia effect.

Chronic myeloid leukaemia. The situation pertaining to chronic myeloid leukaemia (CML) is, if anything, even more complicated. CML is incurable with conventional therapies but carries a median survival of about four years with good quality life. BMT is potentially curative for CML but for the maximum chance of cure the transplant must be carried out early in the disease course prior to the onset of accelerated phase or blast crisis. The dilemma facing the patient and clinician is thus whether to risk sacrificing possibly many years of healthy life for an approximate 50% chance of cure carrying a 30–40% chance of procedure-related death in the first year after transplantation and severe acute morbidity and the possibility of longstanding late sequelae.

Lymphomas. As discussed above, the rationale for transplantation in lymphoma is to allow the dose of chemotherapy to be escalated above the limits of marrow tolerance. As the marrow is generally not affected, autologous grafting is usually employed. At present it is unclear whether this form of therapy offers a genuine advantage over alternative methods of dose intensification, such as the use of intensive weekly alternating schedules like MACOP-B. The introduction of recombinant colony-stimulating factors such as granulocyte-macrophage colony-stimulating factors (GM-CSF) may allow the further intensification of such regimens, further reducing the indications for autologous BMT. At present the technique is usually reserved for patients with disease refractory to conventional chemotherapy regimens.

Aplastic anaemias. Patients with severe aplastic anaemia of whatever cause have a poor life expectancy. BMT is probably the treatment of choice for such patients and should be performed as early as possible in the disease course as the regular blood product support required by such patients with its consequent allosensitisation makes graft rejection increasingly likely with delay.

Other marrow disorders. Diseases such as thalassaemia major and sickle-cell anaemia have been successfully treated with BMT. It is difficult to justify the procedure at present in the light of its considerable mortality and morbidity and the long life expectancy of sufferers. It is also possible that in the future it will become possible to genetically manipulate the patient's marrow in order to restore normal haemoglobin production. At present there are considerable technological problems to be overcome before this dream can be realised. Obstacles include the paucity of stem cells in human marrow (at present unidentified, a further problem), transfecting the functional gene to the correct region of the genome, ensuring expression of the gene under circumstances that allow assembly of intact haemoglobin molecules (otherwise, for example, a new form of thalassaemia may be substituted for the existing disorder) and the establishment of the new stem cell in preference to the defective one. Furthermore, even if the above constraints could be met, gene expression may also occur in all marrow cell lines as the genetic engineering would have to be done at the stem cell level.

Inherited enzyme defects. Patients with diseases such as Hurler's syndrome and osteopetrosis have been shown to benefit from allogeneic BMT, presumably due to cells such as macrophages transplanted with the marrow. Such transplants should be carried out early in life as they can be shown to correct, for example, the enzymatic abnormalities associated with Hurler's syndrome, and it is hoped that subsequent mental retardation may thus be avoided.

Other malignant disorders. With the exception of lymphomas, dose escalation with autologous marrow transplantation has proved disappointing and has not found an established role.

Gene therapy

The possibility that inherited single gene haematological disorders may be treated by genetic manipulation of the marrow stem cell population, presumably coupled with ablation of abnormal haematopoiesis, has been touched on above. A more suitable potential candidate for such an approach is a disease like severe combined immunodeficiency disease (SCID) in which the requirements of gene expression (in this case adenine deaminase) are less stringent and thus more attainable. In this case, the expression of the gene would probably be sufficient to correct the disorder, without the constraints of coordinated expression with other genes that apply to the haemoglobinopathies, as outlined above.

Colony stimulating factors

The recent cloning and expression of the genes for granulocyte-macrophage colony stimulating factor (GM-SF) and granulocyte colony stimulating factor (G-CSF) has allowed the use of these agents with the aim of reducing the duration of neutropenia post-transplant; they have shown promising results. Paradoxically, the use of such agents may reduce the indications for autologous BMT as their use may allow more intensive conventional chemotherapeutic regimens to be utilised.

Polymerase chain reaction

The polymerase chain reaction (PCR) is a recently developed technique that allows the specific amplification of predetermined regions of the genome for subsequent biochemical analysis. The technique can be used to identify an abnormal DNA sequence in a single cell. The potential use of the technique lies in its ability to detect an abnormal cell amongst large numbers of normal ones. Already the PCR has been used in CML post-transplant to assess the presence of *bcr-abl* gene rearrangement (present in the Philadelphia chromosome) in marrow samples from patients in haematological remission. As indicated above, part of the problem in selecting patients for allogeneic BMT with acute leukaemia is identifying patients at risk of relapse. The PCR may allow the identification of patients haematologically in remission but harbouring small numbers of leukaemic stem cells, allowing more precise targeting of post-remission therapy.

CONCLUSIONS

Bone marrow transplantation is a powerful technique offering the prospect of cure to patients with otherwise incurable diseases. Major problems remain, however, in that the morbidity and mortality of BMT, especially from unrelated donors, remains high, precluding its use in older patients. Future refinements in technique may be hoped to widen the scope of transplantation and possible avenues of progress have been outlined.

Index